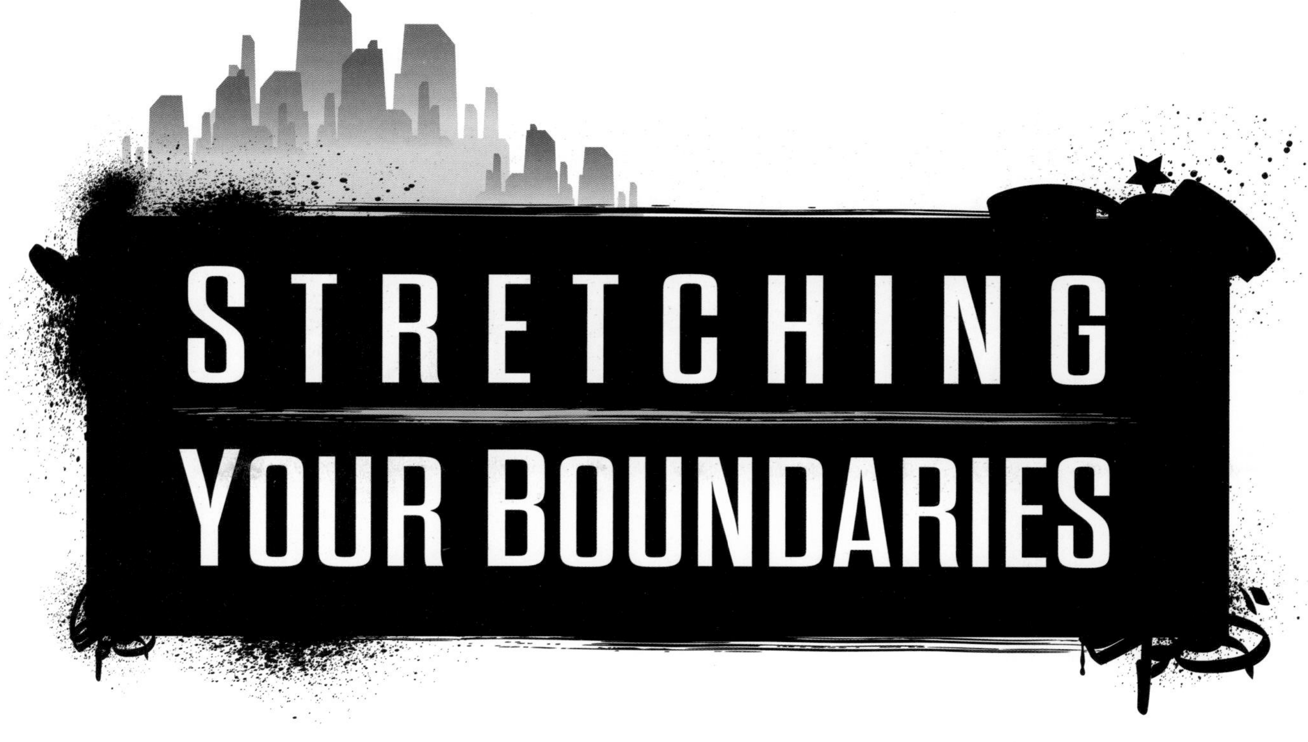


## Flexibility Training for Extreme Calisthenic Strength

Al Kavadlo

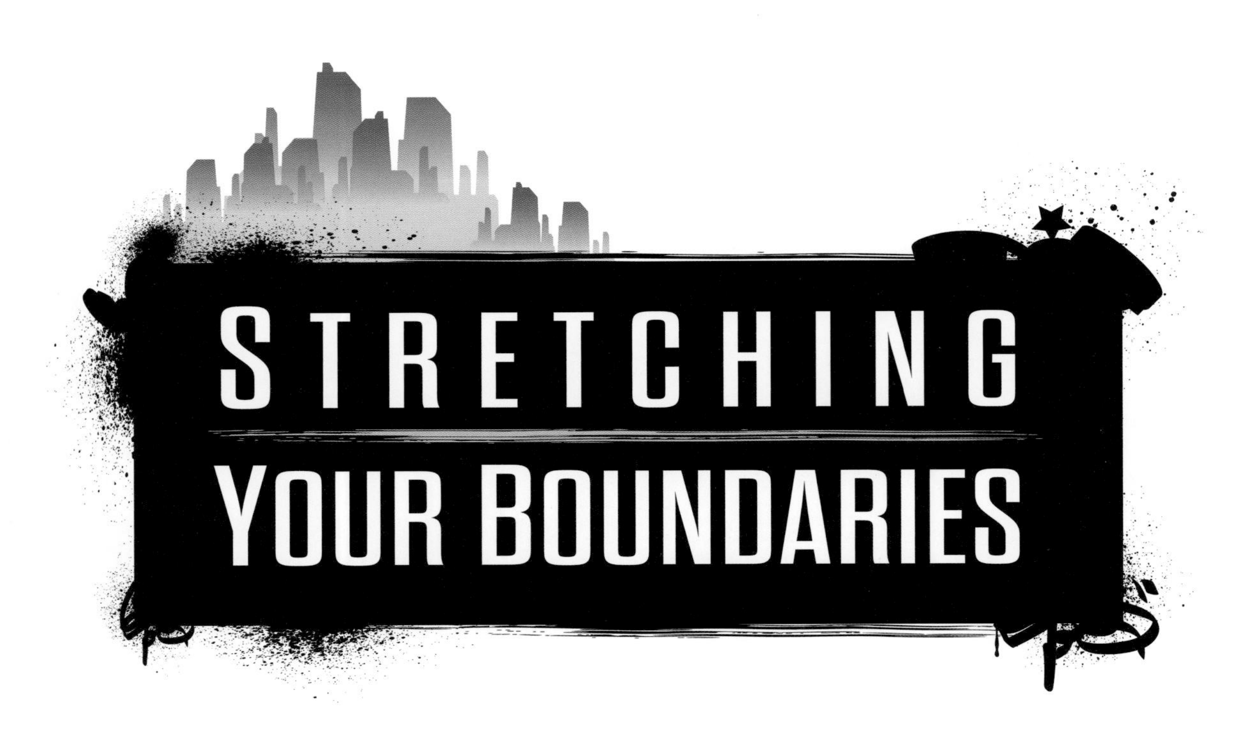



A Dragon Door Publications, Inc production

Published in the United States by: Dragon Door Publications, Inc
5 East County Rd B, #3 • Little Canada, MN 55117
Tel: (651) 487-2180 • Fax: (651) 487-3954
Credit card orders: 1-800-899-5111 • Email: support@dragondoor.com • Website: www.dragondoor.com

ISBN 10: 0-938045-91-1 ISBN 13: 978-0-938045-91-5

This edition first published in January, 2014
Printed in China



Book design and cover by Derek Brigham • www.dbrigham.com • (763) 208-3069 • bigd@dbrigham.com

Photography by Jordan Perlson
Models: Jack Arnow, Norris Baichan, Jasmine Brooks, Angelo Gala, Meng He, Al Kavadlo, Danny Kavadlo, Rachel Kuhns, Keith McDermott, Ted Michalek, Jeff Montfleury, Bob Rothchild, Wes Sanchez, Lauren Sison, Kim Wong

Additional photography by Al Kavadlo, Danny Kavadlo, Rachel Kuhns and Wes Sanchez

# -Table of Contents -

Foreword by Elliott Hulse

**PART ONE- Stretch Manifesto**

→ Stretching For Strength .......... 1
→ Taking Your Medicine .......... 9
→ Kid Stuff .......... 15
→ Mobility Matters .......... 21
→ Breath is Life .......... 29

**PART TWO - The Stretches**

→ Preface .......... 39
→ Dynamics .......... 41
→ Standing Statics .......... 49
→ Grounded Statics .......... 95

**PART THREE - Programming and Sample Routines**

→ Standards of Practice .......... 153
→ On Mats .......... 161
→ Symmetry .......... 163
→ Hypothetical Training Splits .......... 171
→ Sample Routines .......... 177

Acknowledgements .......... 185
About the Author .......... 187

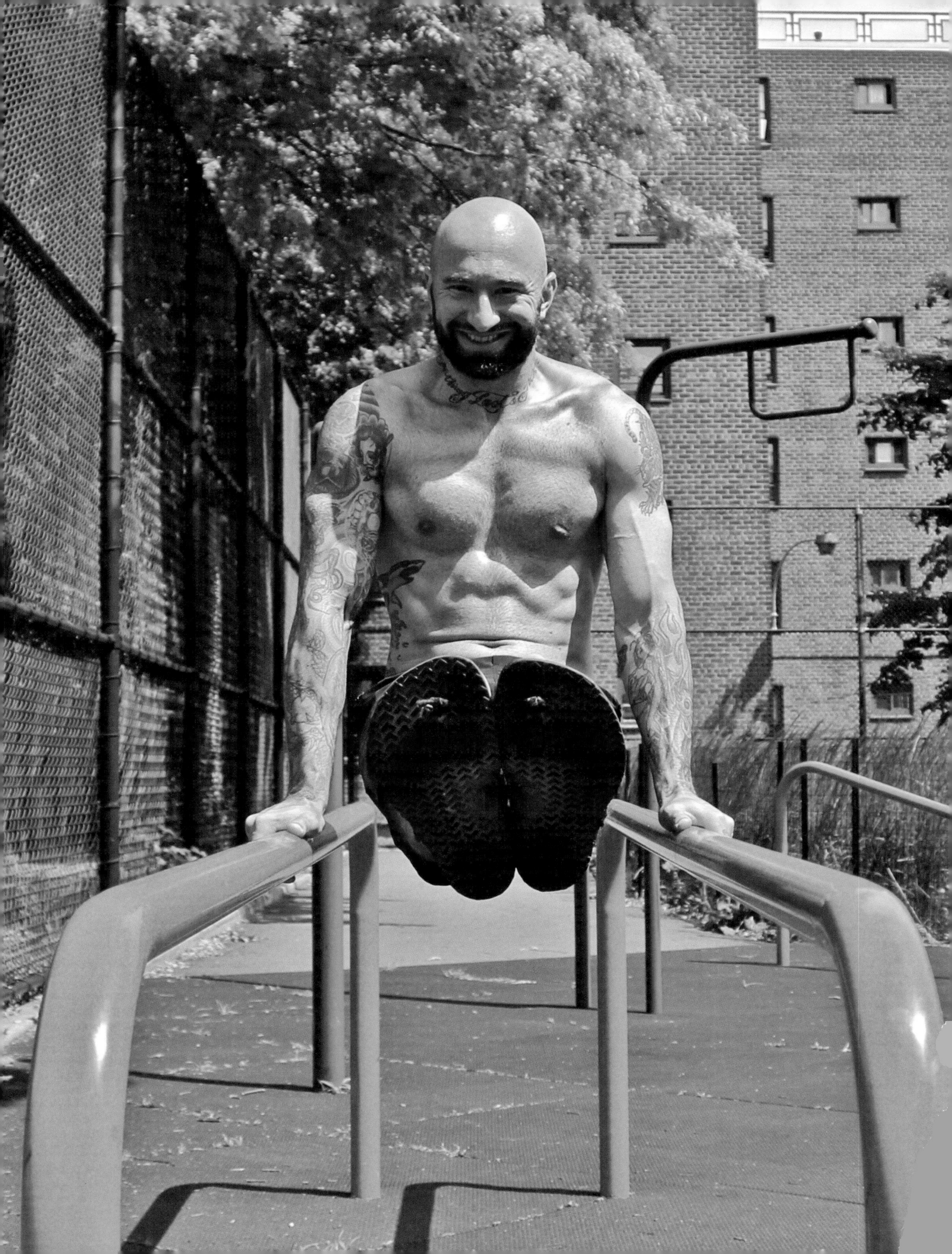

# Foreword:

## By Elliott Hulse

Every tradition, religion and science recognizes that the human being balances between the world of Matter and an intangible, yet mysteriously palpable and somewhat measurable world of Energy. The building blocks of human form, whether you scientifically refer to them as atoms, or poetically refer to them as dust, are impelled towards movement by a primal impulse we call breath. We are the movement of breath through the body.

Just as beautiful music is produced when the skilled musician blows through a well-crafted flute, so too does man's life become a beautiful song when the breath of the Universe moves smoothly and softly through his body. But unlike the flute, which holds its creator's form the duration of its existence, the human body is constantly in flux. It is always growing, reacting and responding—it is a sensitive "thinking body" that is highly malleable.

From the very first slap laid upon the baby's backside by the doctor, the soft, supple, spiritual conduit we call "body" begins taking the form of the demands pressed upon it by its Earthly existence. From this point onward, the once unobstructed respiratory wave begins to exhibit defensive, utilitarian and even neurotic restrictions created by and held on to by the muscular system.

According to the late Wilhelm Reich there are several bands of muscular tension that regularly manifest throughout the core of the body, all of which restrict the capacity to breathe deeply. Muscles in the face and skull, the jaw and neck, the chest, the belly, and finally the pelvic floor all contribute to the subtle flexion and extension of the physical human core that he called the respiratory wave. As a psychoanalyst, Reich determined that each of these muscular restrictions is created by the organism as a physical defense against a psychological pain. He asserted that by helping his patients release their muscular tension and restore their capacity to breathe deeply that they not only felt better mentally, but obviously they will look better!

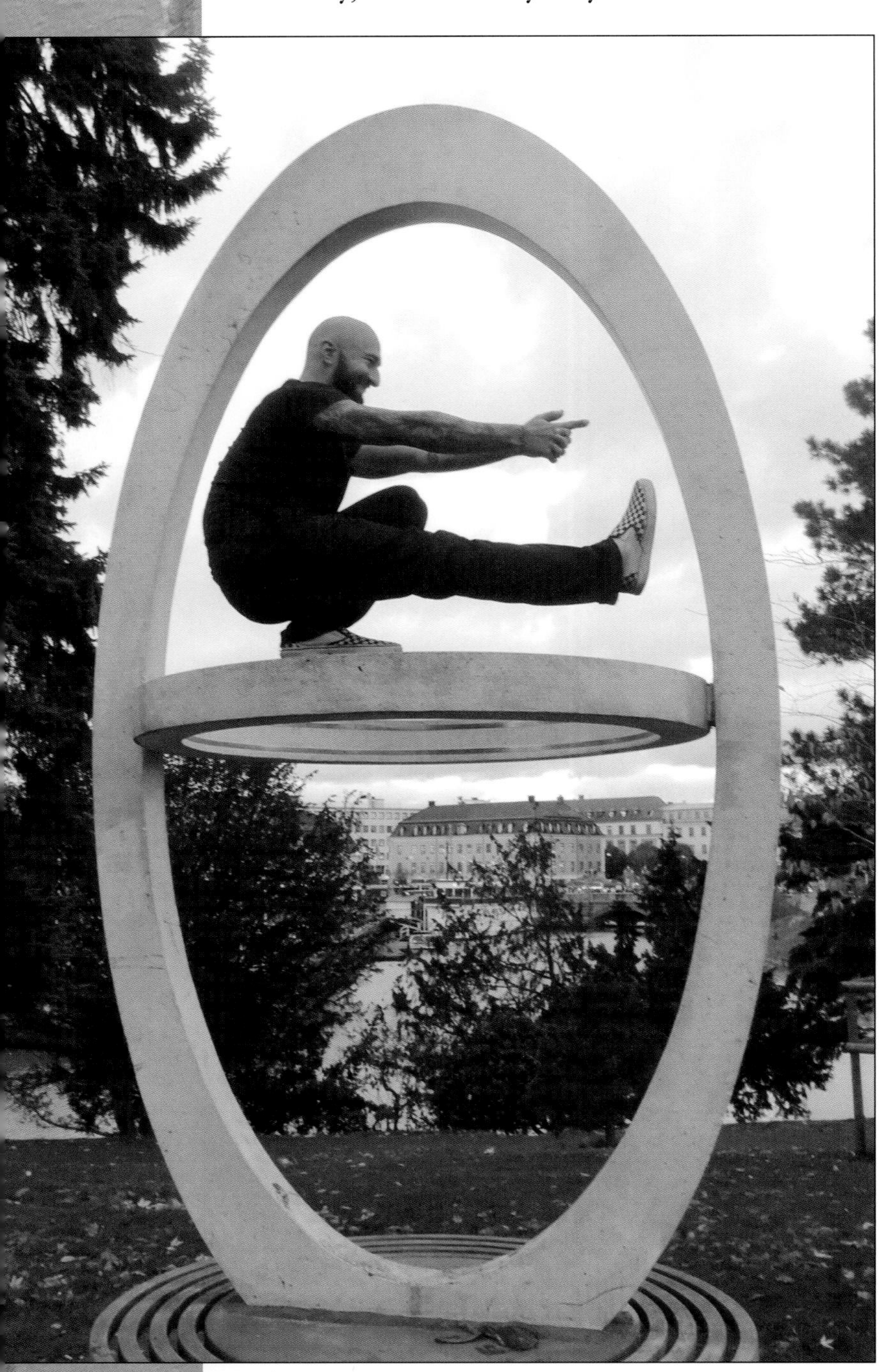

A body free from muscular tension breathes deeply, allowing a fuller expression of the spirit energy to pass through it; also this body will stand taller and move better though properly aligned joints and sound human biomechanics.

In the past it was the Tai Chi and Yoga masters who understood and became practitioners of bringing about the physical alignment which allowed full spiritual or psychological expression though the human form. Just like the instrument repairman who might fix the damaged or mistreated flute, allowing the musician to once again breathe into the instrument creating beautiful music, so too does the practitioner who brings physical alignment back into the human form allow his client to once again produce beautiful music though his life.

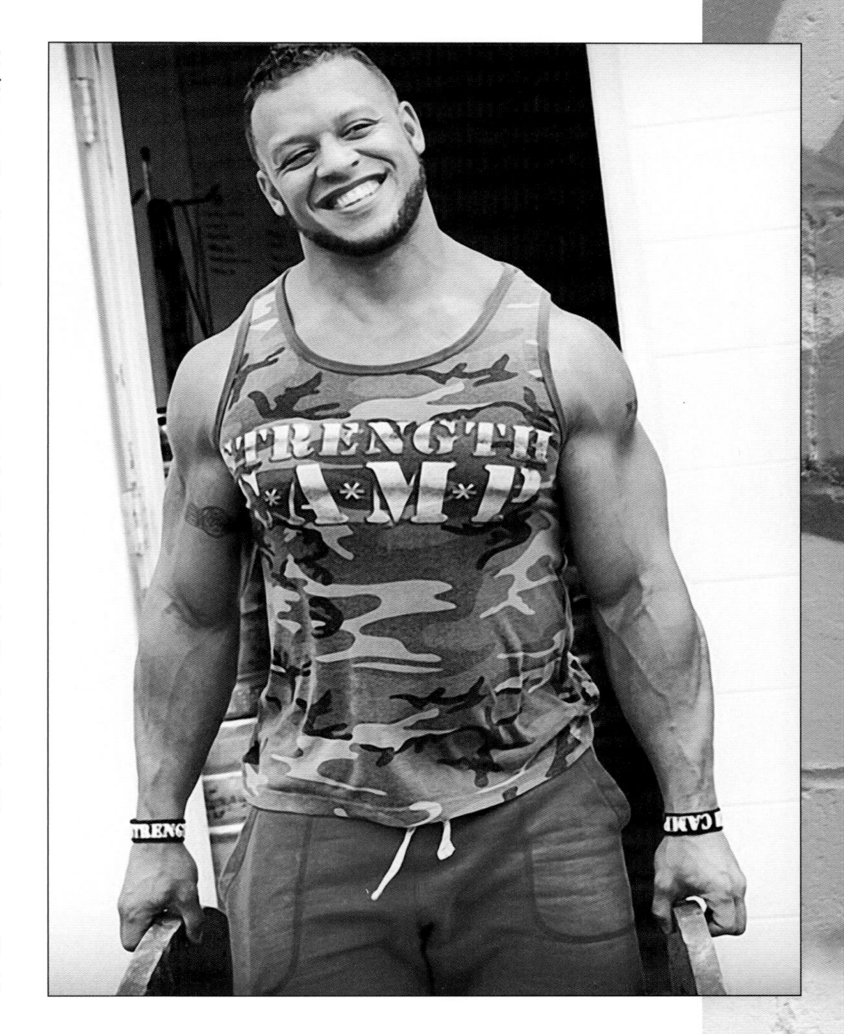

Al Kavadlo is a fitness trainer who not only recognizes the physical benefit of stretching and breathing, but also recognizes how working with his clients in this way changes their lives—from the inside, out. In ***Stretching Your Boundaries*** you'll sense Al's deep understanding and love for the human body.

You will experience Al's appreciation for poetry and practicality. In this book, Al invites you to take a deeper look at the often overlooked, and sometimes demonized, ancient practice of static stretching. He wrestles with many of the questions, dogmas and flat-out lies about stretching that have plagued the fitness practitioner for at least the last decade. And finally he gives you a practical guide to static stretching that will improve your movement, performance, breathing and life.

Thank you Al, for helping to bring awareness to perhaps the most important aspect of physical education and fitness.

Grow Stronger,

Elliott Hulse

Elliott Hulse

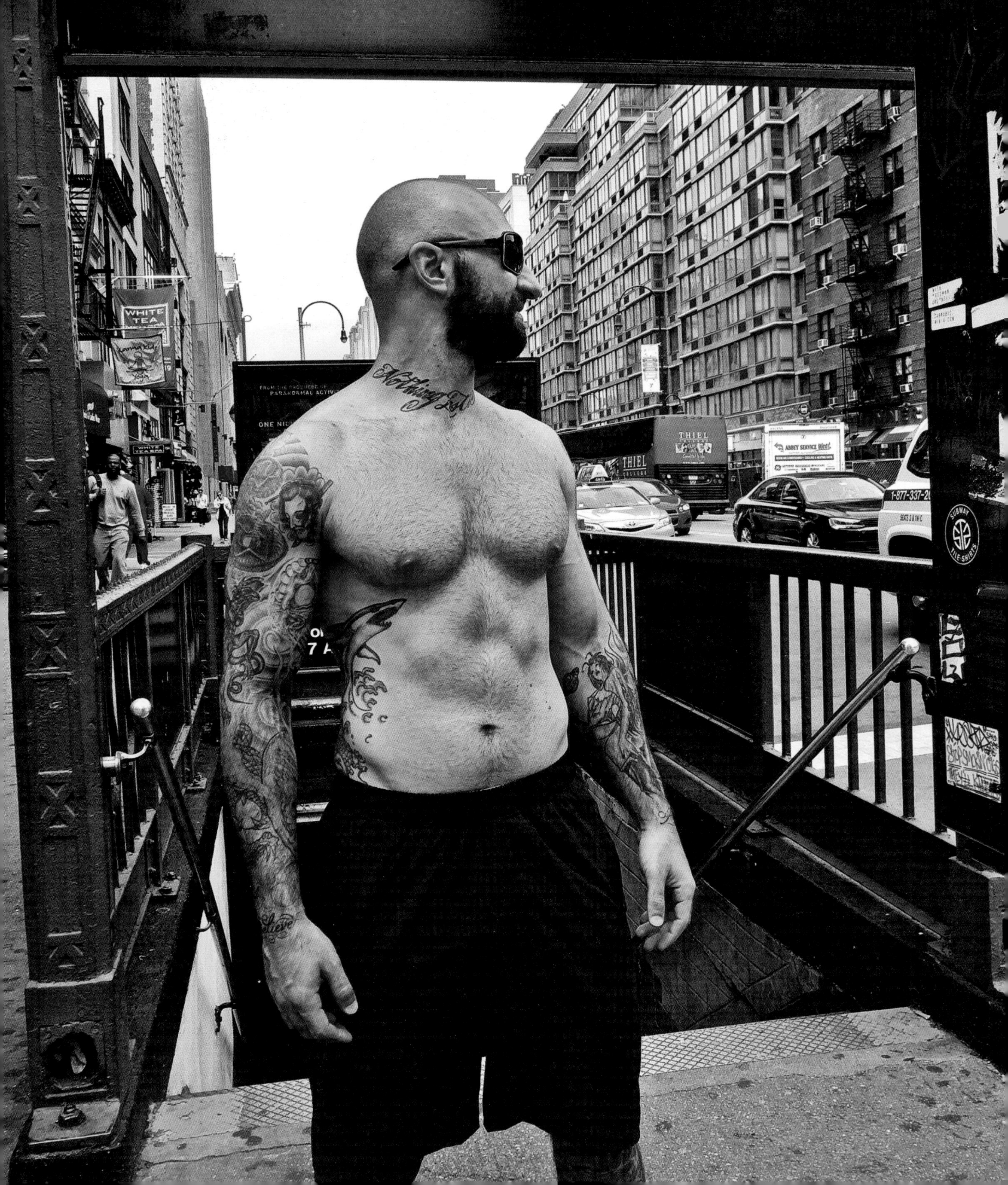
Subway-PATH Trains

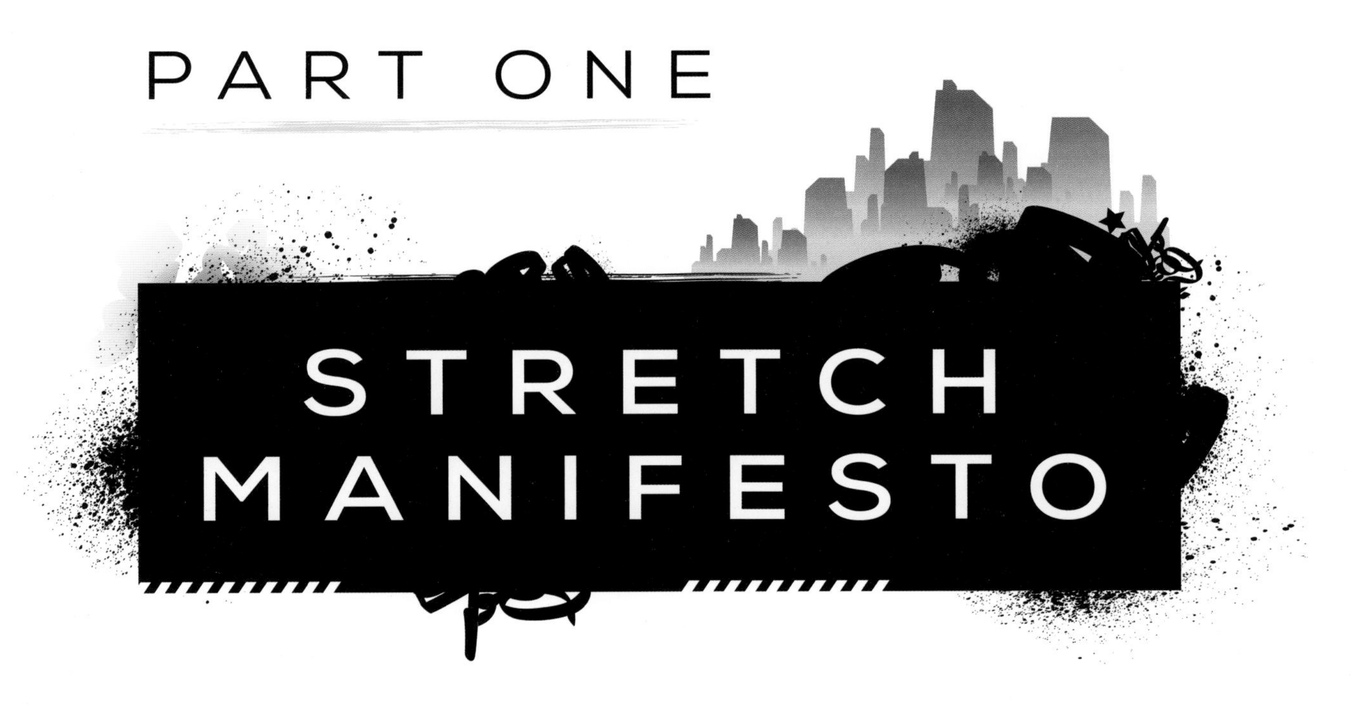


"You have your way.
I have my way.
As for the right way, the correct way,
and the only way, it does not exist."

*-Friedrich Nietzsche*

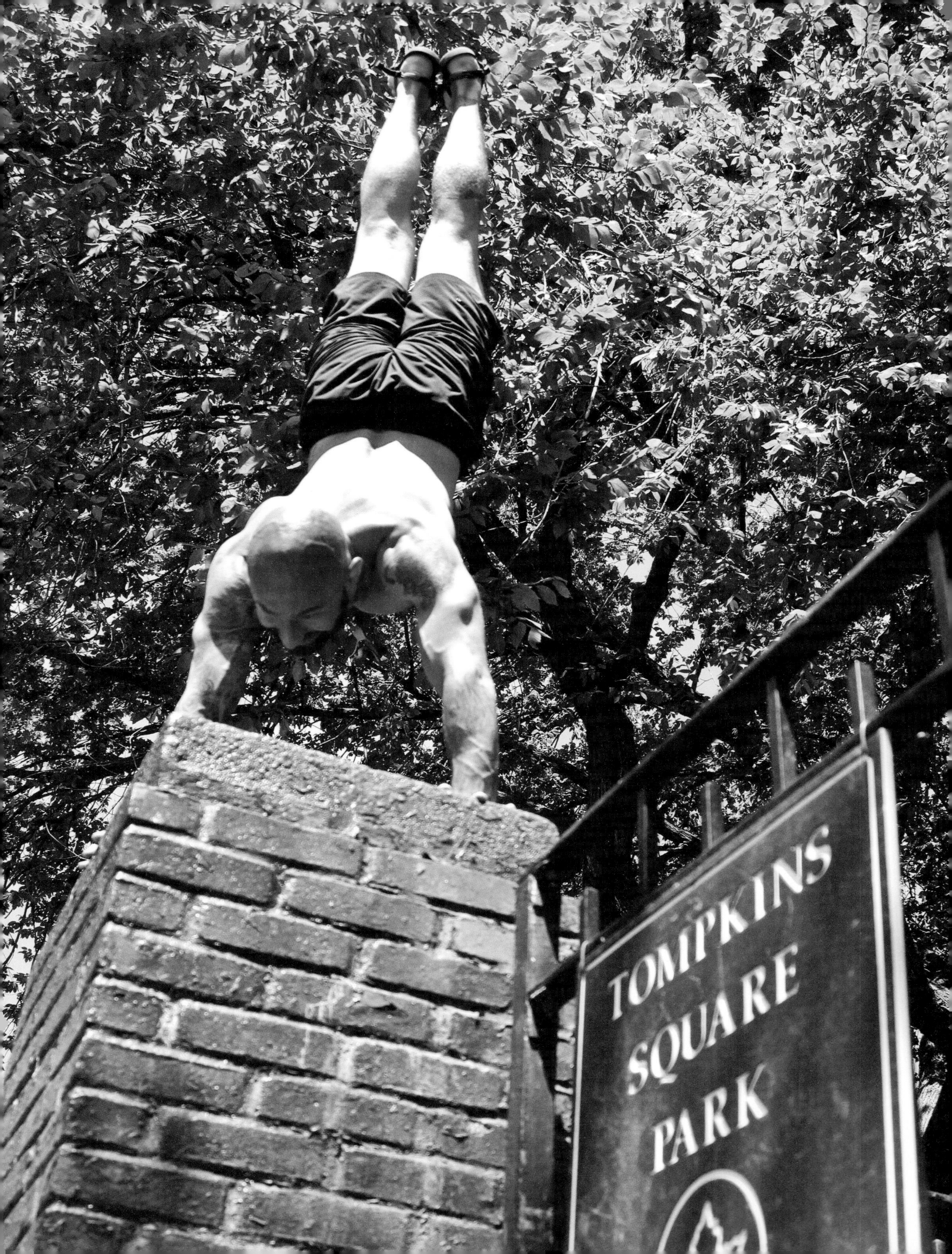
TOMPKINS
SQUARE
PARK

# STRETCHING FOR STRENGTH

"Change is only possible through movement."

*-Aldous Huxley*

If you look around any commercial gym, you're likely to see a wide variety of activities taking place: strength training, aerobics, simulated bicycle riding, people doing god-knows-what on a vibrating stability platform, and of course, good ol' stretching. Most gyms even have a designated stretch area. Though you sometimes see serious-minded folk in these rooms, the stretching area in many fitness facilities seems to be primarily for people who want to bullshit around, be seen at the gym and feel like they accomplished something productive.

For this reason (as well as others), a lot of serious strength training enthusiasts are quick to overlook or even decry flexibility training. I've heard several professional fitness trainers proclaim stretching to be a waste of time. Some even argue that static stretching will actually hinder your strength gains and athletic performance. Though I believe stretching is generally more helpful than harmful, there is some truth to these claims. Let's get this out of the way quickly so we can move on.

First off, a lack of effort leads to a lack of results. If you just sit there and slump over toward your toes without any real intention behind it, you probably won't do much to affect change in your hamstrings. You reap what you sow. Stretching to increase your range of motion is simple in theory, but it is not easy in practice. It requires concentration, patience and strength.

Additionally, not every stretch is appropriate for every individual. Some people will naturally be tighter in some places while others will achieve a full range of motion with little effort. If you're not tight in a given area, you may not feel any need to stretch there at all. I've seen a handful of adults who can comfortably get into a full butterfly stretch or lotus pose without really working on it. Though these same folks are sometimes tight in their upper back or hamstrings, hip openers are probably not necessary for them.

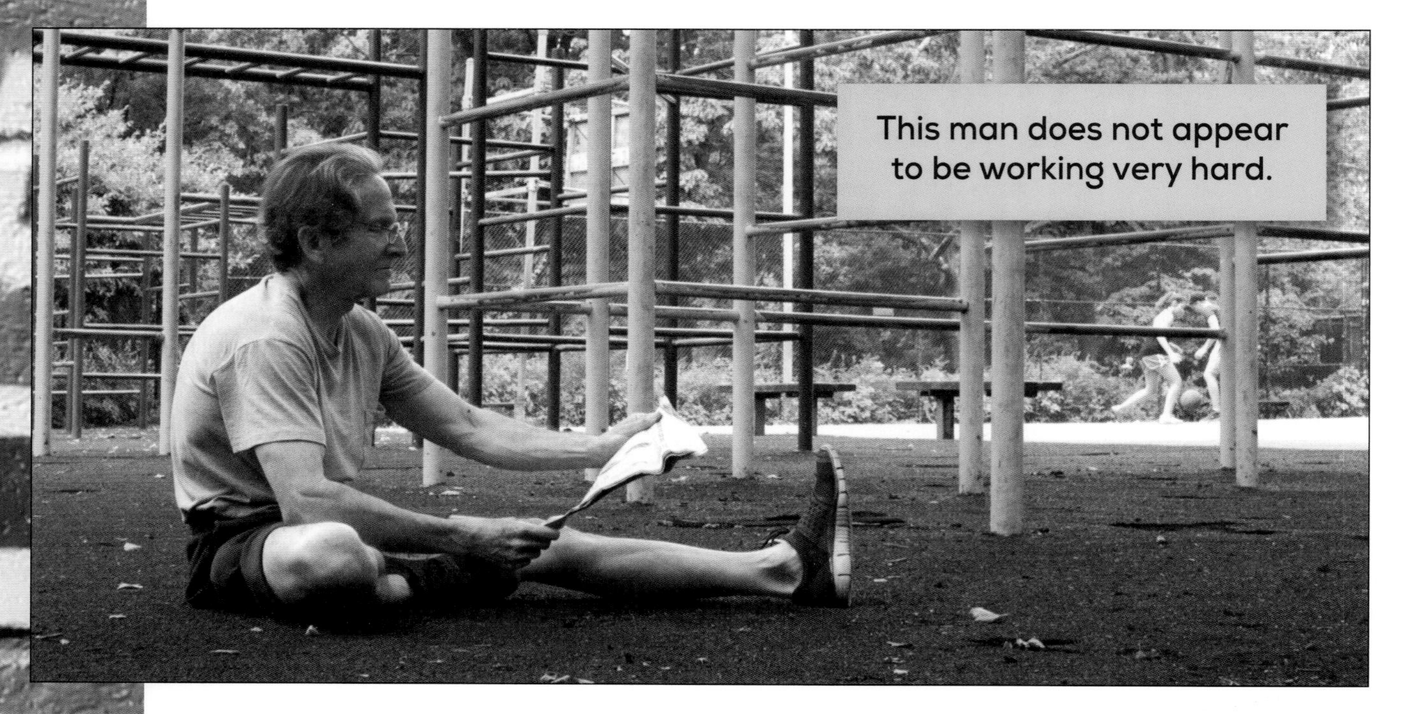
This man does not appear to be working very hard.

Furthermore, under certain circumstances, specific stretches may be contraindicated or harmful for certain individuals. For example, a person with a lower-back injury may exacerbate that situation if they engage in excessive hamstring stretching, while another with a frozen shoulder may have trouble with moves that require placing the arms overhead. Folks in these situations may have to progress very slowly or modify some of the poses to better suit their individual needs. As I often remind my clients, you've got to listen to your body.

Everything has its time and place. It's usually a bad idea to eat right before swimming, but eating is generally pretty important. Along those same lines, prolonged static stretching immediately prior to intense dynamic movement can be a recipe for injury. For example, performing ten minutes of static hamstring stretches right before a set of plyometric jump squats may relax your legs too much, temporarily reducing their ability to explosively contract. When you suddenly go into that jump, you may pull a muscle or land poorly. For this reason, intense flexibility training is usually best performed after a strength workout or on a separate day entirely. However, a brief dynamic stretch sequence can serve as a nice warm-up prior to your strength work (see Part Three for specific routines).

Also consider the specific needs of the individual: gymnasts, dancers and martial artists require greater range of motion than the average person simply looking for general fitness. Although there may be no apparent reason to train for hypermobility if you are not in one of these specialized groups, you might find enjoyment in it. Any sort of disciplined practice offers the opportunity for personal development. However, the range of motion required for healthy day-to-day living is far less than what is requisite for any of the aforementioned disciplines. The stretches and routines in this book were designed for total body mobility as it applies to calisthenics training - not contortionism.

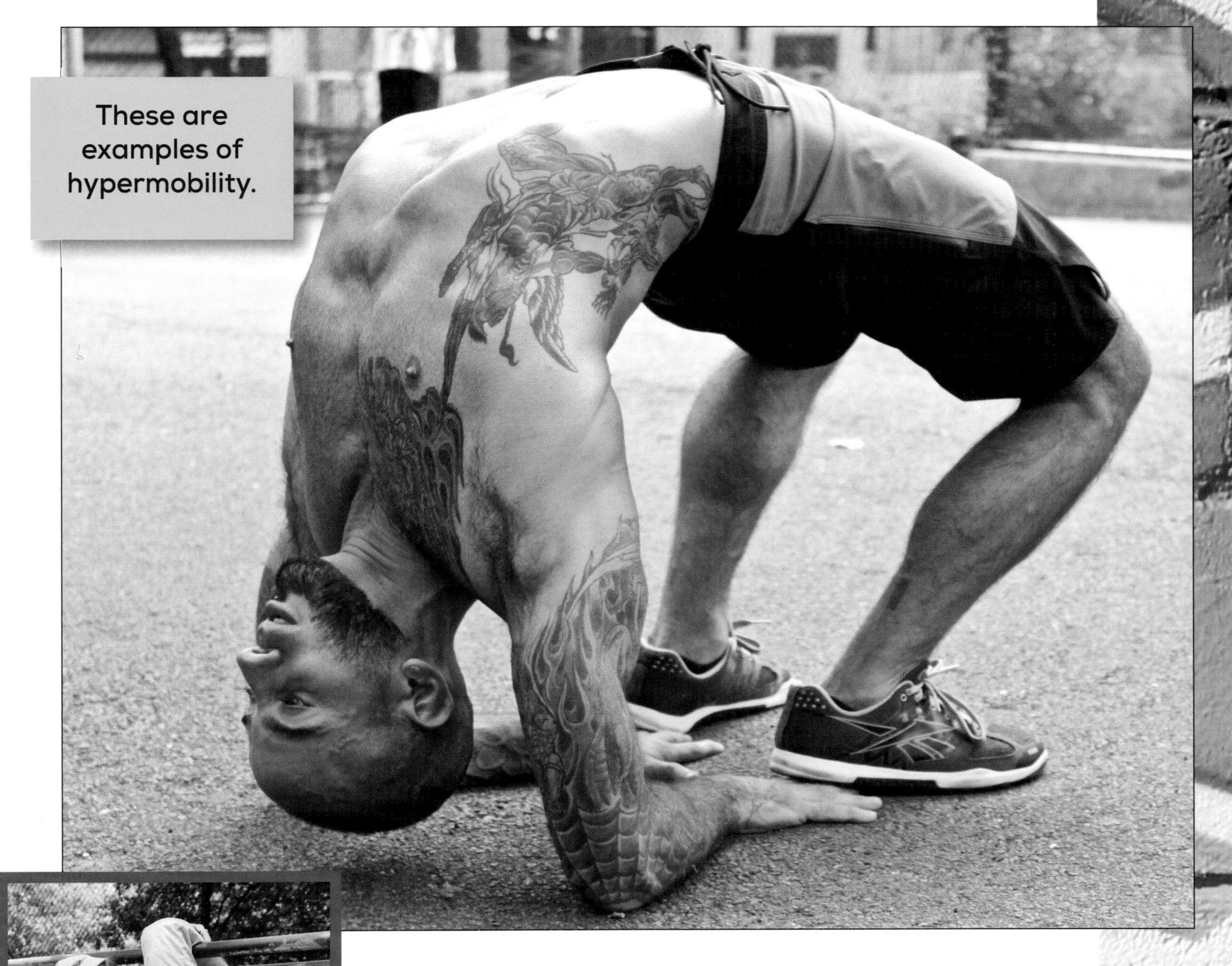

These are examples of hypermobility.

As for the claim that mobility training is detrimental to your strength gains, this can be true. After all, there is only so much training the body can handle at once. Focusing simultaneously on multiple challenging, yet unrelated endeavors makes it difficult to improve at any of them. It can also lead to burnout, but this doesn't mean stretching is bad for the average person looking for overall calisthenic fitness. Sometimes you have to give up something to get something else. You can have anything you want, but you can't have everything you want. If you've prioritized strength training too much or for too long, it might be most beneficial to devote a few weeks or months of your training toward improving your mobility, while shifting your strength training into maintenance mode.

Additionally, it's possible that a lack of mobility may be holding you back from reaching your potential. Without a full range of motion, fundamental exercises like squats, bridges and even push-ups can't be fully utilized. In the long run, focusing on mobility may ultimately improve your strength.

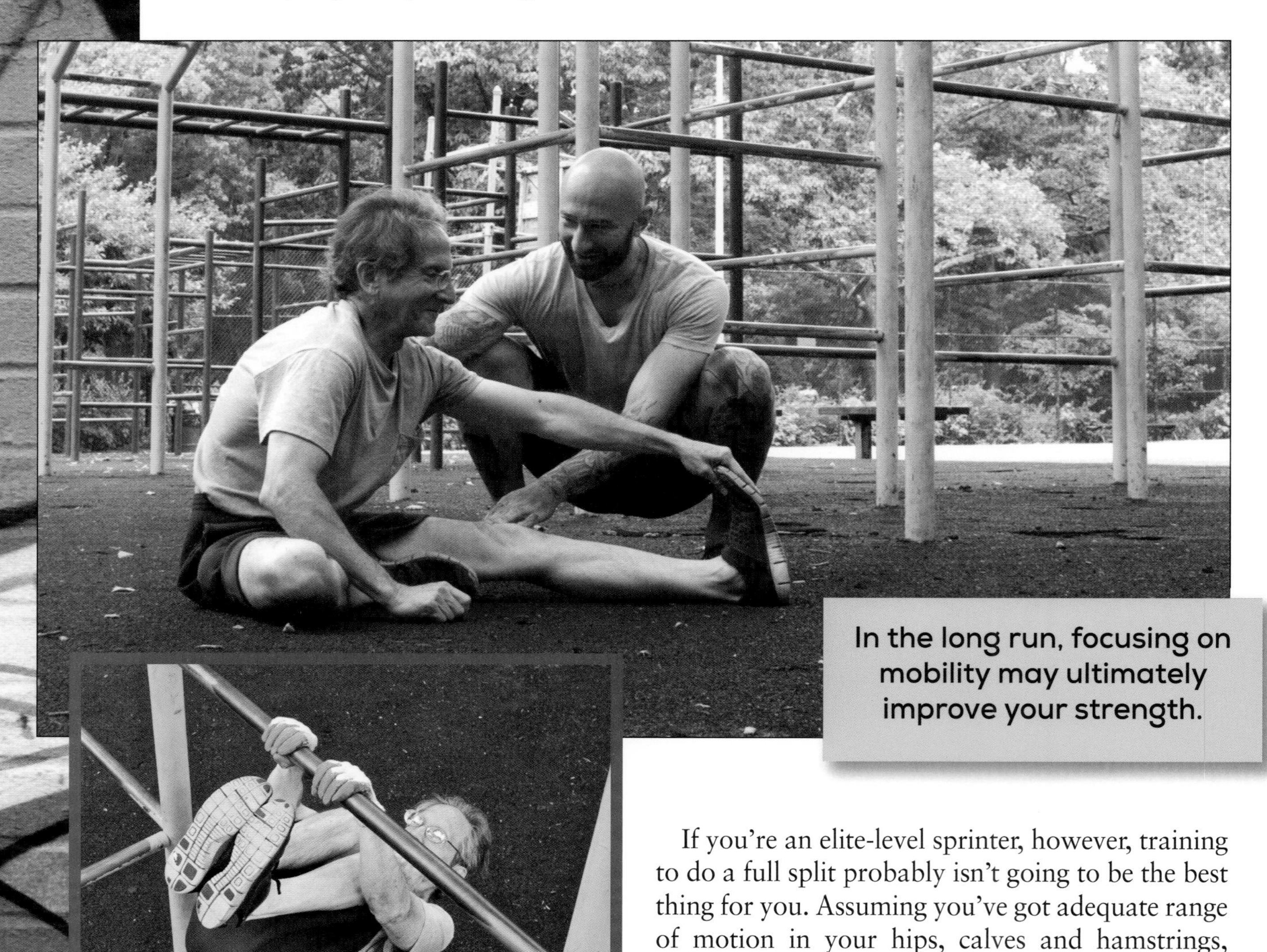

**In the long run, focusing on mobility may ultimately improve your strength.**

If you're an elite-level sprinter, however, training to do a full split probably isn't going to be the best thing for you. Assuming you've got adequate range of motion in your hips, calves and hamstrings, your time would likely be better spent specifically practicing toward increasing your strength and speed. For the rest of us, stretching our hips, groin and hamstrings is most likely going to help us more than harm us.

Genetics play an undeniable role in everything, including flexibility potential. Some people really don't need to stretch much at all, but they are the outliers. Let's be very clear however: your genetics don't give you an excuse to be inflexible. While the spectrum of mobility is quite large, we all have the potential to achieve a full, healthy range of motion in all of our joints.

Though a few folks may naturally be tight, the cause of most peoples' stiffness is simply years of neglect. Your body adapts to your actions (or inactions). If you move often, you will get good at moving, but if you've spent most of your life sitting in a chair, chances are your hips, hamstrings, shoulders and upper back have tightened up as a result. It takes a long time for this to happen, and it can take just as long to undo. While you might gain some immediate benefits by implementing the techniques in this book, don't expect to magically improve your range of motion with five minutes of stretching twice a week if you've spent the last two or three decades sitting for twelve hours a day. You may need to give extra time and attention to certain areas, as well as making a point to avoid activities that exacerbate the situation.

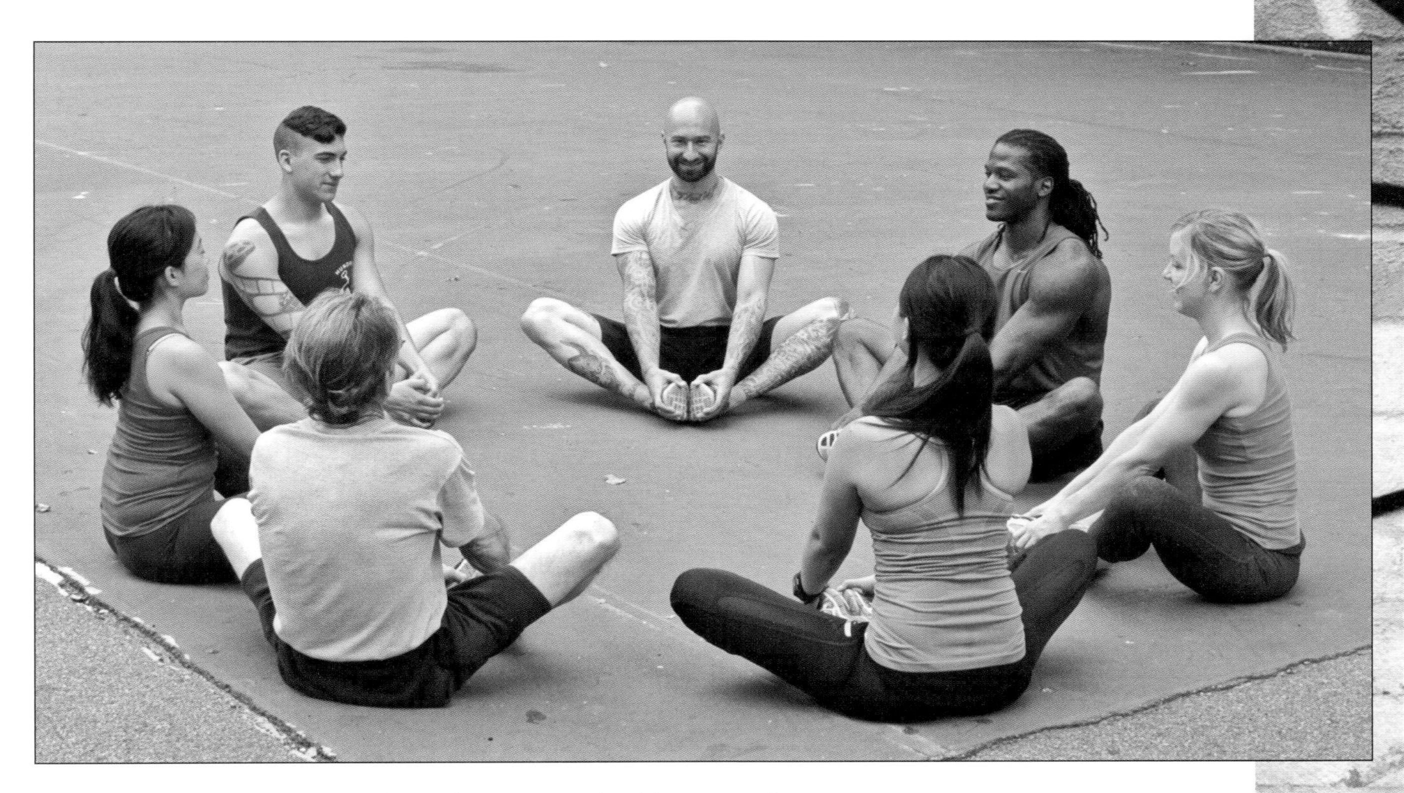

The practice itself should be the most valuable part of your training. Do not get too attached to the idea of achieving any specific goal. Progress is fun and encouraging, but those feelings of excitement are fleeting. No matter how far we come in our training, there are always new skills and poses to work toward or refine. Keeping a humble, joyous attitude about your training is the healthiest way to achieve long-term growth. Aggressive goal-setting can actually do more to hurt your practice than help it. Pursuing a goal too hard may cause you to make short-sighted decisions in the moment. This can lead to injuries or other setbacks.

What happens when you achieve a goal anyway? Your mind immediately creates another. Goals are therefore most valuable once we realize the futility in them. Of course having an objective in mind can fuel your focus and motivation; just don't get carried away. Do what is appropriate and realistic for you and your body. Though human potential exceeds most people's expectations, stretching your boundaries takes time and patience.

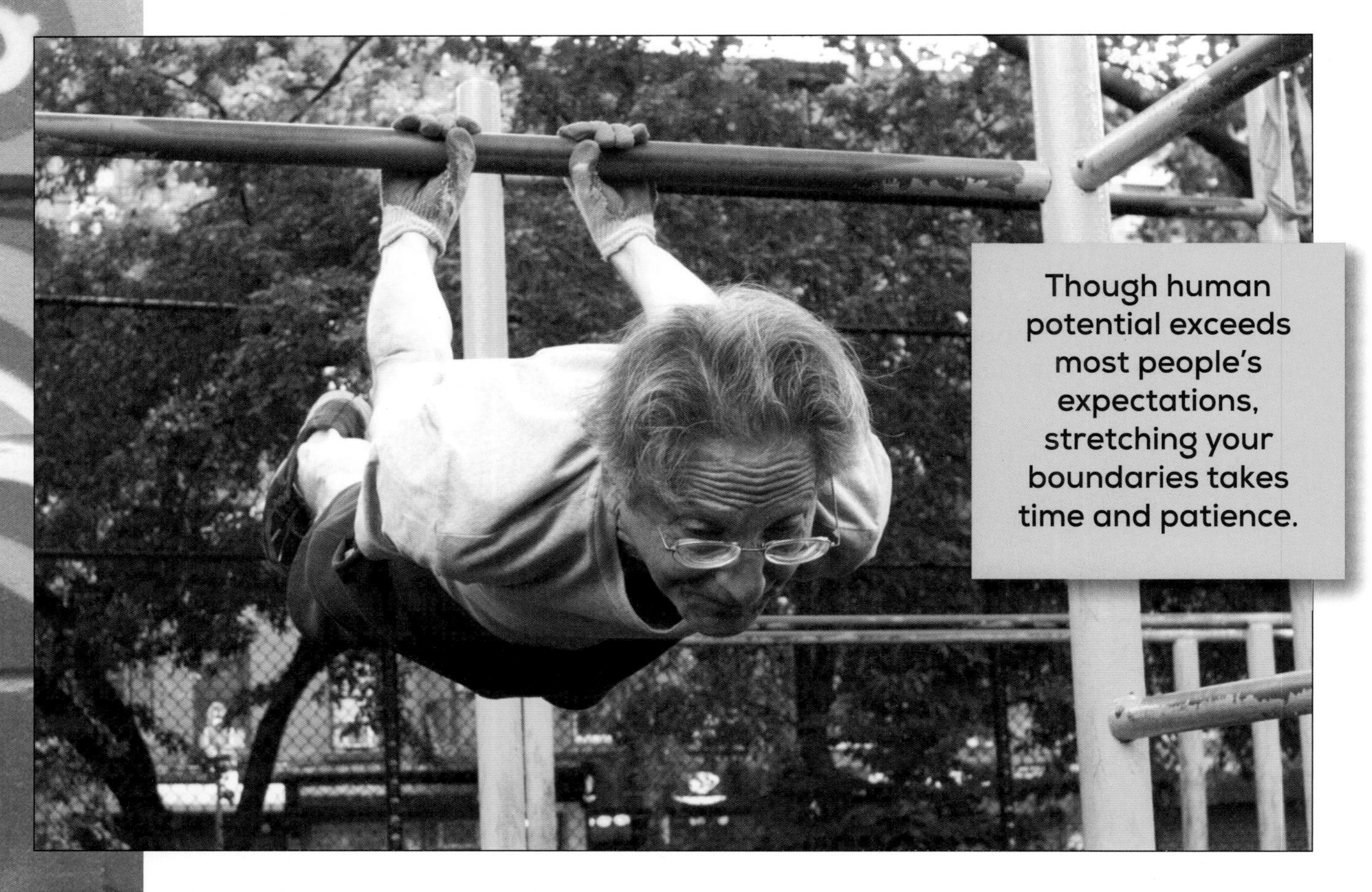

Though human potential exceeds most people's expectations, stretching your boundaries takes time and patience.

The exercises and workouts that you will find in this book focus primarily on flexibility and mobility, though many of them bear an undeniable strength component as well. The more you train with your body weight, the more you may come to find that the lines between strength and flexibility become blurred. Many of the techniques shown in this book are active stretches involving focused breathing and activation of some muscles to stretch others. Do not underestimate active stretching; it can be quite demanding both physically and mentally.

To assemble the most well-rounded bodyweight fitness regimen, I suggest combining the advice within this book along with the techniques and workouts from my previous books ***Raising The Bar*** and ***Pushing The Limits!*** The information in these three books can keep you busy for a long, long time with a diverse range of complementary training tools. You can mix and match different combinations to create unique workouts for yourself for years to come. All that is required is the desire to explore your body's potential.

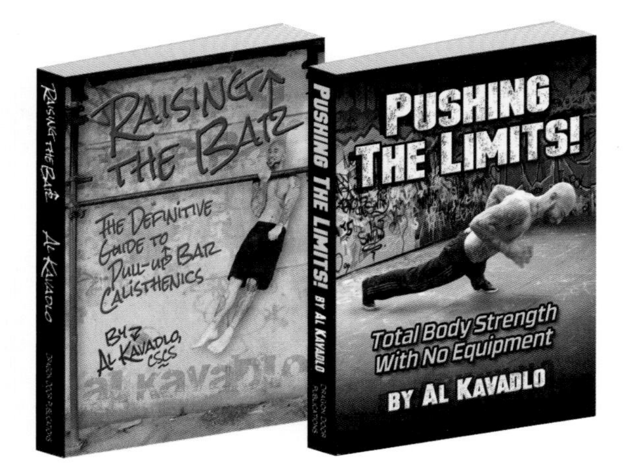

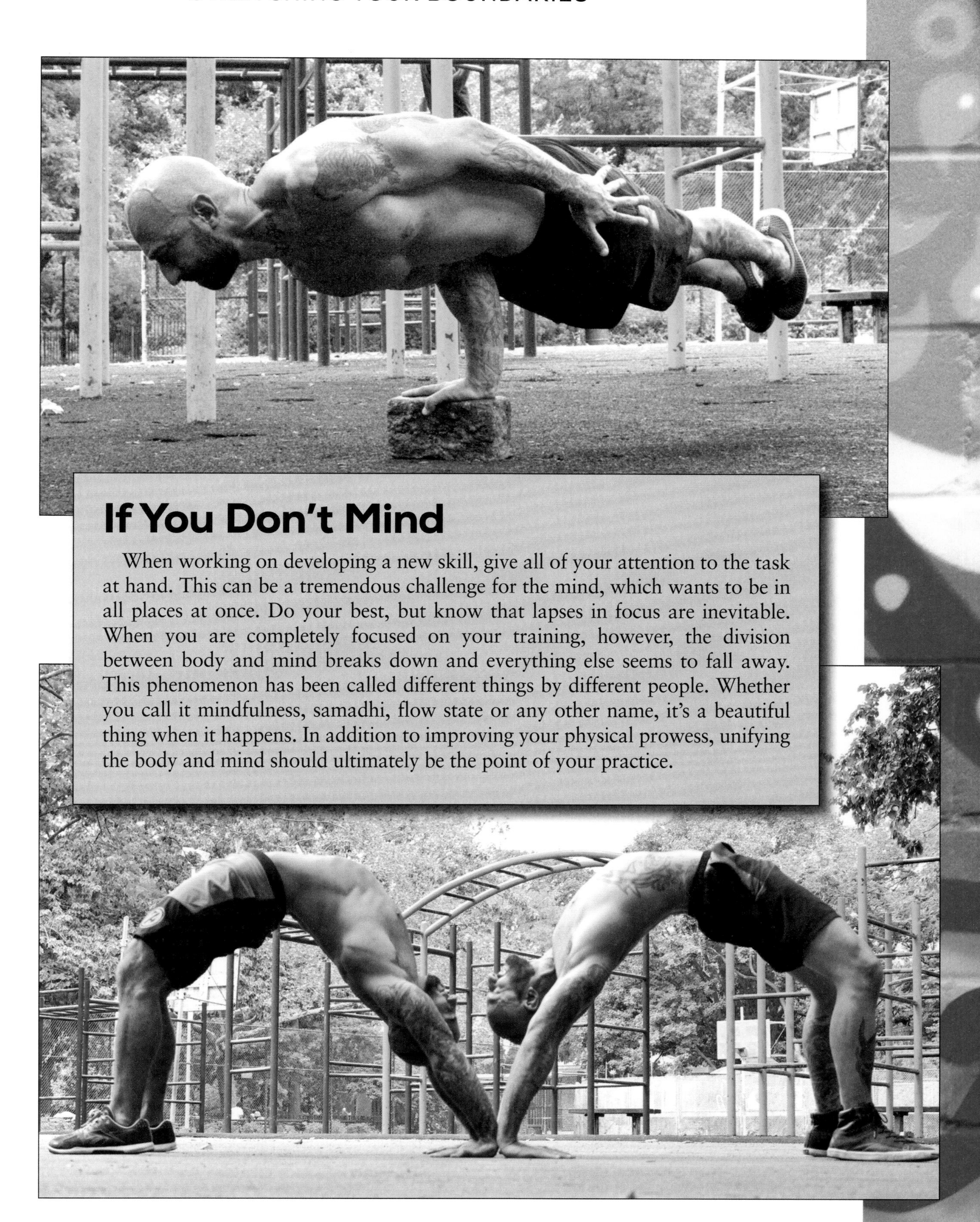

## If You Don't Mind

When working on developing a new skill, give all of your attention to the task at hand. This can be a tremendous challenge for the mind, which wants to be in all places at once. Do your best, but know that lapses in focus are inevitable. When you are completely focused on your training, however, the division between body and mind breaks down and everything else seems to fall away. This phenomenon has been called different things by different people. Whether you call it mindfulness, samadhi, flow state or any other name, it's a beautiful thing when it happens. In addition to improving your physical prowess, unifying the body and mind should ultimately be the point of your practice.

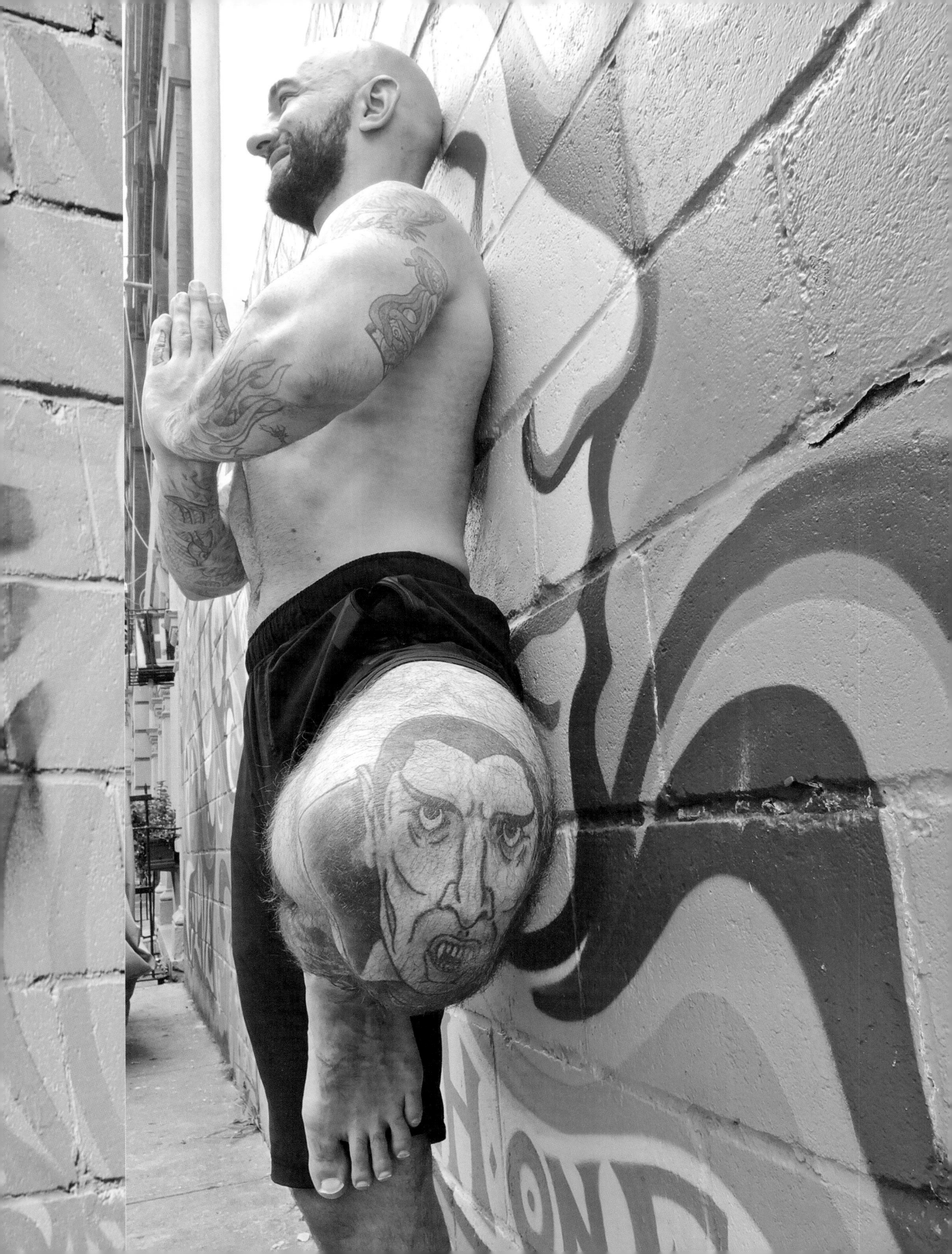

# TAKING YOUR MEDICINE

## "Movement is medicine."

## *-Unknown*

Of course, stretching can be overdone. Too much of a good thing almost always becomes a bad thing eventually - the same is true of strength training - but the idea that stretching in general is useless or even detrimental misses the big picture. If you've got a cold, a couple tablespoons of cough syrup might help you sleep through the night and feel better the next day, but drinking three bottles of the stuff could land you in the emergency room. I could even argue against drinking water because you could overdose on it if you force yourself to drink several gallons in a short period of time. Of course that would be ridiculous though. Drinking lots of water is good for you!

There is an inherent degree of risk to everything, but that doesn't mean we should lock ourselves in a cage and avoid all potentially dangerous activity. We just need to be sensible and put some thought into things. Anyone who's practiced strength training for a significant amount of time has no doubt had to deal with setbacks and (hopefully minor) injuries. In fact, strength training is often blamed for these injuries. This is also ridiculous; blaming strength training for an injury is like blaming your car because you crashed into a tree. Individuals, not their vehicles (automotive or otherwise), are responsible for their actions, as well as the consequences that follow.

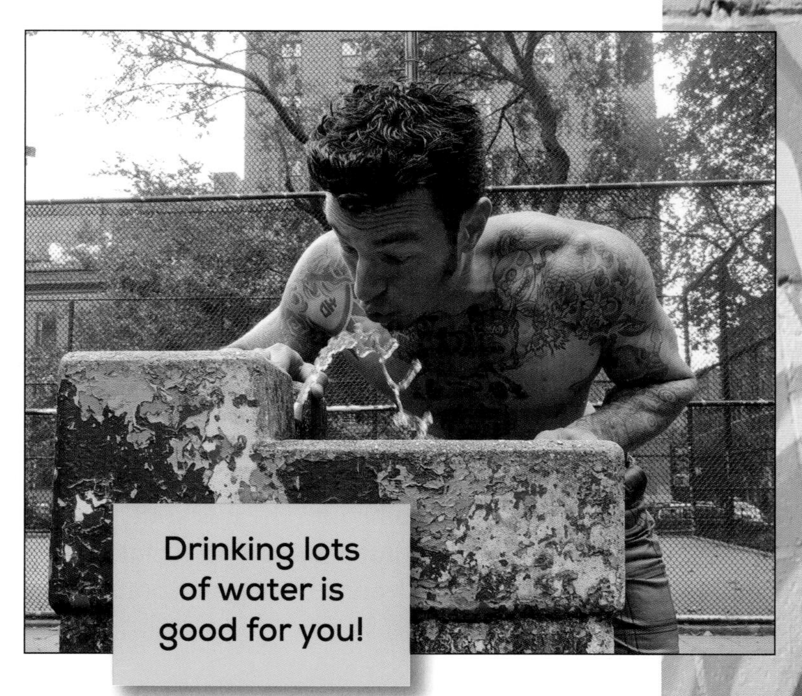

Drinking lots of water is good for you!

Stretching and strength training are no different in that regard. Yes, some people do get hurt by participating in these activities, but both are often scapegoated as the sole cause of injury. If you are diligent and consistent in your stretch routine, you will reap the benefits of your work. If you are foolish and/or short-sighted, you may wind up frustrated and/or injured.

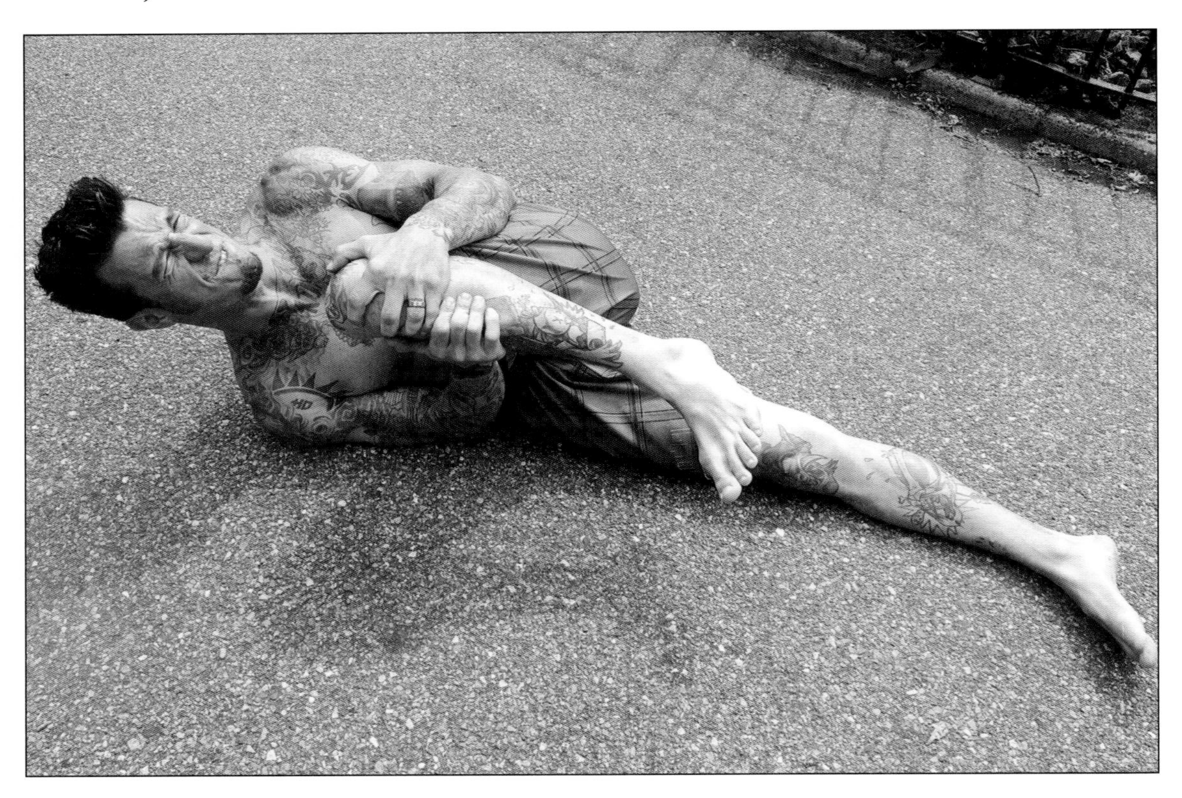

Aside from a few brief bouts of tendinitis, minor sprains, and a couple scrapes and bruises, I've stayed injury-free in spite of working out for the majority of my life. In fact, I believe it's because I've worked out for over twenty years that I have never had a serious injury. Sure I've had my share of bumps along the way (and learned from them), but I've never torn a muscle, dislocated a joint or broken a bone. Other than an emergency surgery due to a freak bout of Meckel's Diverticulitis in my early twenties (a peanut got stuck in my malformed small intestine), I've never needed serious medical attention of any kind.

In those times when we are nursing tendinitis or getting over a strained muscle, movement is the best medicine - you've just got to be careful with the dosage! Light to medium stretching promotes circulation. Getting the blood flowing to your achy areas is the best thing to help them recover. Intense stretching will likely leave you sore, which could impede your recovery. Just like strength training, you can't go all out every time. If you're not 100% going into the workout, then it's fine to take it easy. I want you to stretch your boundaries, but I want you to take your time doing so. This is not a competition; be patient with yourself and your practice. Honor your body and respect your level.

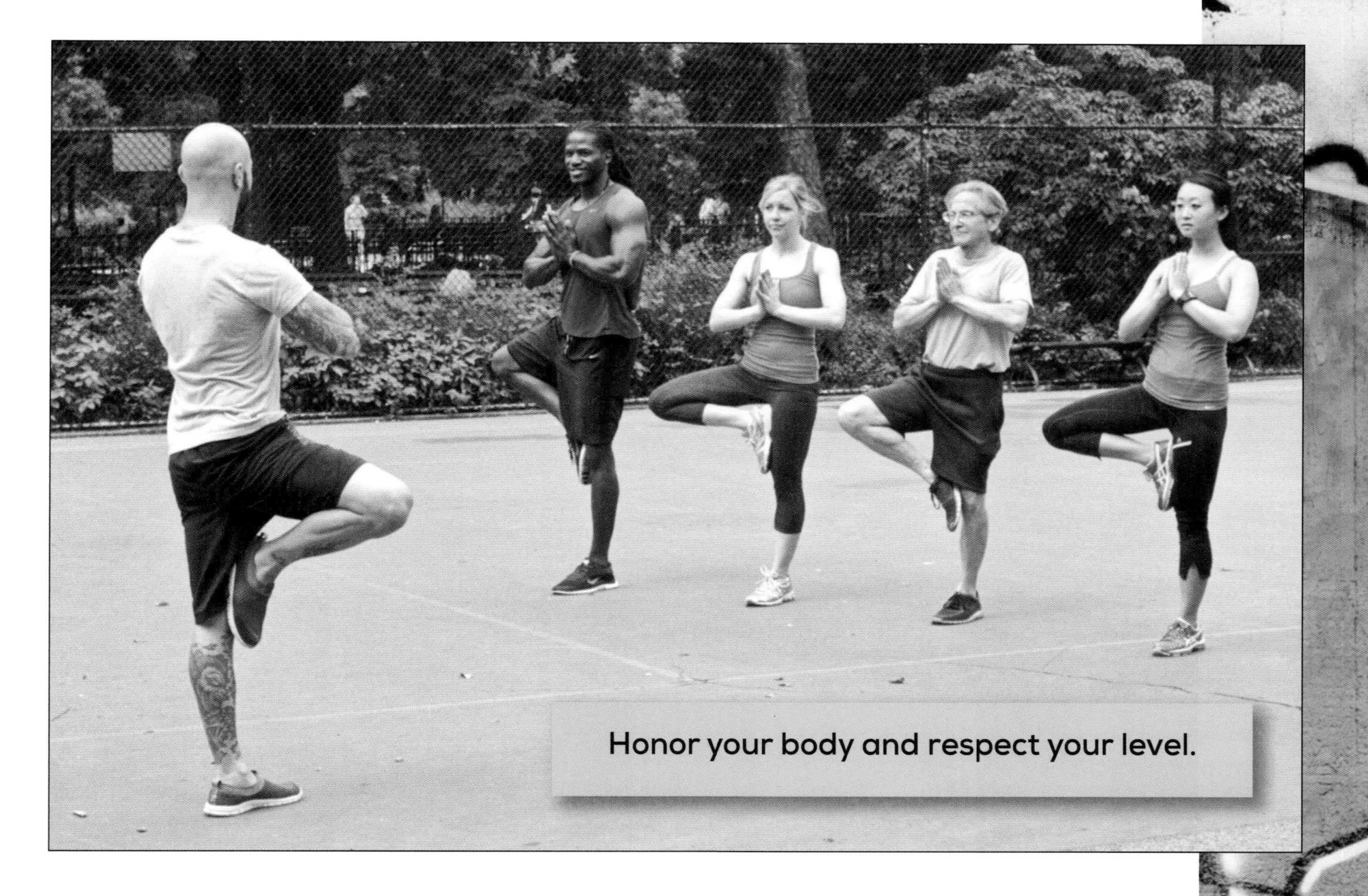

Honor your body and respect your level.

In the last ten years, I've trained people from all walks of life. The ones who took their stretching seriously and approached it with humility (especially the guys who wanted to improve their calisthenics game) have benefitted from it. I've felt and witnessed the rewards of flexibility training in myself and my clients. I've seen it with my own eyes and I know it works. Perhaps that will be the case for you as well.

The more popular any given activity becomes, the more likely there will be detractors looking for ways to cut it down. Reactionary behavior is nothing new. The problem stems from a larger issue in our culture - society's need to force everything into dichotomies of right and wrong, good and bad, healthy and deadly. Things are not always so. In reality, all things are multifaceted and complex. Between black and white, there are many shades of gray.

When we over-analyze things, we tend to lose sight of what information is useful and realistic. I find it interesting that the word "academic" means both "pertaining to a college, school or other educational institution" as well as "not practical." You learn by doing things, not just by studying or analyzing data. Don't read this and simply take my word for it. Try the postures and training routines outlined in this book, experiment with your own variations and see for yourself what works for you. I'm leaving it to you to draw your own conclusions.

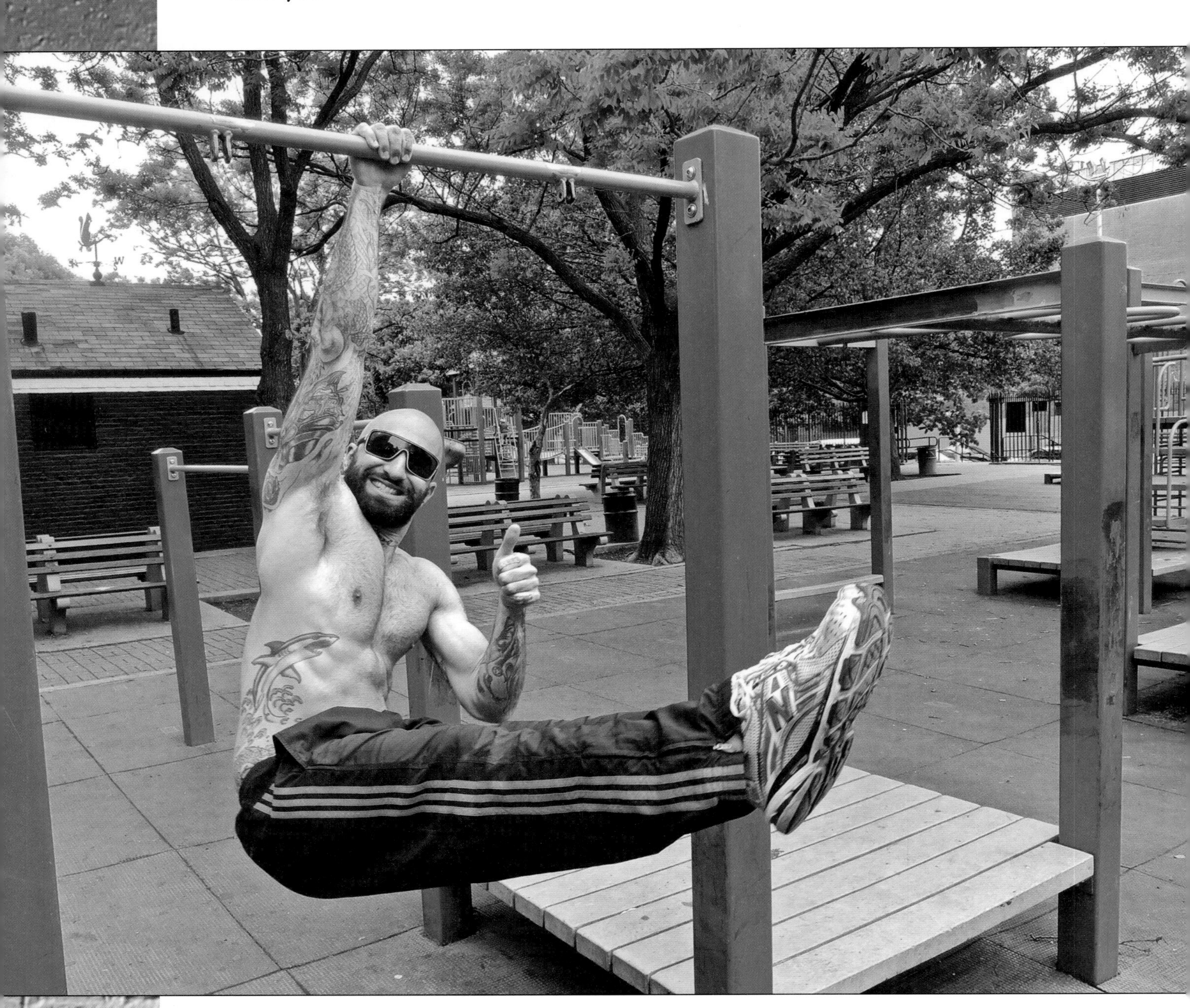

**ac·a·dem·ic [ak-uh-dem-ik]**
***adjective***

1. of or pertaining to a college, academy, school, or other educational institution, especially one for higher education.
2. pertaining to areas of study that are not primarily vocational or applied, as the humanities or pure mathematics.
3. theoretical or hypothetical; not practical, realistic, or directly useful.
4. learned or scholarly but lacking in worldliness, common sense, or practicality.
5. conforming to set rules, standards, or traditions; conventional.

Source: Dictionary.com

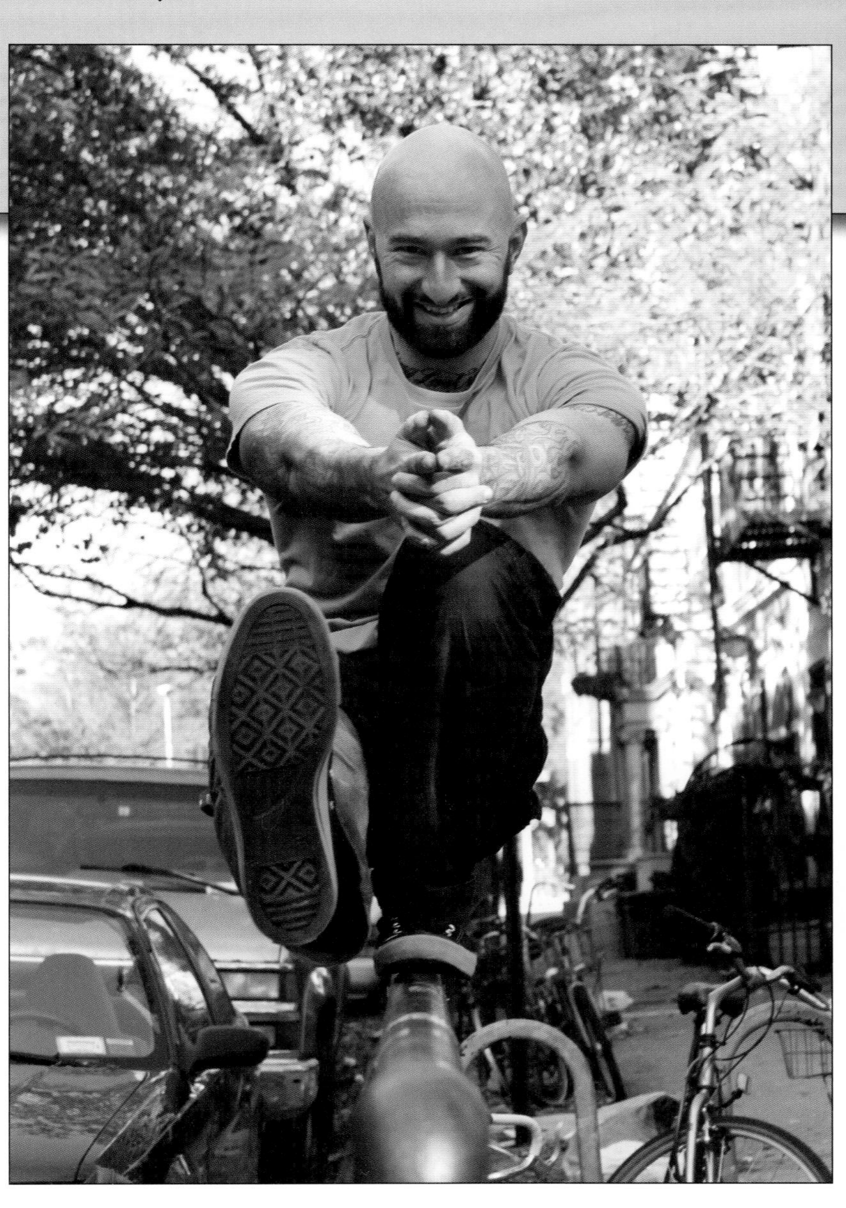

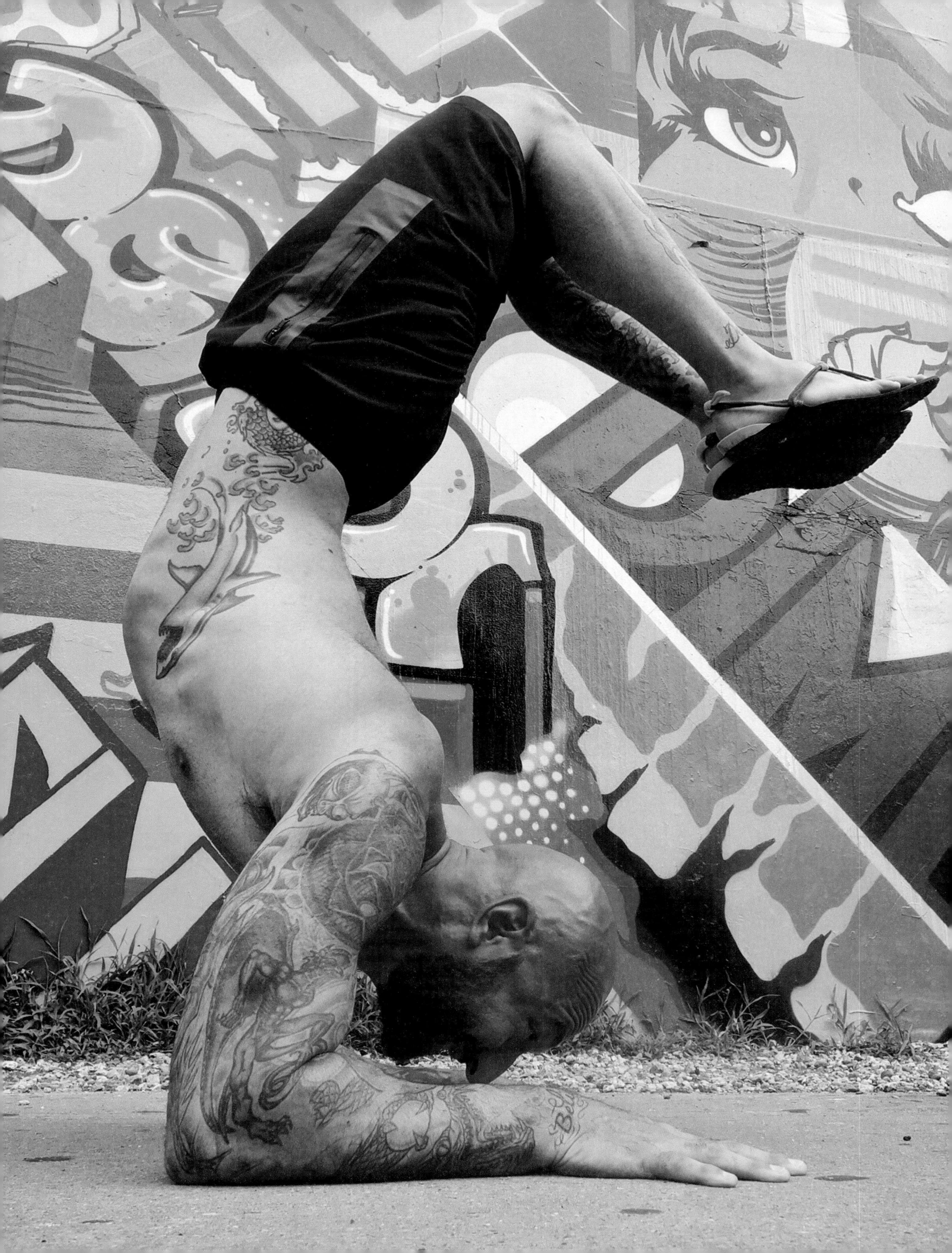

# KID STUFF

**"Over-thinking, over-analyzing, separates the body from the mind."**

***-Tool, "Lateralus"***

When I was a kid, I just wanted to play. I didn't realize I was training! I sure didn't care whether what I was doing was called yoga, calisthenics, stretching or anything else. I just knew that moving my body was a lot more fun and interesting than sitting around all day. Nowadays, I realize that naming things helps with communicating ideas, yet I recognize that splitting hairs over details eventually becomes a trivial pursuit. I've never been a stickler for terminology, so if you find me using words like "yoga" and "stretching" somewhat interchangeably, bear with me. I might also refer to a certain pose or stretch by a different name than what you are accustomed to. Try not to get bogged down in these small details.

Call it whatever you want!

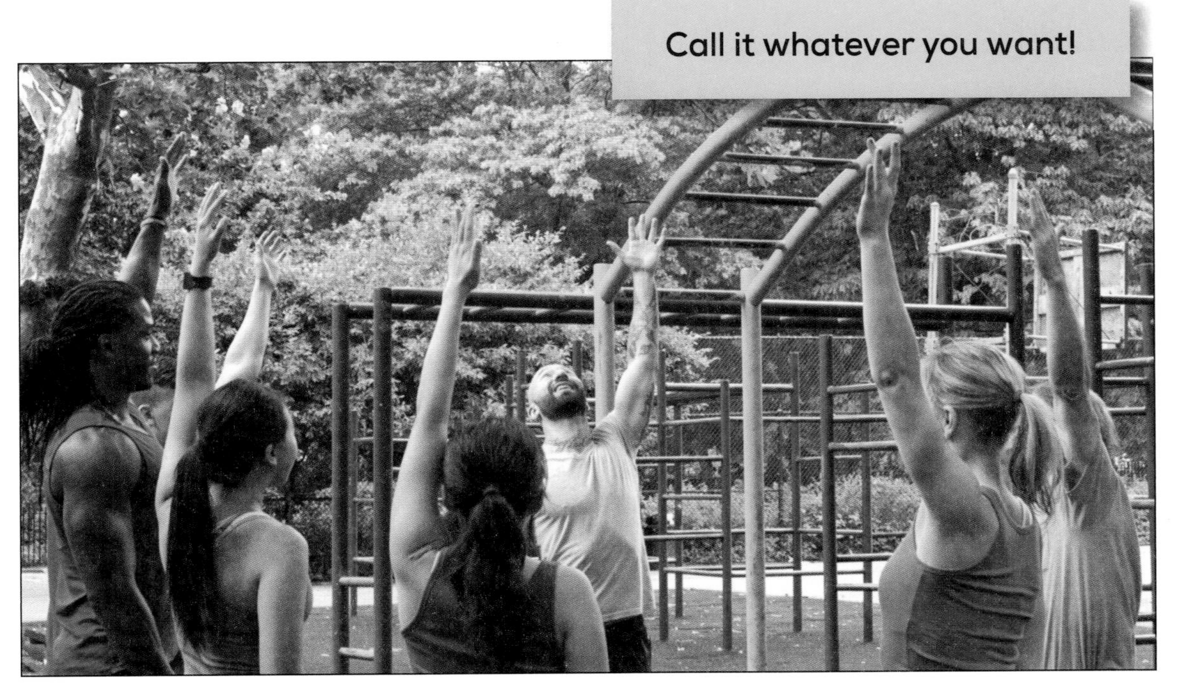

My earliest experiences with yoga were learning to do a lotus pose and headstand when I was around nine years old. I thought they were cool looking and wanted to learn them for this reason alone. I didn't know or care if there were any benefits outside of the simple joy of exploring physical movement. (Incidentally, this was the same motivation later on when I made it my mission in life to learn the human flag at age 27.)

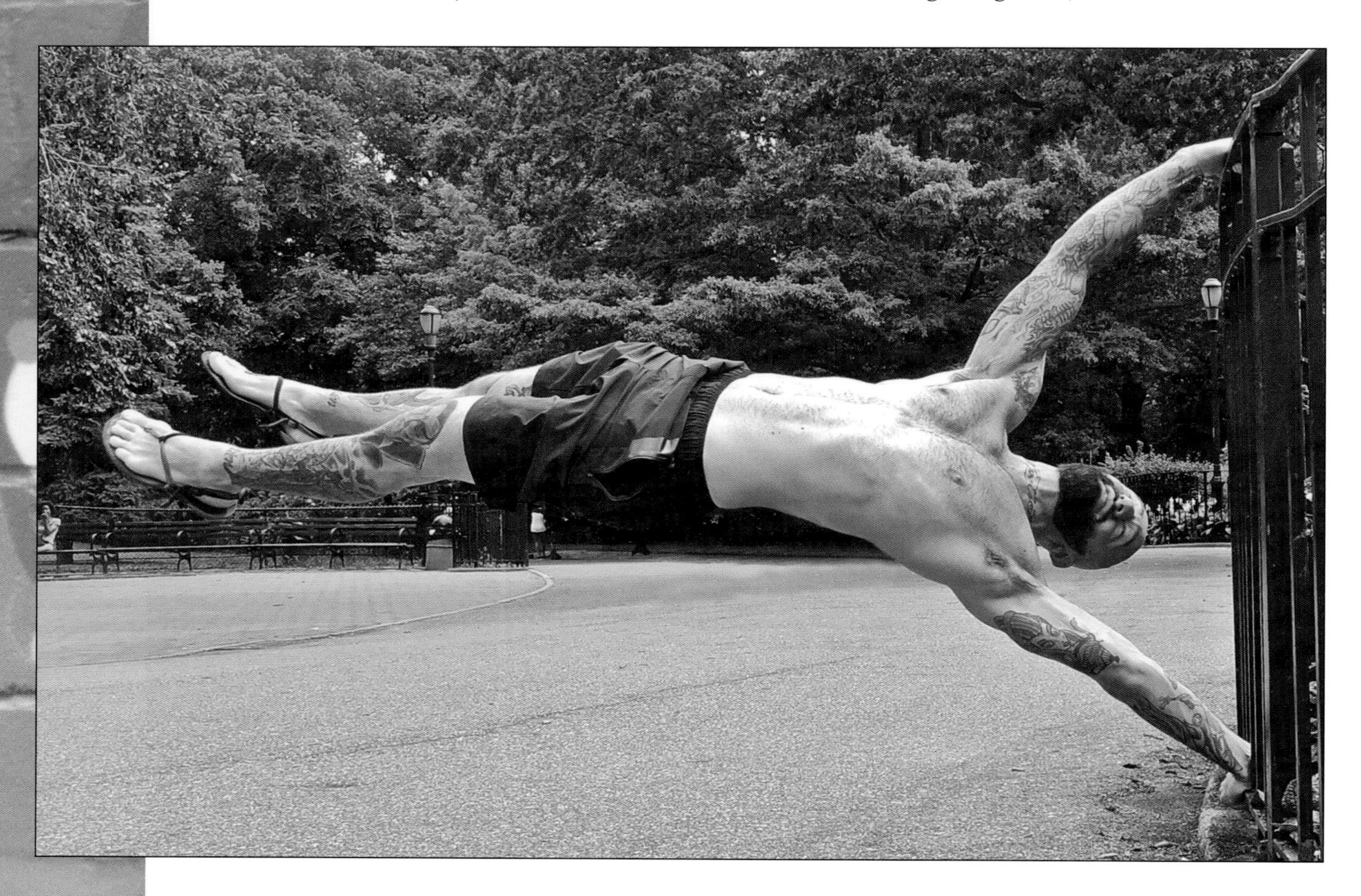

During the '80s, my dad dabbled in yoga. Around that time, I remember seeing a picture of the lotus position in a book that was lying on the dining room table. It looked awesome! I decided to try it and found that it was a bit of a stretch, but if I really went for it, I could hold the pose for a few seconds before it became too uncomfortable. Nobody ever told me, but I knew to back away when I started to feel pain in my knees. I gave myself recovery time between efforts but kept practicing. Since I thought it looked so cool, I really wanted to get good at it. This is honestly still a big part of my motivation for much of my training today. As I was young and supple, I trained myself to hold the lotus position for extended periods of time without discomfort in only a few weeks. The older you get, however, the longer it can take to improve your mobility. If you're lucky enough to be reading this while you are young, consider yourself very fortunate. Regardless of your age, take your time gradually progressing through these exercises.

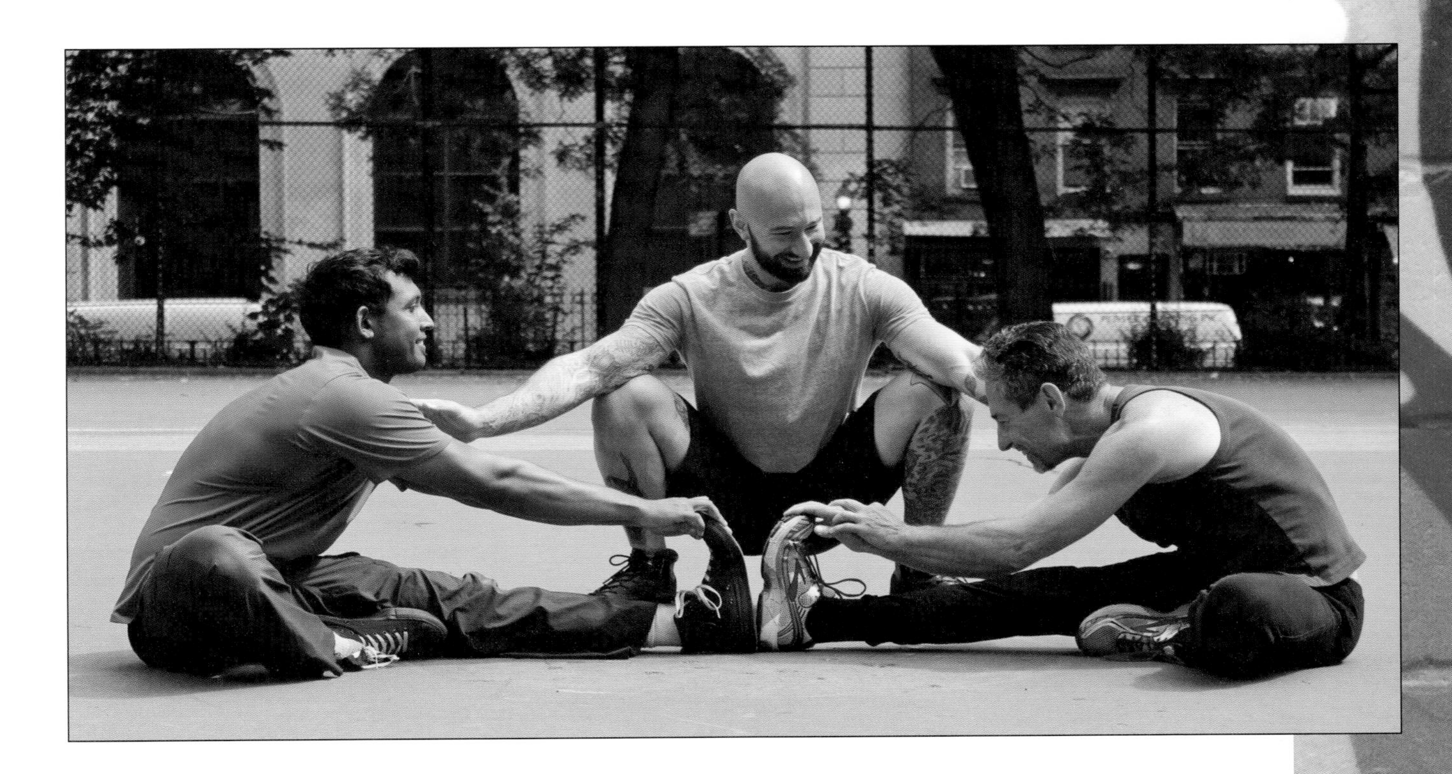

Around the same time as my early lotus training, I saw my dad doing a headstand for the first time. Like most kids, I thought it looked really cool so I decided to try it myself. Though it took a bit of practice, I got the hang of the headstand fairly quickly. I think it's easier when you're only four and a half feet tall. I still love seeing children's reactions to headstands. While adults are often nervous about inversions, kids almost always want to try them without a second thought.

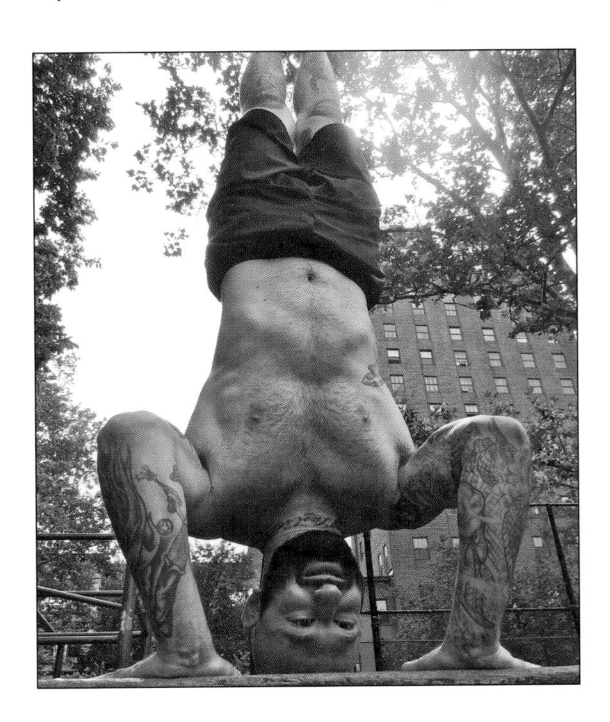

My reason for learning the lotus and the headstand was never about core strength, balance or hip flexibility. Like I said before, I really just wanted to do them because I liked how they looked. Also, it was fun! Without being aware of any real benefits, I was simply drawn to the moves for their own sake. In retrospect, I'm glad I found that lotus picture as a kid and thought that it was neat looking. I credit that for my current hip mobility. Though I didn't realize it until fairly recently, those informal childhood yoga sessions were actually when I started exercising. I didn't begin strength training until I was a teenager, but messing around with yoga poses was the beginning of my fitness journey.

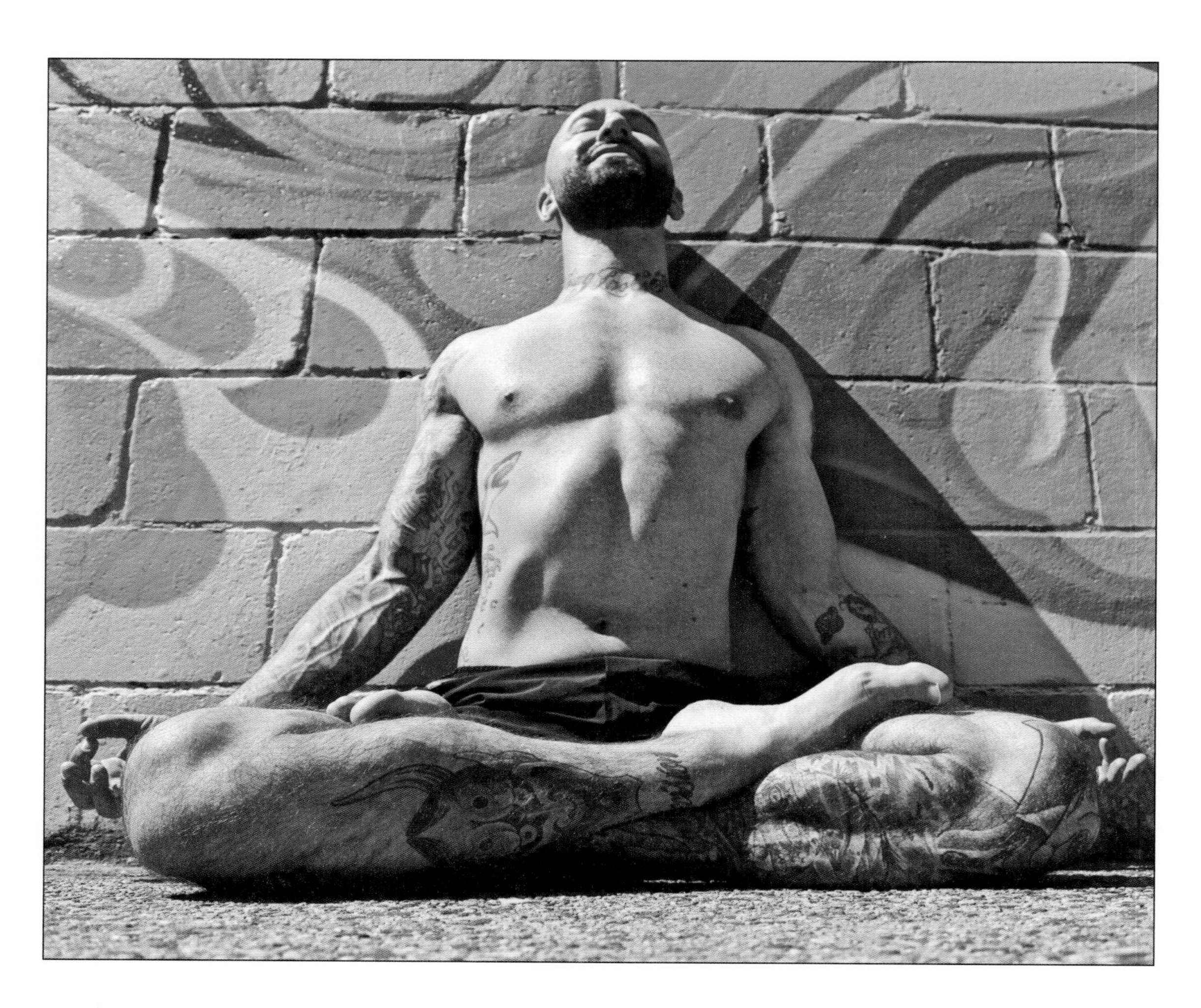

Though I can't hold a lotus position as comfortably as I did when I was a child, I have maintained the ability to perform the pose simply by practicing it regularly. Of course I still back off if it starts to bug my knees. My headstands are better than ever, although I did have to relearn the skill in my early twenties. I hadn't done a headstand in over a decade at that point, but it returned to me fairly quickly once I started practicing again.

There's a concept in exercise science called the "specificity principle" which is just a fancy way of saying that you get good at the things you consistently do. If you want to acquire new skills, you have to work specifically toward those skills. You can't improve your flexibility without dedicated practice.

There's also something colloquially known as "muscle memory" which refers to the body's amazing ability to build on previous experience, even if that experience was acquired a long time ago. The first few sessions back might be a bit rusty, but it takes less time to relearn a skill than it takes to learn it the first time. These two factors are both key reasons why I can still do a lotus and headstand in my mid-thirties.

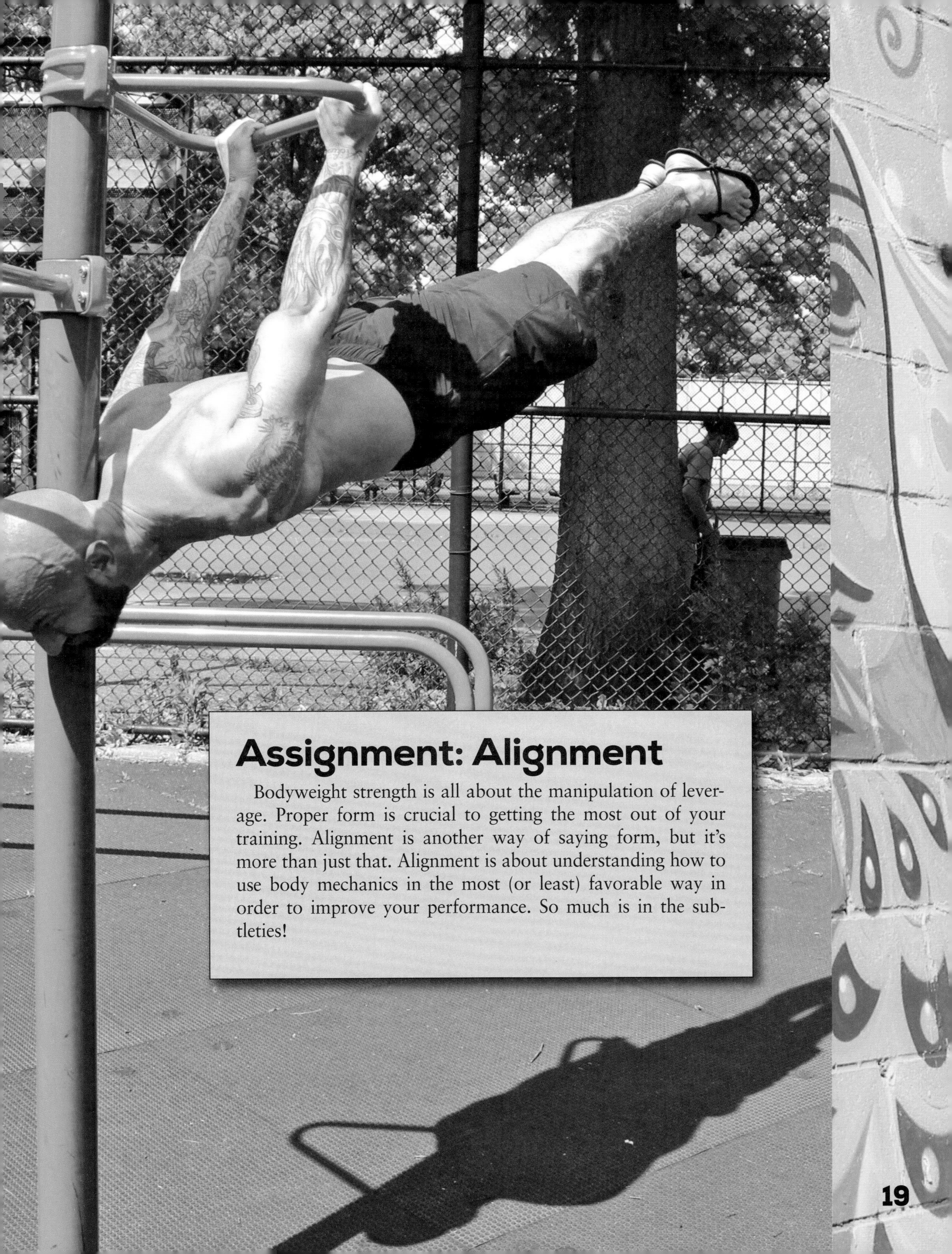

## Assignment: Alignment

Bodyweight strength is all about the manipulation of leverage. Proper form is crucial to getting the most out of your training. Alignment is another way of saying form, but it's more than just that. Alignment is about understanding how to use body mechanics in the most (or least) favorable way in order to improve your performance. So much is in the subtleties!

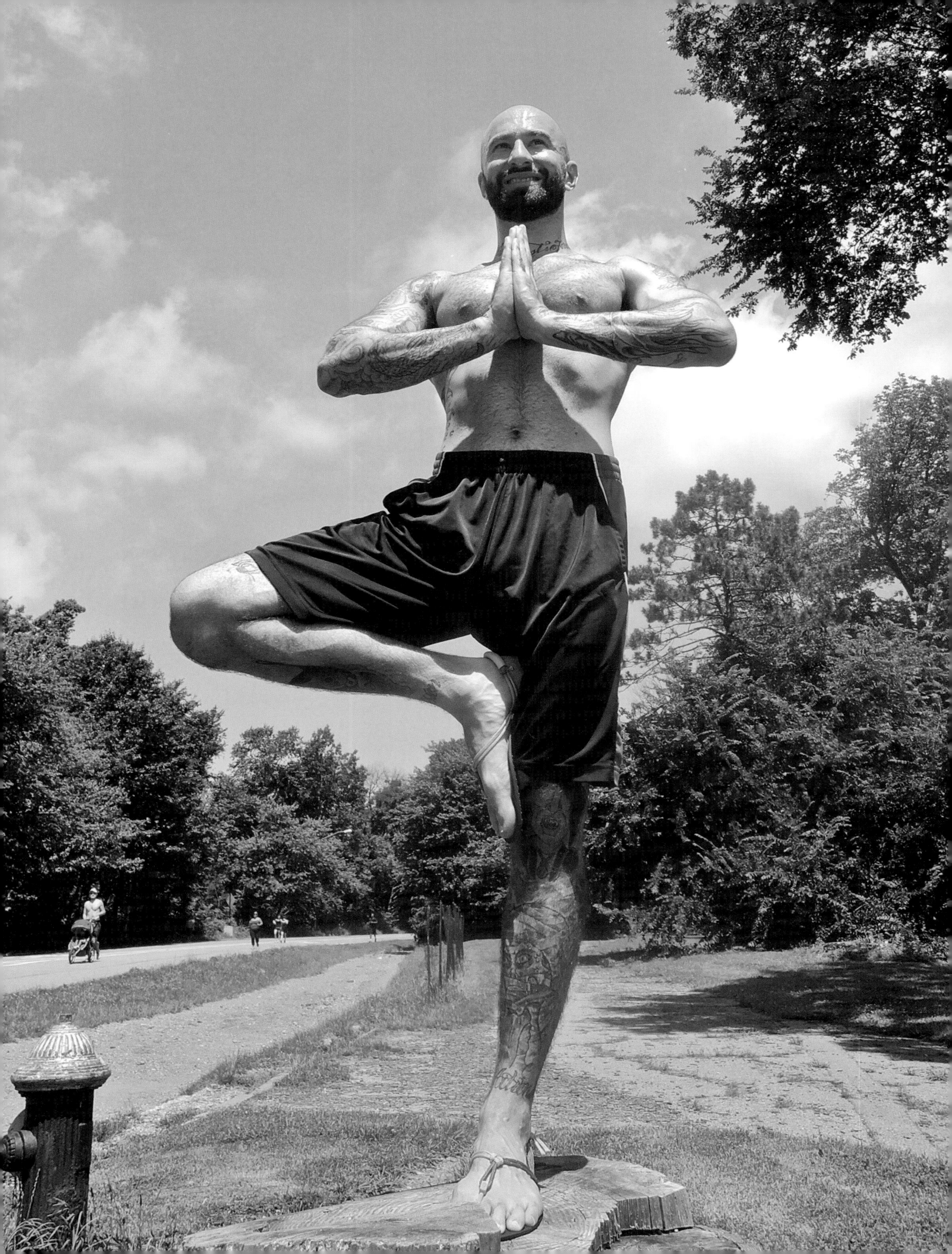

# MOBILITY MATTERS

"What are these barriers that keep people from reaching anywhere near their real potential? The answer to that can be found in another question and that's this: Which is the most universal human characteristic: fear or laziness?"

*-Louis H. Mackey*

Trends will come and go but mobility will always matter in bodyweight training. There's no way to perform high-level calisthenics moves like handstands, back bridges, pistol squats or elbow levers without establishing a full range of motion in your joints. I'm used to the mainstream media using fearmonger tactics to frighten people away from living life to its fullest, but I'm dumbfounded by how often I come across fitness professionals decrying stretch techniques that have been proven effective for thousands of years. These same hucksters who want to tell you stretching will hurt your athletic performance are often the ones who peddle empty promises and fake quick fixes. They cater to two of the most universal human emotions: fear and laziness. Don't allow yourself to be duped. If something seems too good to be true, it probably is. Always question things that defy your common sense. Definitely question me if you think I'm ever blowing smoke up your ass. A healthy dose of skepticism can do wonders!

People like to believe that newer means better - and sometimes that is true. However, with regard to movement, I believe the ancients had it right the first time around. Yoga is one of the oldest forms of bodyweight training that's ever existed - and if you practice calisthenics, yoga (or stretching or whatever you like to call it) is probably the best way to supplement your practice. It's something I've been doing myself for over a decade.

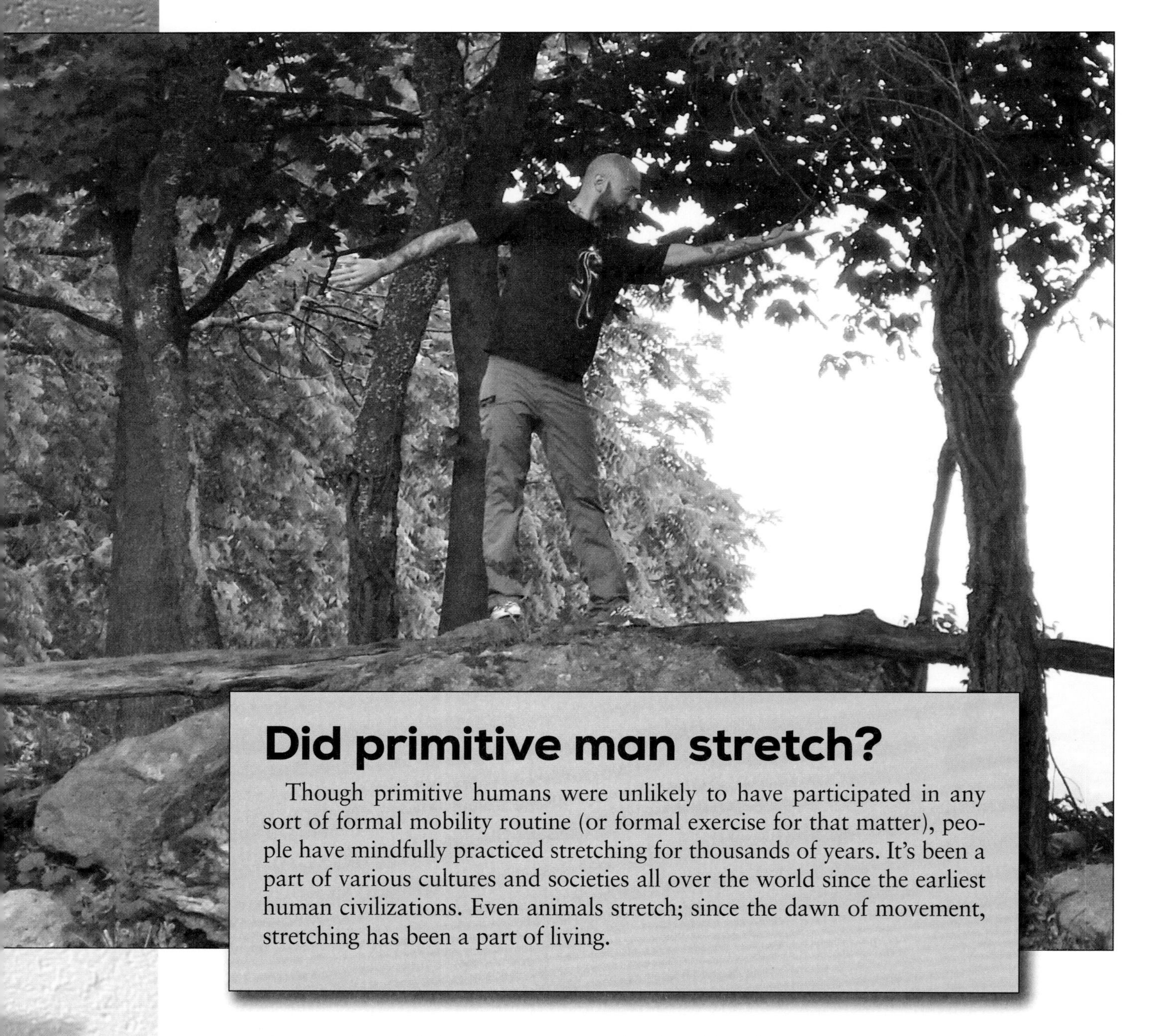

## Did primitive man stretch?

Though primitive humans were unlikely to have participated in any sort of formal mobility routine (or formal exercise for that matter), people have mindfully practiced stretching for thousands of years. It's been a part of various cultures and societies all over the world since the earliest human civilizations. Even animals stretch; since the dawn of movement, stretching has been a part of living.

Along with tribal dancing, yoga may be the oldest form of ritualized human movement that's ever been recorded. Drawings of yoga poses have been found in archeological artifacts dating back over five thousand years. Though it's more popular nowadays than it's ever been, yoga is a timeless practice, not just a fancy way to stretch. To purists, yoga transcends the physical practice entirely, extending into emotional, spiritual and all other facets of being. It's an entire belief system.

To me, yoga is simply another form of bodyweight training - another item to keep in my proverbial toolbox. As you'll see, there are a lot of parallels and similarities within the poses, postures and holds seen in traditional yoga and calisthenics. Both are essentially about getting in touch with your body through movement. No matter which style you prefer, the fundamental movements of the body transcend labels and categories. Whether you call it a push-up or chatturanga dandasana, the subtle differences are insignificant when the larger spectrum of human movement is taken into consideration. There's no need for different schools of movement to be at odds with one another when they have so much in common.

Just like yoga, calisthenics is simply a workout to some, while for others it is an entire lifestyle. For many of us, the physical benefits of working out are just a small piece of the pie compared to the mental, emotional and spiritual rewards. It doesn't matter if we're yogis, traceurs or calisthenics practitioners, movement is still medicine - and the benefits remain the same.

The word calisthenics comes from the ancient Greek words "kallos" and "sthenos," which roughly translate to "beauty" and "strength" in English. Calisthenics therefore can be interpreted to mean "beautiful strength." Of course, the beauty of calisthenics is not just physical - it encompases those deeper spiritual qualities that the ancient yogis sought to get a glimpse of through their practice. The word strength can also refer to mental power as well as physical prowess. The division between body and mind is an illusion.

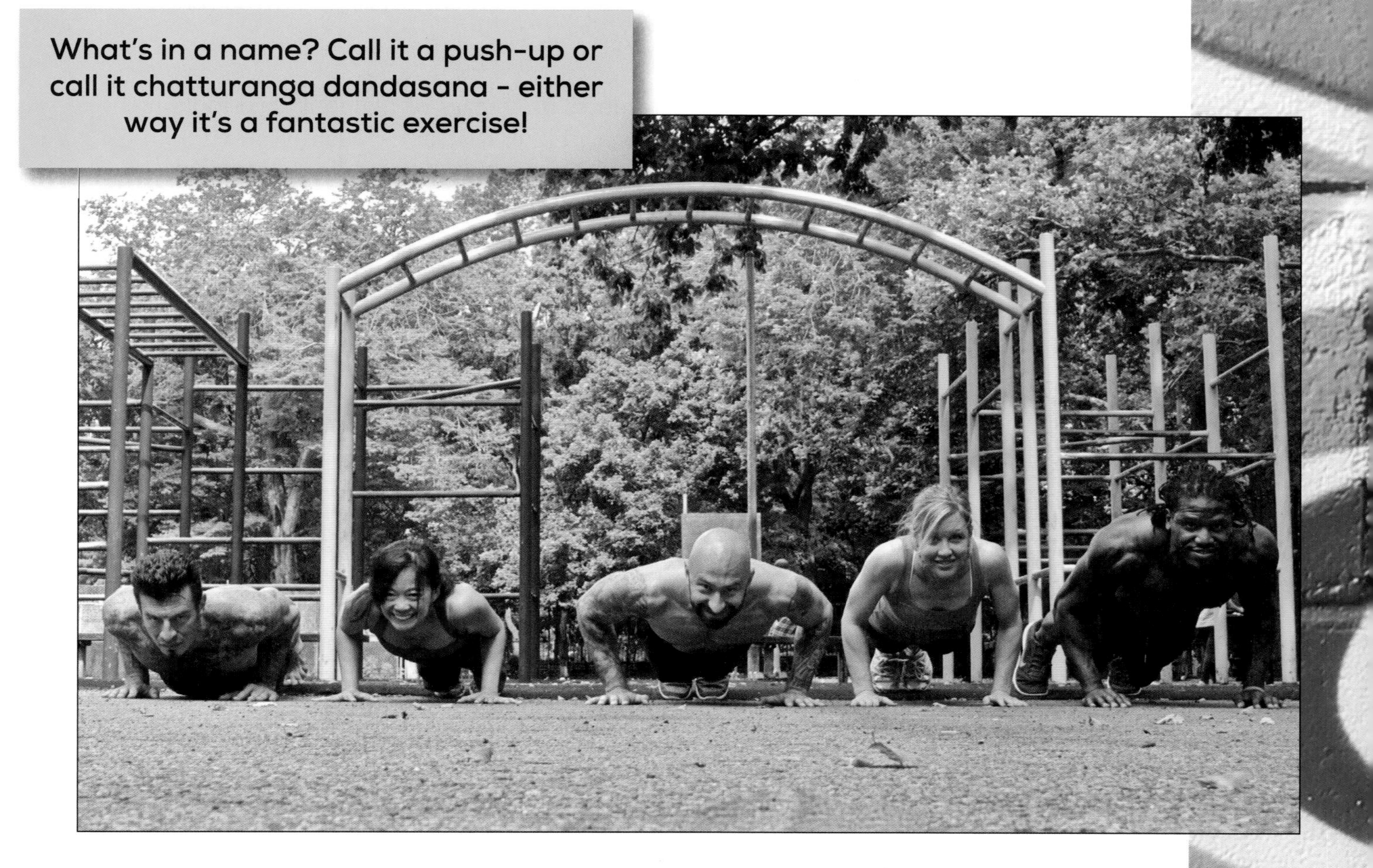

**What's in a name? Call it a push-up or call it chatturanga dandasana - either way it's a fantastic exercise!**

**beau·ty** [byoo-tee]
*noun*

1. the quality present in a thing or person that gives intense pleasure or deep satisfaction to the mind, whether arising from sensory manifestations (as shape, color, sound, etc.), a meaningful design or pattern, or something else (as a personality in which high spiritual qualities are manifest).

**strength** [strengkth, strength]
*noun*

1. the quality or state of being strong; bodily or muscular power; vigor.
2. mental power, force, or vigor.
3. moral power, firmness, or courage.

Source: Dictionary.com

For a lot of people, the word yoga conjures up images of malnourished-looking folks contorting themselves into esoteric positions. Either that or a bunch of poseurs thinking they're spiritual because they burned some incense and followed some stretches along with a DVD. While those stereotypes are not totally without merit, the yoga community encompasses so much more! Don't be so quick to dismiss its value or you'll miss out on a great deal of physical wisdom. Though I've brought my own take on things to the table, many of the stretches and postures presented in this book come directly from various schools of yoga.

I often talk about using your whole body as one cohesive unit in order to achieve calisthenic greatness. Coincidentally enough, the word yoga is derived from the ancient Sanskrit word for "union." Calisthenics and yoga are two sides of the same coin. On the surface, it may seem that one focuses more on strength, while the other is more concerned with flexibility. The reality is that both are primarily about finding harmony between strength, alignment and flexibility by unifying all the parts of the body.

The first time I ever took a yoga class I was 24 years old. I had been working as a personal trainer at a commercial gym for a little while and decided it would be good for me to get firsthand experience at some of the classes we offered. I went to my first class with the expectation that it would be very easy and very boring. I was wrong on both counts! The class challenged me in new and exciting ways, leaving me humbled, yet thirsty for more.

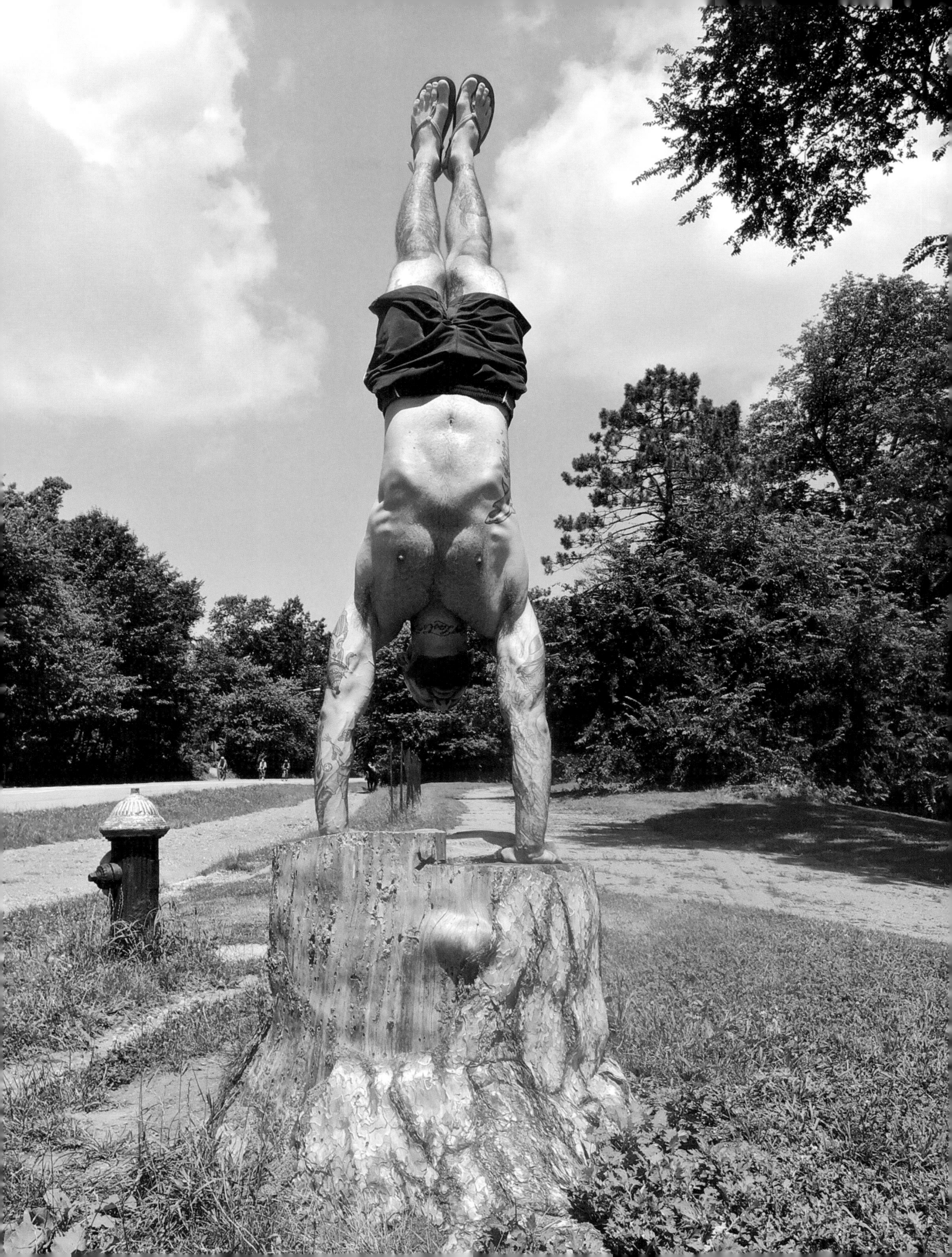

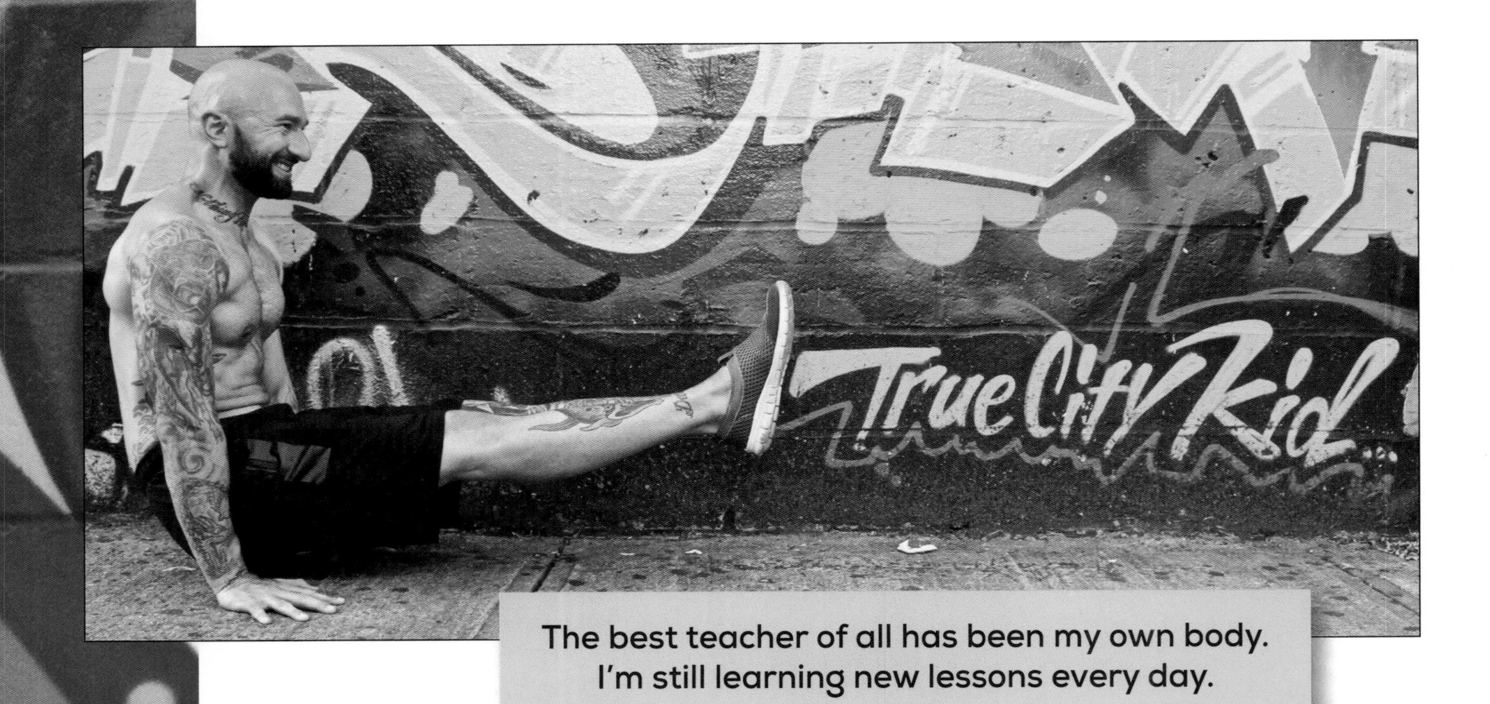


The best teacher of all has been my own body. I'm still learning new lessons every day.

I kept going back week after week - eventually bringing some of the things I was learning from yoga class into my workouts. I was enjoying the new challenges and it was a nice change of pace from my usual routine, which at the time included a lot of weight training along with some basic bodyweight exercises like pull-ups and dips. After some time, I started trying out different classes, different styles and different teachers. Though many of the basic poses ("asanas" as yogis call them) transcend styles, I soon found out there is a lot of variety within the world of yoga! Over the years, I've taken hundreds of yoga classes and learned from dozens of different teachers. The best teacher of all, however, has been my own body. I'm still learning new lessons every day.

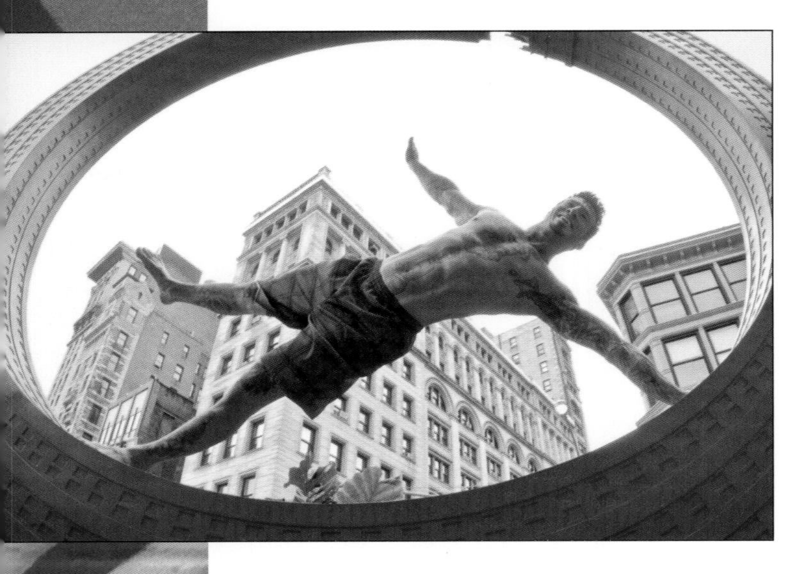

Although I'm not a yoga expert, I am a guy who's practiced on and off for much of his life. I've also done a lot of other styles of training and worked as a personal trainer to a diverse group of clients. I've always subscribed to Bruce Lee's philosophy to take what works for you, discard what doesn't and bring your own spin to it (I'm paraphrasing a bit.) In keeping with that, I've developed a few routines that compliment my bodyweight strength training in a manner that's just right for me. I'm excited to share these sequences with you in the pages ahead - but first, you've got to learn how to breathe!

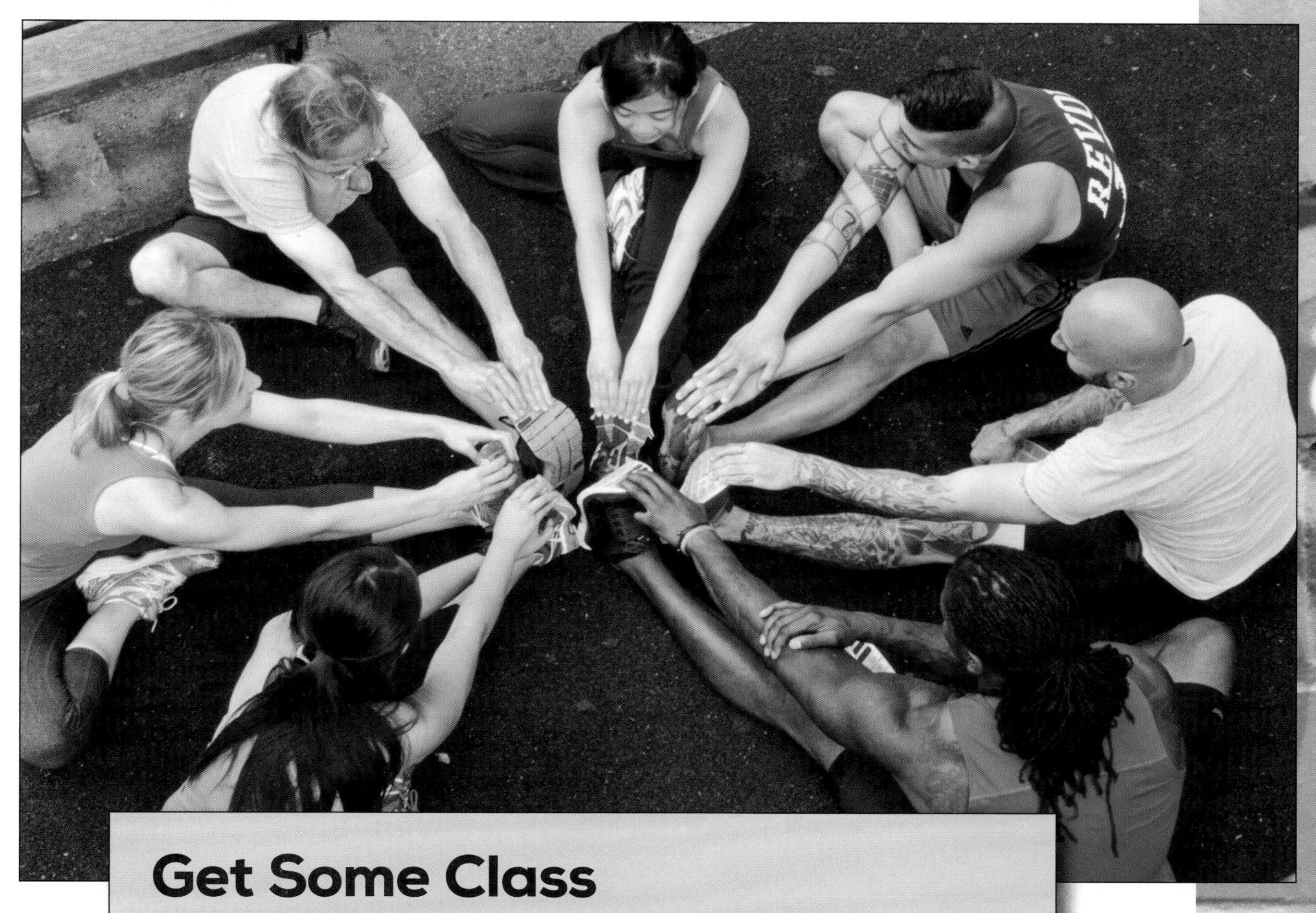

## Get Some Class

If you're new to flexibility training, I urge you to take a yoga class or one-on-one session with an experienced instructor. Though it can be tough to take that first step, it almost always winds up being worth it. Having an instructor there in person adds a lot to the training. You'll receive guidance, encouragement and lots of useful cues about things you may have overlooked. You may also make new friends who share your interest in fitness. Additionally, the structure of the class will help you adhere to longer periods of intense stretching. As you build your practice, you may feel more equipped to go it alone.

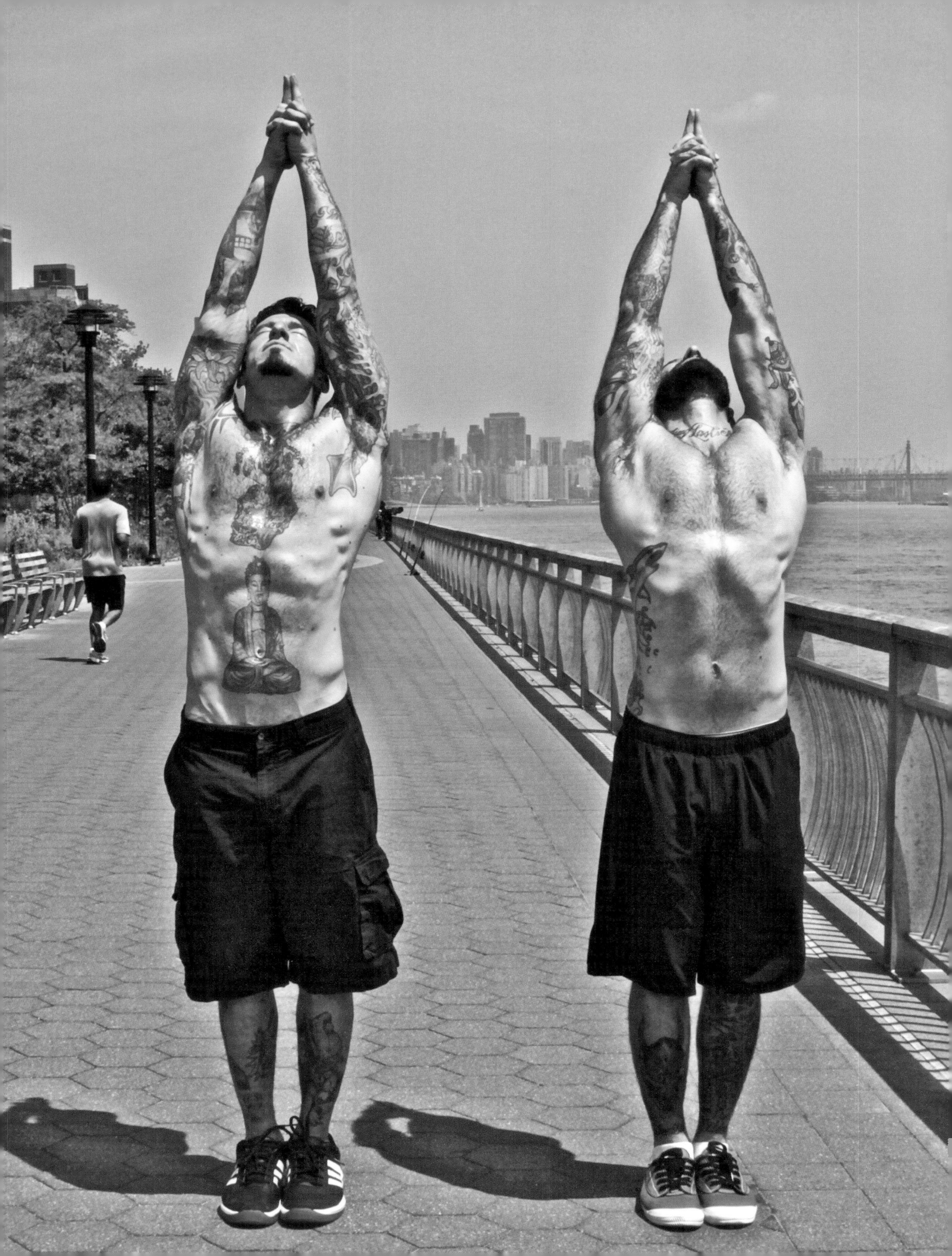

# BREATH IS LIFE

"An intellectual says a simple thing in a hard way, an artist says a hard thing in a simple way."

*-Charles Bukowski*

When I say breath is life, I'm not trying to sound poetic or profound - I mean it in the most literal way possible. Oxygen is an essential element required for proper bodily function. People can go weeks without food and days without water, but it only takes a few minutes without oxygen for the brain and other organs to completely shut down. Without breathing we would all be dead very quickly, yet breathing is something most of us tend to take for granted. I want you to bring a heightened sense of awareness to your breathing during your flexibility training. Pay attention to every inhalation and exhalation you take. Make each one as full and deep as possible.

Utilizing deep breathing during your training encourages blood flow and neuromuscular activation in parts of the body that don't typically receive much attention in our day-to-day lives. Focusing your mind and your breath on one part of your body while moving in such a way to increase blood flow to that area will help bring awareness to your practice. You will wake yourself up to the subtleties of basic human movement patterns, including many that may be in a dormant state in your body. Doing so will allow you to spread new life throughout all of your moving parts. Deep, controlled breathing helps your body relax into each pose, while simultaneously providing a focus point to calm the mind. Our internal world does a lot more to shape our external bodies than most people realize. It all starts with your mind and your breath. Everything I've achieved in fitness (and life) has been borne from the inside out.

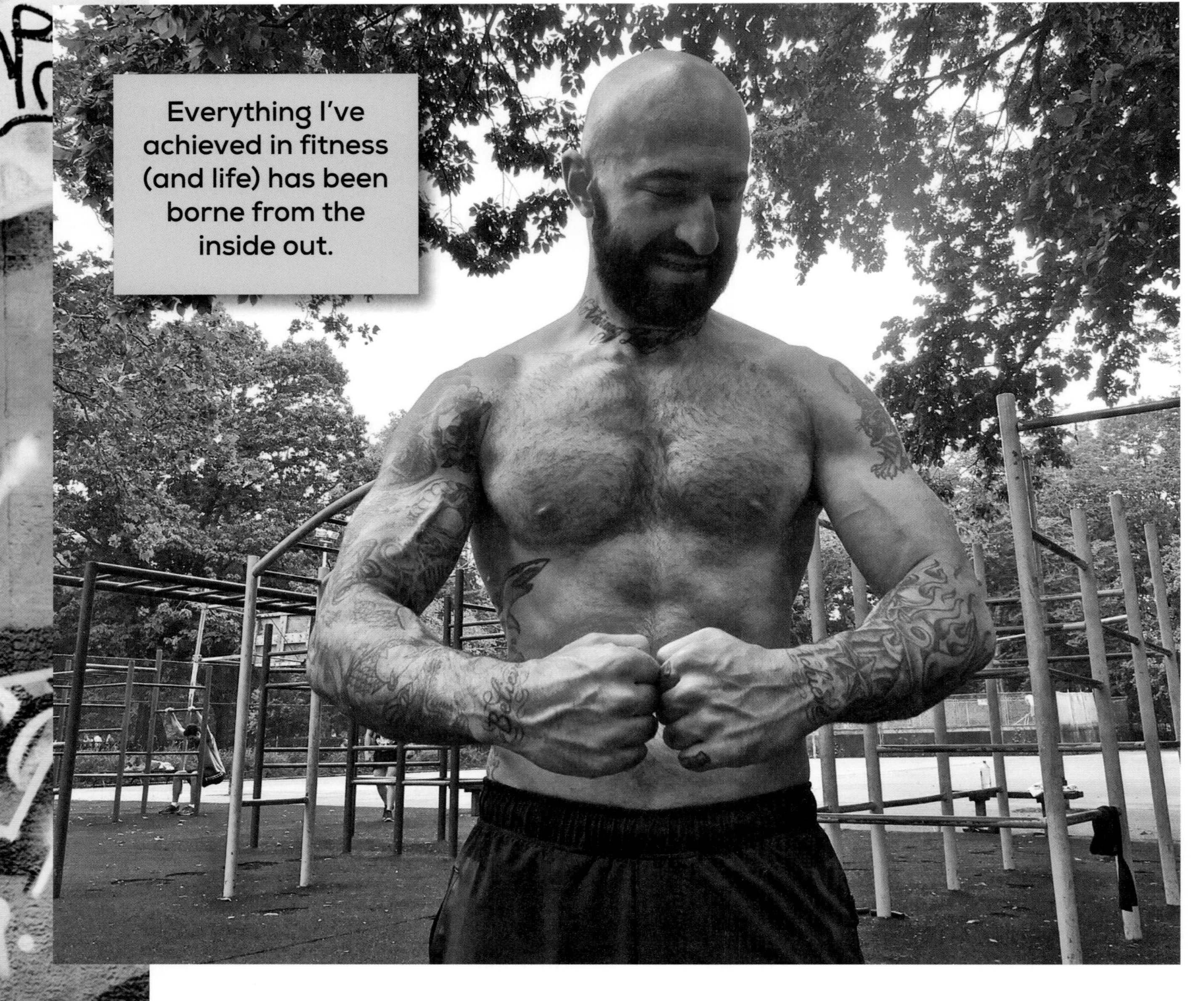
Everything I've achieved in fitness (and life) has been borne from the inside out.

Almost everyone acknowledges the significance of strong abdominal muscles, and people who train in calisthenics are probably aware of the role of the obliques. Clever trainers will also point out the importance of the lower back muscles in overall core strength, as they act as an antagonist to the abdominals. However, there is another antagonist to the abs that most people forget which also plays a crucial role in core strength - the diaphragm. Just because you can't see a muscle in the mirror, doesn't mean it's not important. Your diaphragm is in charge of your body's air supply, which makes it even more crucial than your abs!

It may sound ridiculous, but most people don't know how to breathe properly. Sure you get enough air in your lungs to keep you alive, but when was the last time you filled them close to capacity? How about emptied them fully? There is a world of power in your breath! Learn to harness it, and you'll be one step closer to bodyweight mastery.

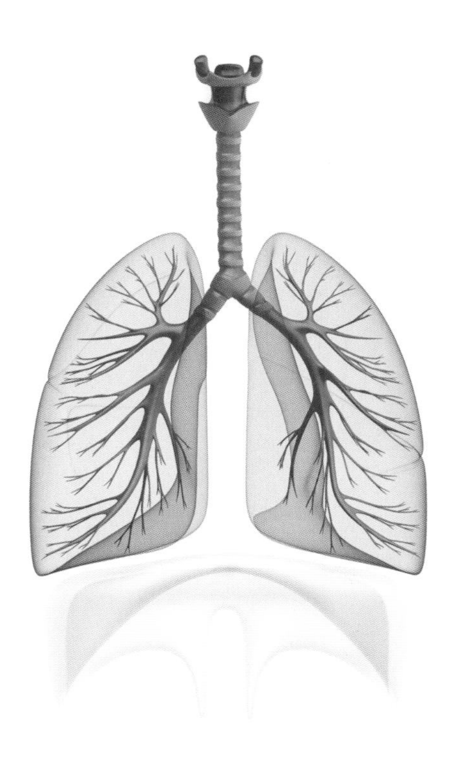

During inhalation, the diaphragm contracts, creating space for your lungs to expand. As you exhale, your diaphragm relaxes, expelling carbon dioxide and other toxins from the body. Whether you realize it or not, your diaphragm is keeping you alive. Like your heart, your diaphragm knows what to do whether you're thinking about it or not. Unlike your heart, however, it's not hard to learn to control your diaphragm. Fostering diaphragmatic control will lead to a greater sense of how all of your body's muscles are intimately intertwined, allowing you to use them together. This is key to total body control and extreme calisthenic strength. Furthermore, actively engaging your diaphragm can help stabilize your spine during many difficult movements, leaving you less likely to strain or injure yourself.

Go ahead and take a deep breath right now. Did your chest rise? It shouldn't. Proper activation of the diaphragm draws the breath deep into the belly.

If you're having a hard time figuring out how to breathe into your belly, it can help to practice the technique lying on your back with one hand on your stomach. From this position, take a deep breath while focusing on expanding your abdomen against your hand. It may take some trial and error to figure out how to accomplish this, so if your chest or shoulders rise, just breathe out and try again. This technique will come easier to some than others. It may be very different than what you're accustomed to. Eventually you should be able to take a big breath into your belly without your chest or shoulders moving at all. Once you've figured out how to do that, the next step is to exhale while deeply contracting your core from the inside. Gradually let the air seep out as you tighten your abdominal contraction, releasing it slowly and steadily to quiet your mental chatter and sink deeper into your practice.

You might find yourself making a hissing sound as you exhale - this is good. In yoga training this type of breathing is called Ujjayi breathing, which translates to "victorious" breathing. This technique is also sometimes called "ocean breath," "cobra breath" or "Darth Vader breath." Whatever you call it, deep diaphragmatic breathing relaxes the mind, allowing for deeper focus while simultaneously expelling toxins from the body. Furthermore, this type of breathing can help raise your body's core temperature, which facilitates a fuller range of motion in your joints.

Once you've gotten the hang of this technique while lying on your back, try it standing. With practice, you'll soon be able to apply deep belly breathing to any physical posture. Once you've tapped into the power of your breath, you'll be able to take your flexibility to new levels!

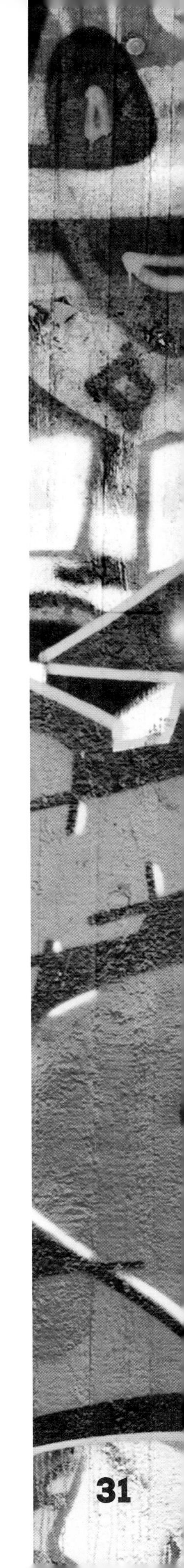

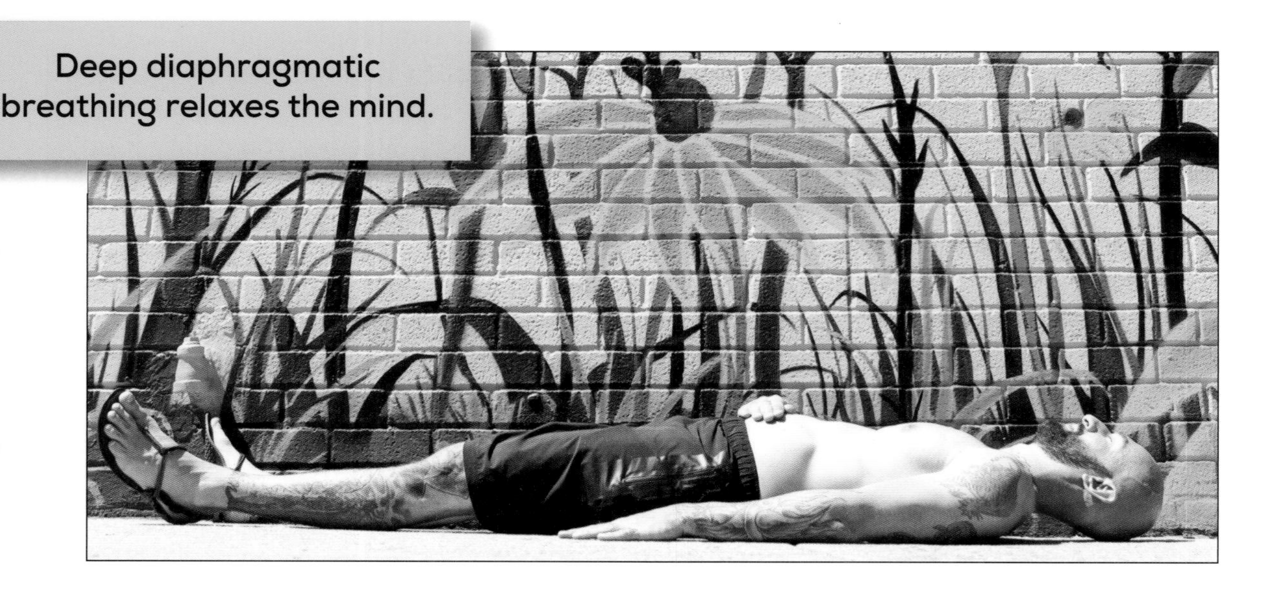

Deep diaphragmatic breathing relaxes the mind.

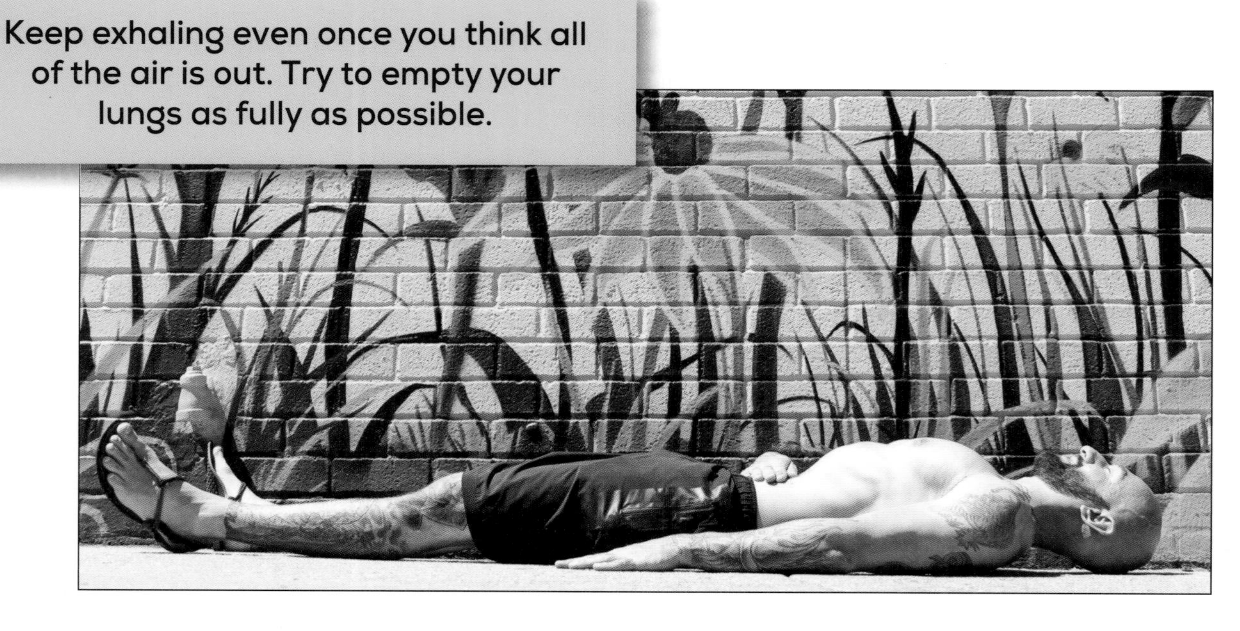

Keep exhaling even once you think all of the air is out. Try to empty your lungs as fully as possible.

In strength training it is common for people to count reps. You aim for a set of twenty push-ups or ten pull-ups or whatever else may be appropriate depending on your fitness objectives and current training level. However, when you perform static stretches, you're not moving much, so I find it best to count your breaths instead. Just like when you rep out on push-ups, however, make sure you're focused on quality over quantity. In the same way that doing ten slow, controlled push-ups will do more for you than ten push-ups performed as fast as possible, I encourage you to focus on making every breath as full and controlled as you can in order to make the most of your stretch training. Take that oxygen deep into your lungs. Savor each drop as you feel it slowly leaving your body. Keep exhaling even once you think all of the air is out. Try to empty your lungs as fully as possible. You might be surprised how long you can keep exhaling even once you thought you were ready to take in more air. Make every breath count!

## Don't Be Nervous

In addition to stabilizing your spine and giving you a point of focus, deep, controlled breathing can also alleviate anxiety and calm the mind. Belly breathing sends the signal to your nervous system to relax. Calm the mind, calm the body.

Muscular tightness is often a neurological issue as much as a physical one. Your body tenses up to protect itself from what it believes to be a potentially dangerous or unstable position. Stretch inhibitors are turned on by your nervous system when the body perceives instability. This is not necessarily a bad thing. Your stretch reflex is designed to keep you safe from injury, and it's very good at doing its job. The problem is that sometimes this mechanism is too good at its job! As your stretch reflex responds to fast changes in muscle length, I urge you to ease into static stretches very slowly. Before holding a pose for an extended period of time, it's often best to ease in with a few shorter holds of just a few seconds. This will prime your nervous system for the movement pattern. Once you get into longer holds, use your diaphragm to stabilize your spine and control your breath. Doing so can communicate to your body that it's okay to ease up a little on its natural tendency to contract when it reaches the fringes of what it perceives to be a safe range of motion. Over time, your nervous system will get the message and your stretch reflex will begin to back off, allowing you to gradually expand your range of motion.

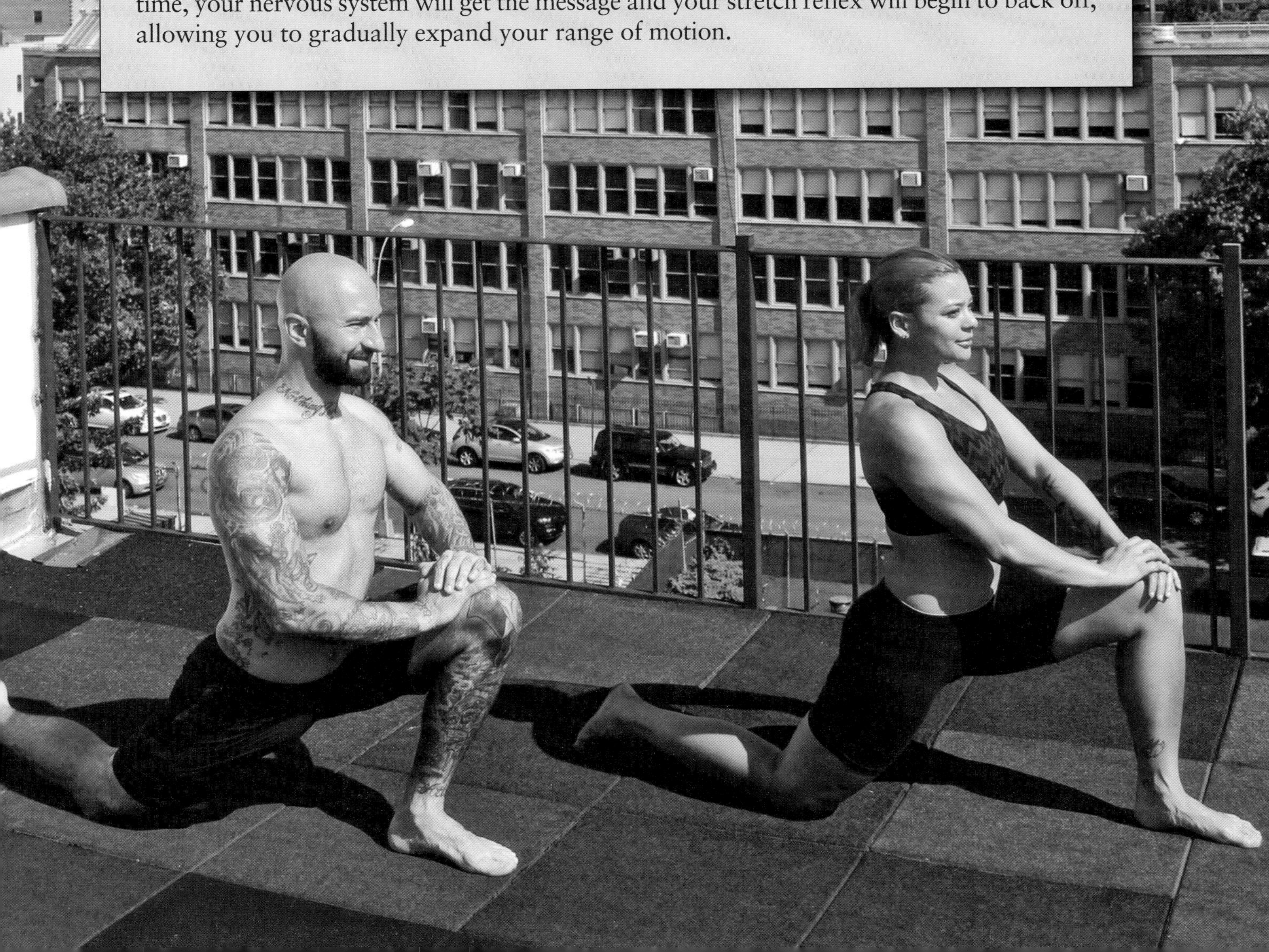

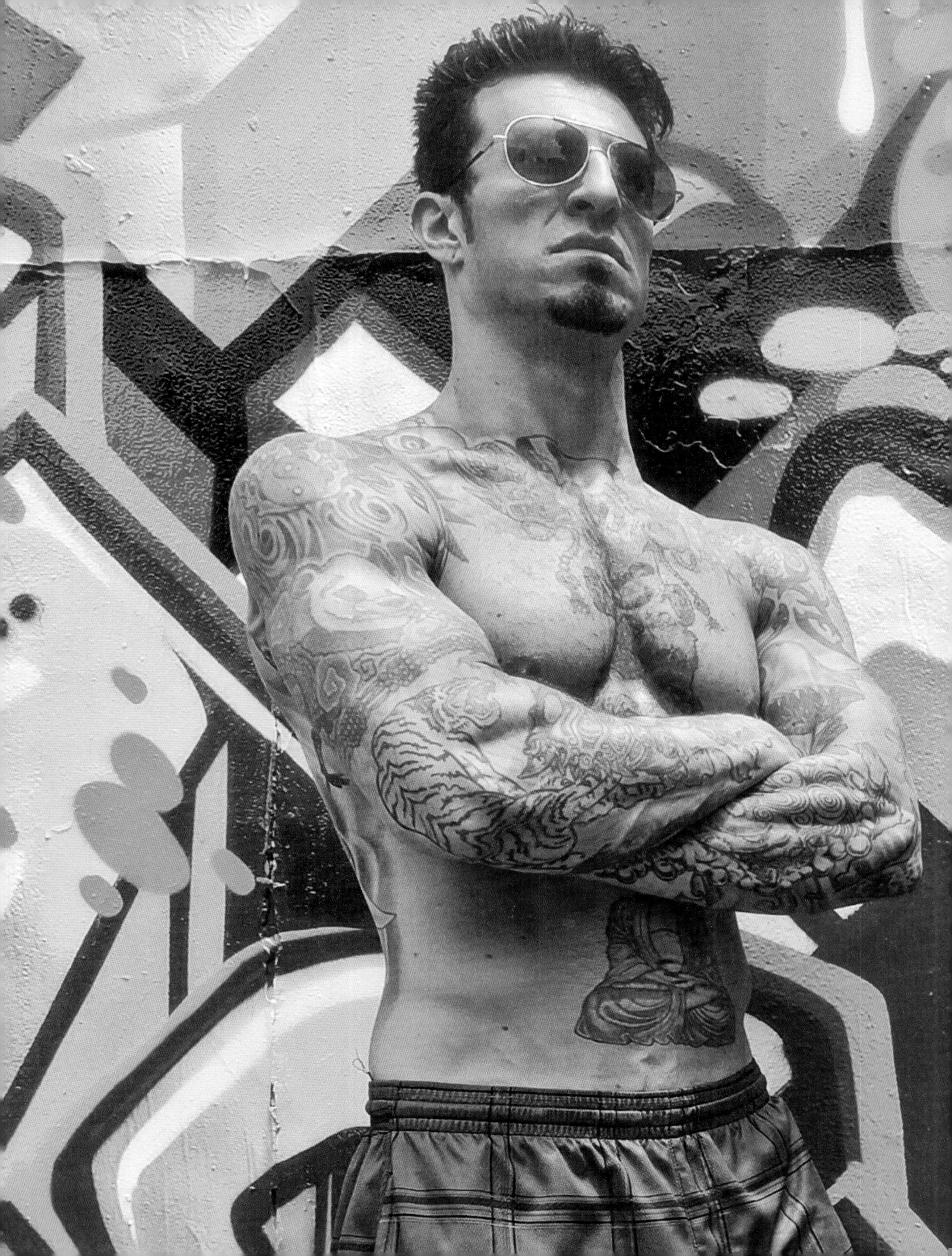

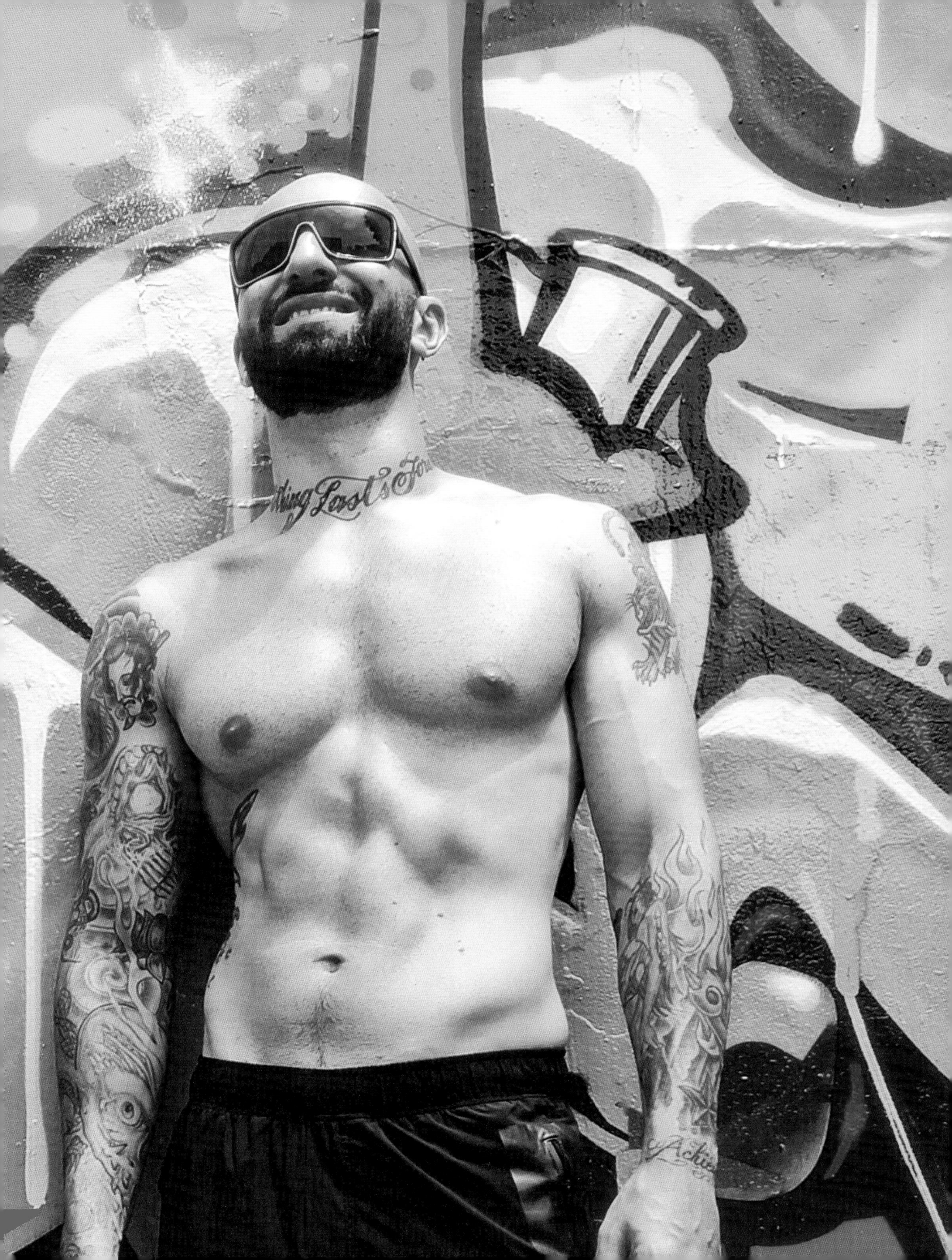

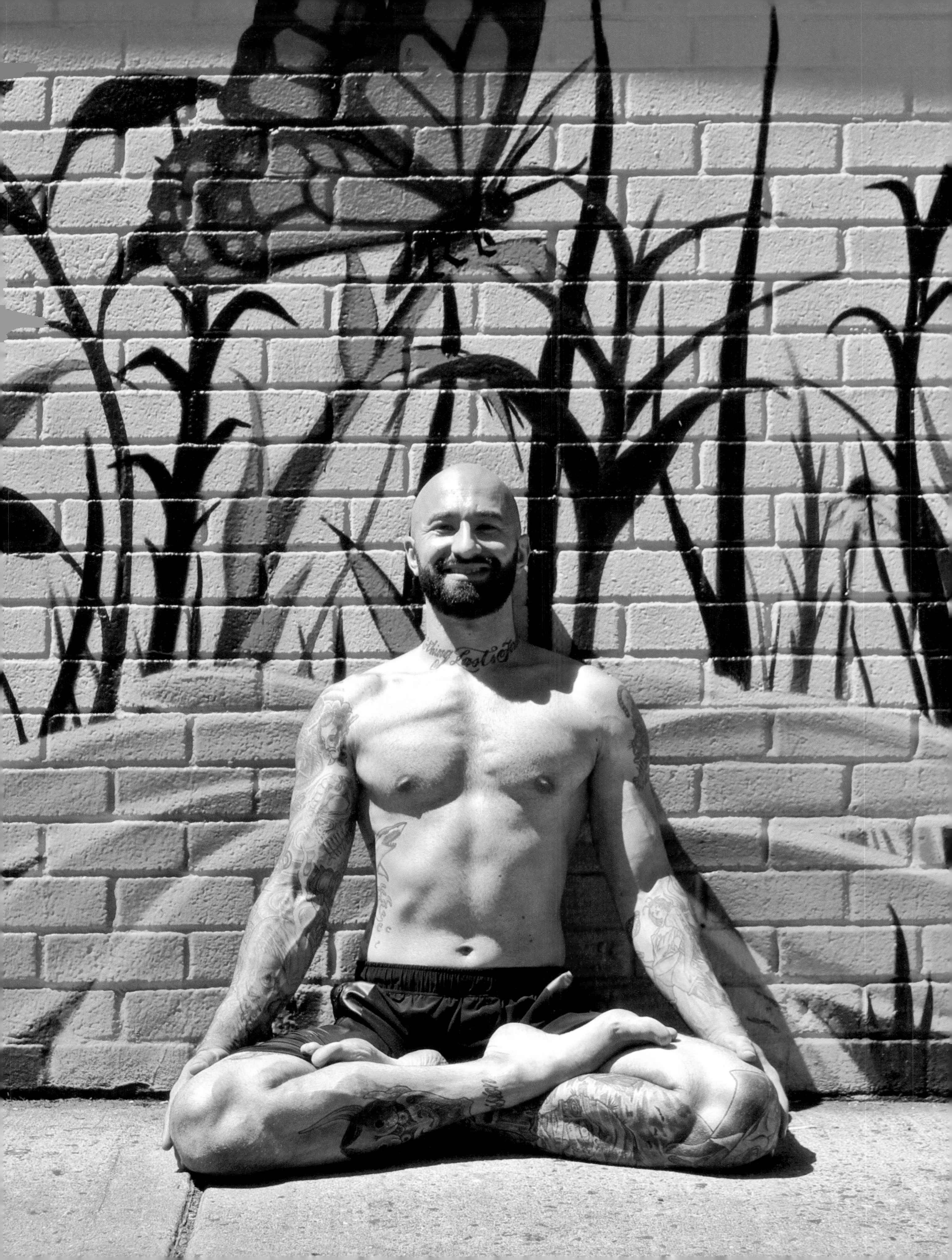

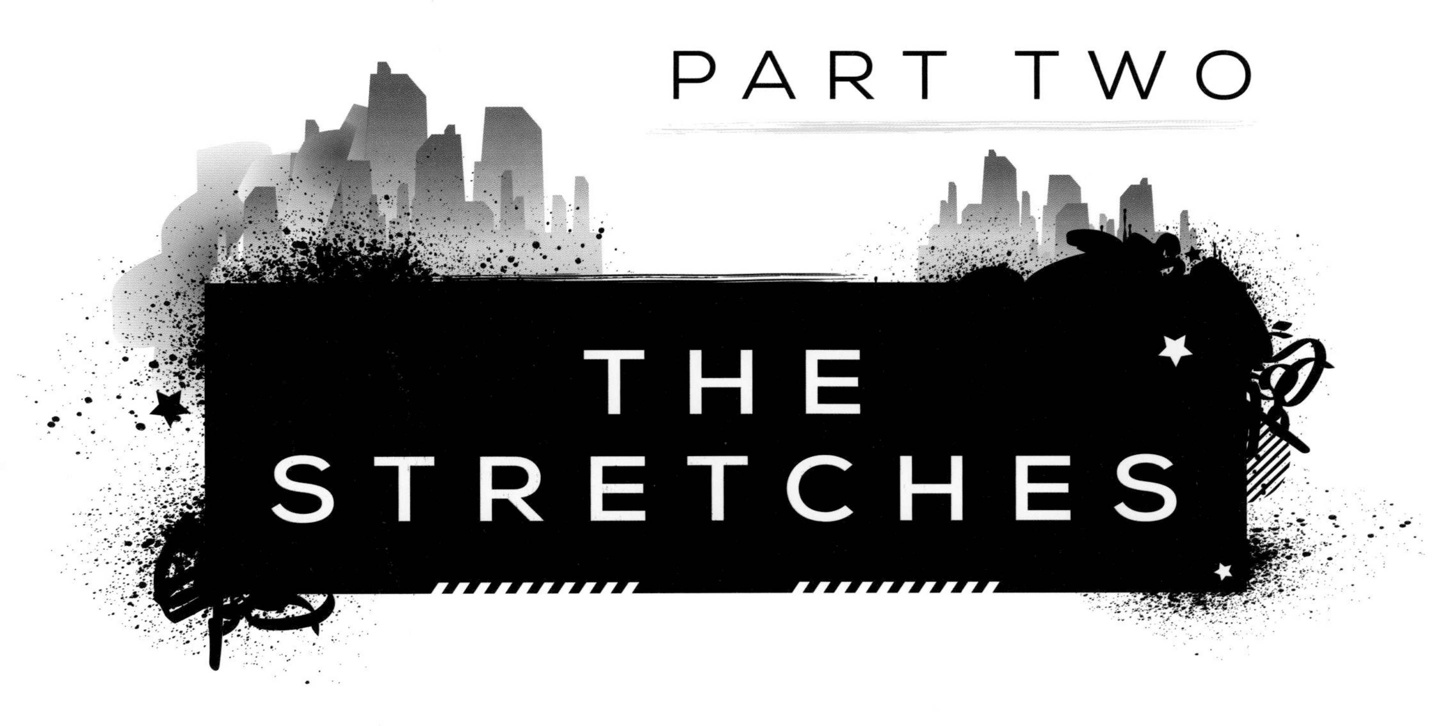

# PART TWO
# THE STRETCHES

"The best way to vanquish an enemy
is to make them a friend."

*- Abraham Lincoln*

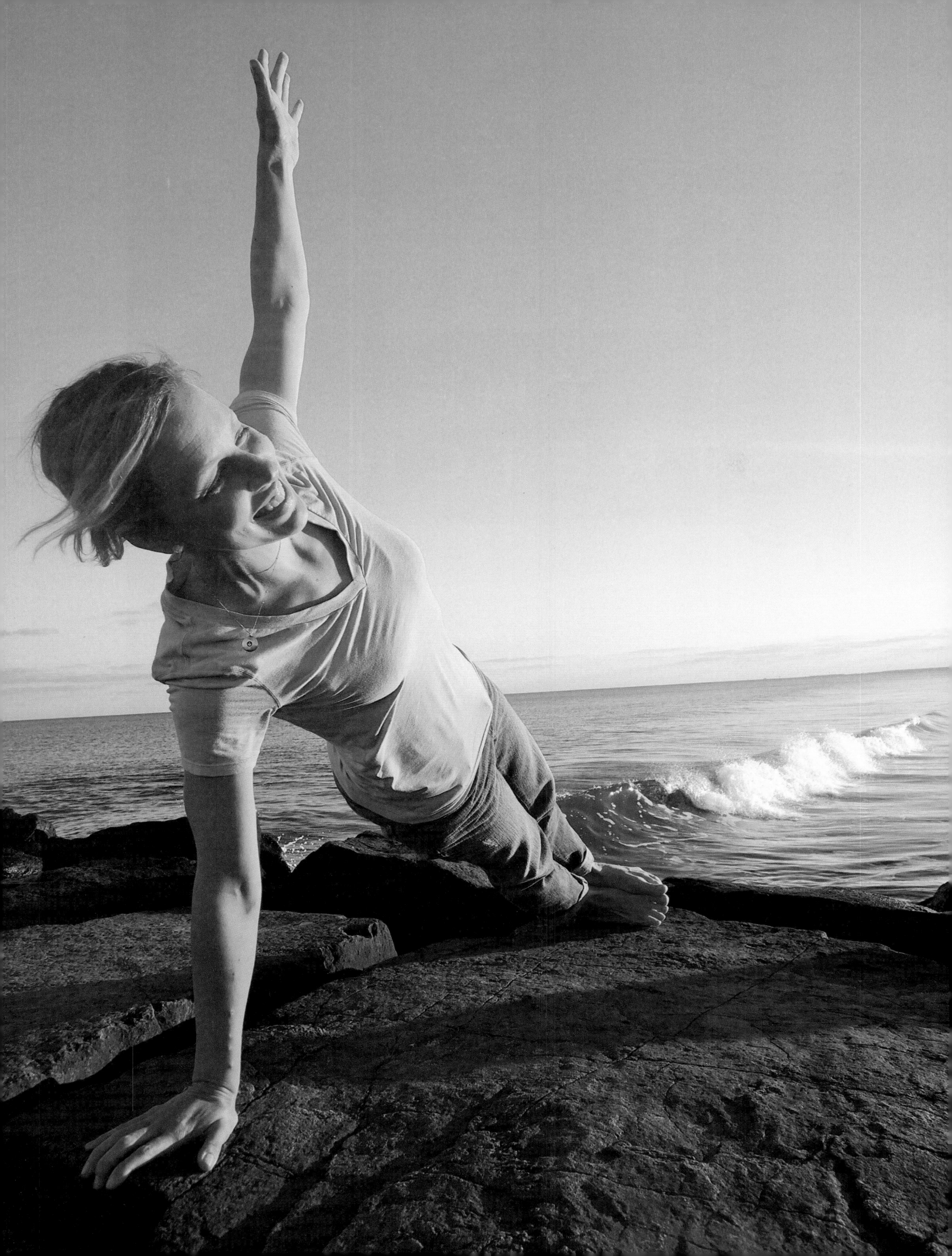

# PREFACE

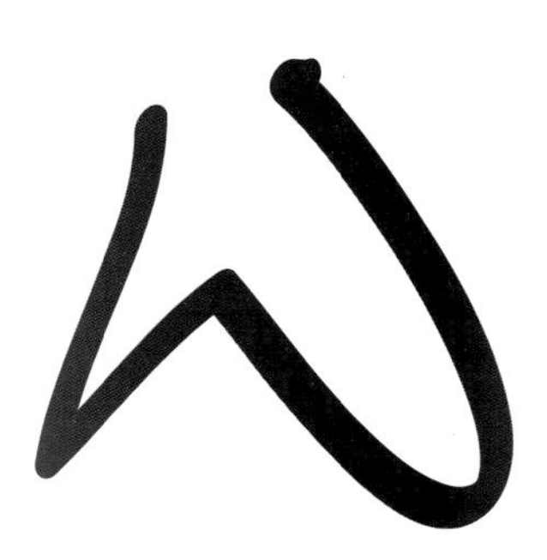

hen you are stiff and inflexible, it can feel like your body is your own worst enemy. It may make you feel frustrated or angry. This can lead to further destructive behavior!

Like honest Abe advises, you've got to open up communication in order to get back on the right path. It can be a slow process but ignoring your body's signals is not going to help. Make friends with stretching and flexibility will no longer be your kryptonite. In fact, you might even learn to enjoy it!

In this section, I've included descriptions of more than fifty of my favorite stretches and postures for flexibility, alignment and ultimately, bodyweight mastery. Though there is plenty of overlap between categories, I've arranged them into three sections to make them easier to absorb: Dynamic Stretches, Standing Statics, and Grounded Statics. Feel free to explore these movements at your own pace and remember to be open to what comes up in the moment.

Greatness arises not from the pursuit of greatness, but rather from doing simple tasks one at a time with care and attention.

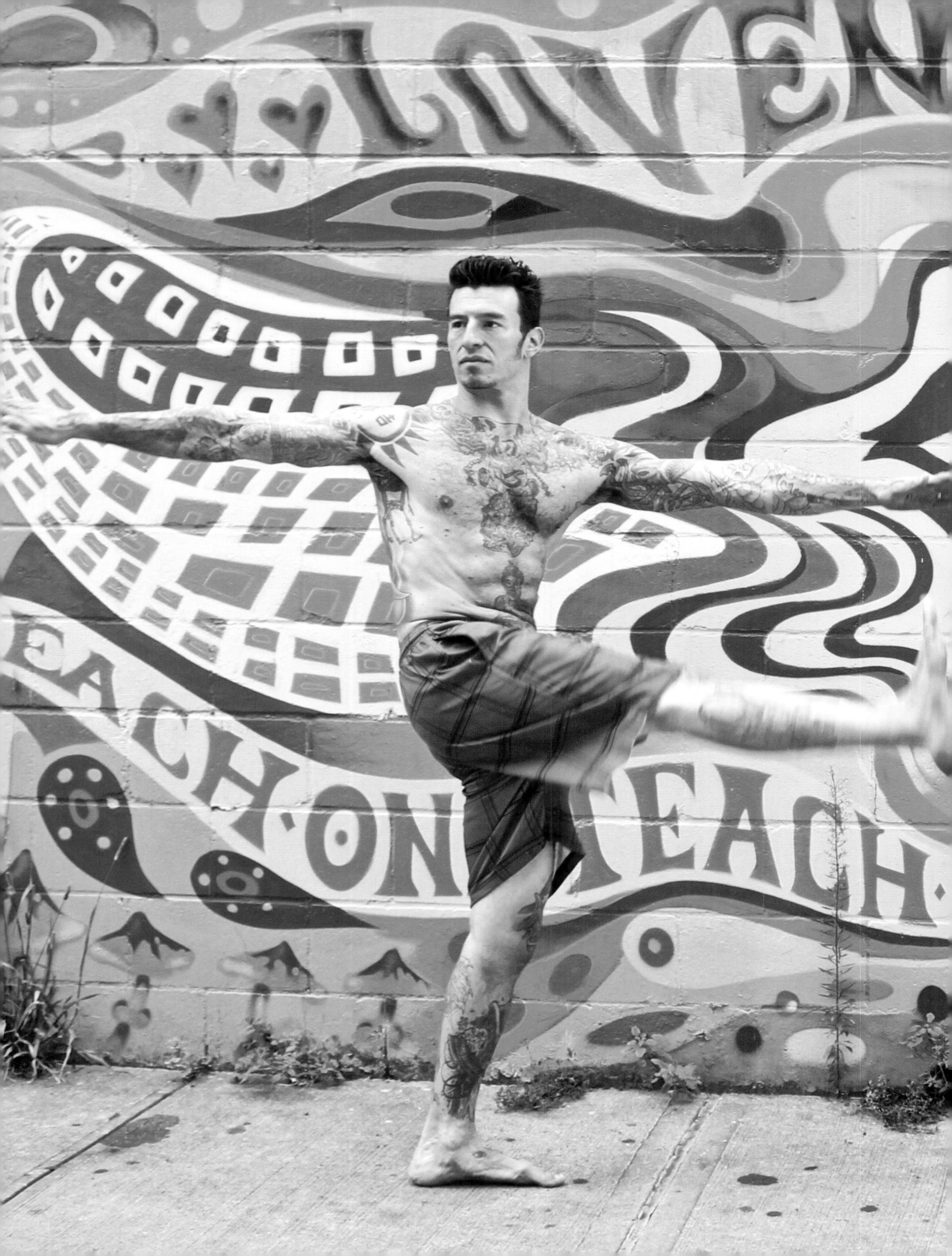

# DYNAMIC STRETCHES

When we think of stretching, most people typically picture holding a static position for an extended amount of time. While there are plenty of those types of stretches to be found later on in this book, the dynamic stretches presented in this section are the complete opposite. Instead of remaining in a fixed position, these dynamic stretches involve moving quickly through a full range of motion by utilizing momentum. That's what makes them dynamic!

When performed properly, dynamic stretching can increase your range of motion and encourage blood and oxygen flow to muscles and connective tissues prior to exertion. Additionally, dynamic stretching can help improve your proprioceptive awareness; practicing these moves is a fantastic way to get a better sense for the different ways in which your body can move through space.

As dynamic stretching is also a great way to quickly increase your heart rate and internal body temperature, I recommend using these dynamic stretches to warm up before your calisthenics training, prior to participating in sports, or any other time you see fit.

# Arm Circle

Arm Circles are a great warm-up and a fun way to work on shoulder mobility. From a standing position, reach one arm overhead and begin circling it behind your body. Point your thumb behind your back as you rotate your arm in as large of a circle as possible. Go slowly at first but feel free to pick up the speed after a few rotations. When you've completed several full circles, reverse direction. When doing forward circles, point your thumb down toward your toes. You can do both arms separately or at the same time.

**Common Mistakes:** Moving too fast, too soon; bent elbows

**Primary Muscle Groups:** Shoulders, chest

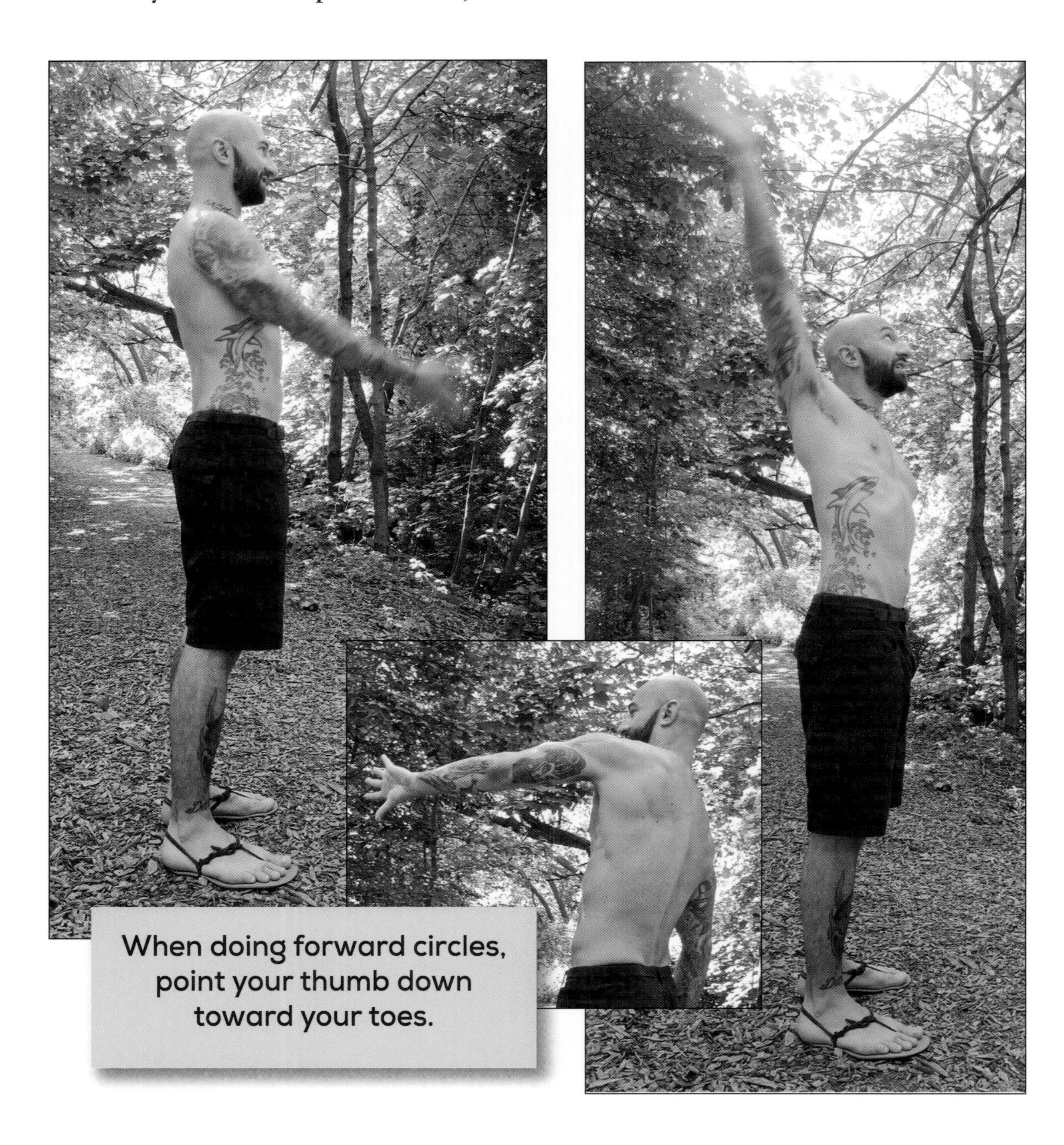

When doing forward circles, point your thumb down toward your toes.

# Shoulder Roll

The Shoulder Roll is essentially the same as the arm circle, only with an exercise band or other object held between the hands to facilitate a deeper stretch in the chest and shoulders.Though arm circles may be done one arm at a time, the shoulder roll is done with both arms moving in unison. Go very gently at first as this can be quite challenging for folks with a stiff upper-body. If you are tight, start out with your hands placed wide. As you warm up, you may gradually bring your hands closer. In time, your range of motion should start to improve.

**Common Mistakes:** Moving too fast, too soon; bent elbows

**Primary Muscle Groups:** Shoulders, chest

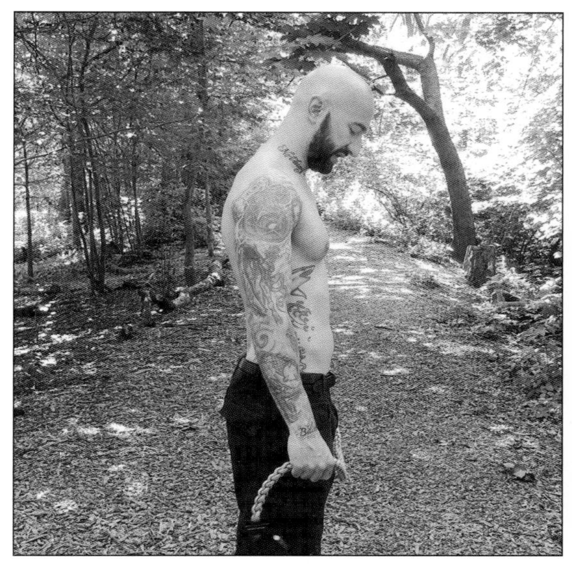

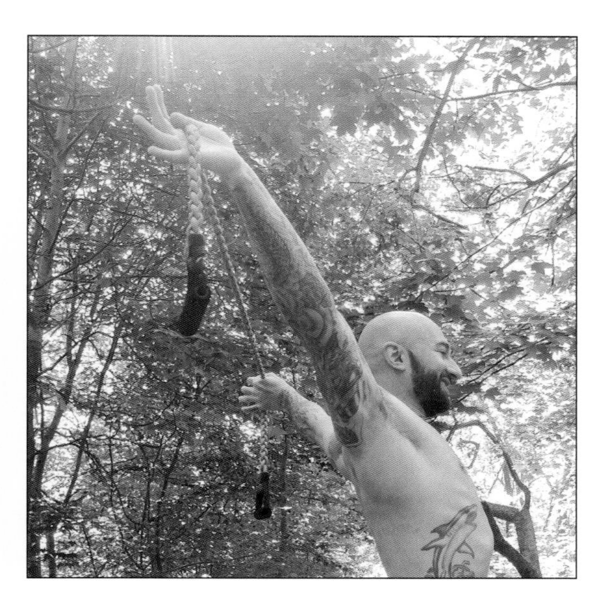

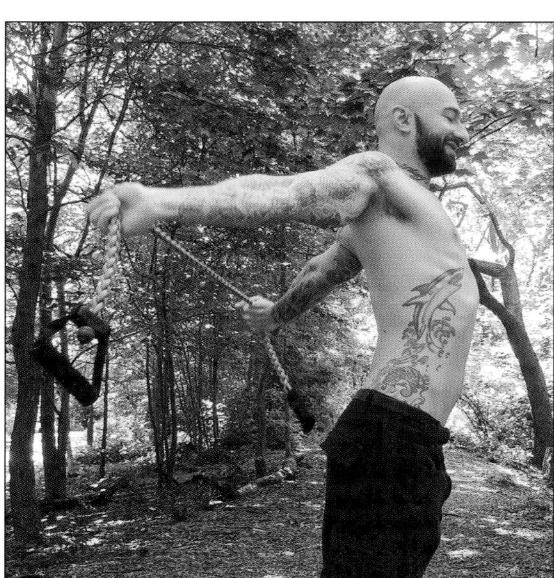

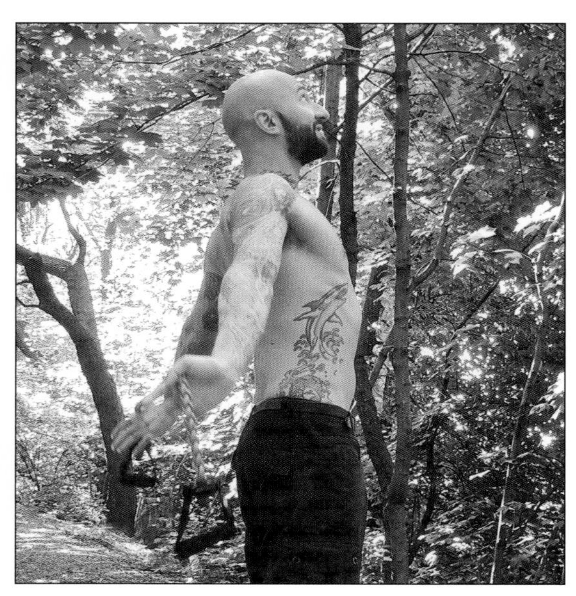

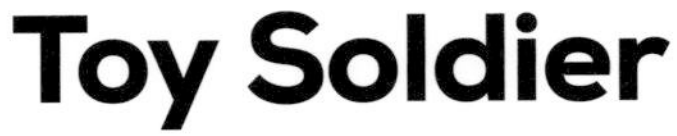

# Toy Soldier

The Toy Soldier is a great dynamic stretch for the hamstrings, hips and trunk. From a standing position, perform a quick front kick while reaching your opposite hand toward the toes of your kicking leg. Focus on keeping your back straight while twisting through your trunk to reach your toes. You can perform this move on alternating legs while traveling forward or do them one leg at a time while standing in place. For an added challenge, try going up onto the toes of your standing leg at the top of your kick.

**Common Mistakes:** Excessive spinal flexion, lack of trunk rotation

**Primary Muscle Groups:** Hamstrings, hips, sides of trunk

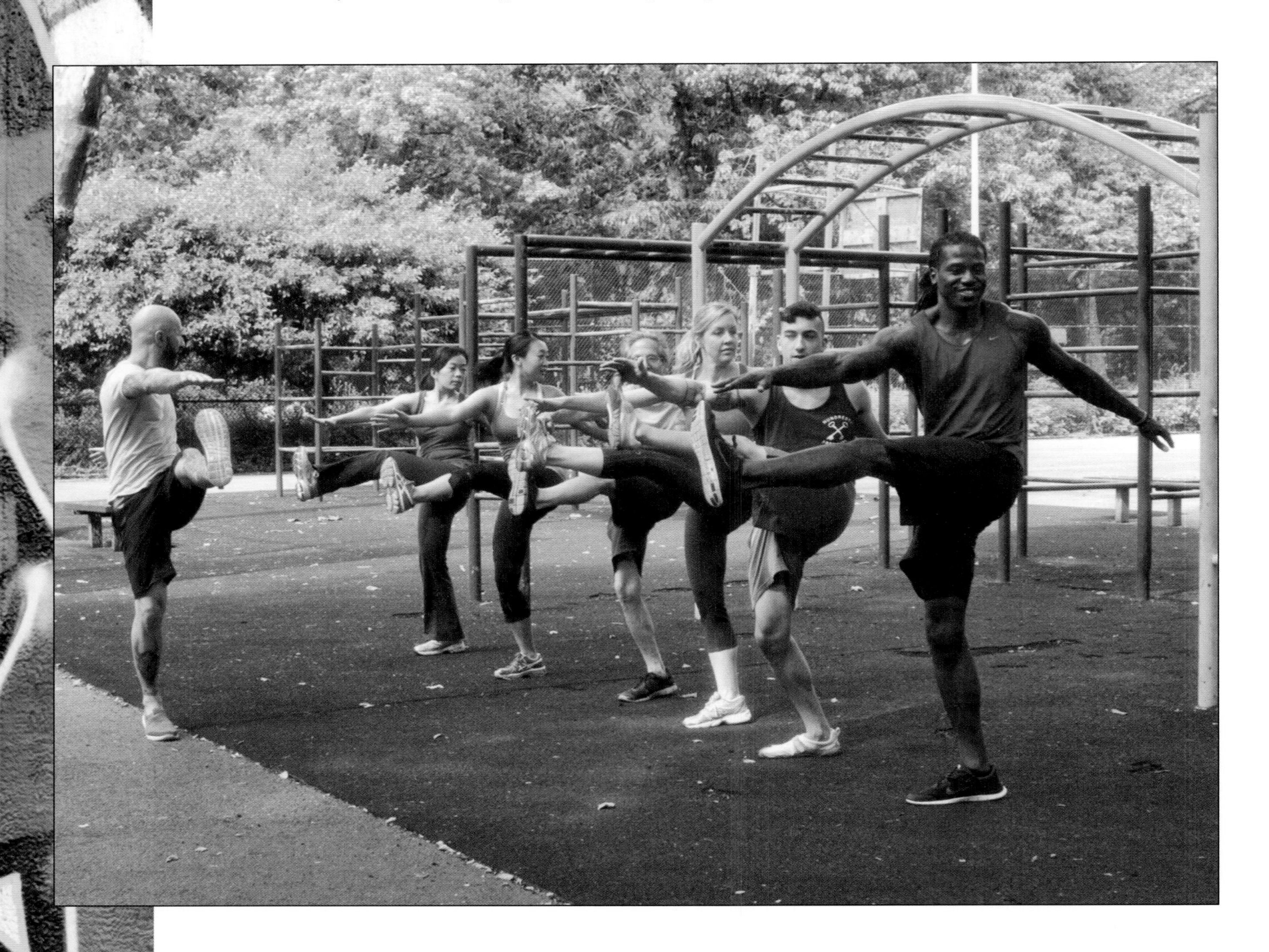

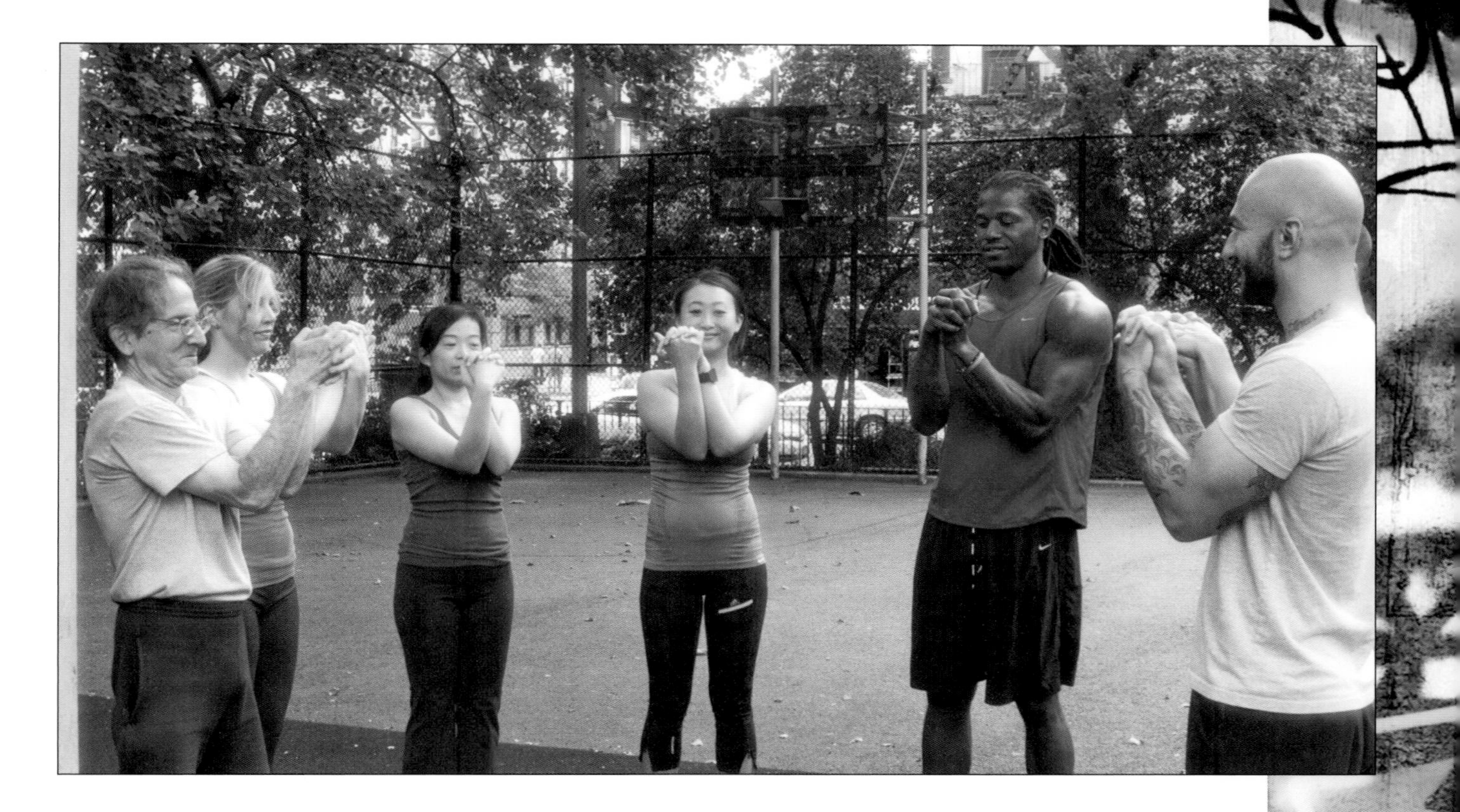

## Wrist Roll

Wrist Rolls are one of the best way to prepare for push-ups, handstands and other exercises that involve bending back at the wrists. Clasp your hands together with your palms facing each other and your fingers interlaced. Keep your arms loose as you begin to flex and extend your wrists in a circular motion. Stay relaxed as you roll your hands up, down, in and out. Alternate which hand is on top after several repetitions, as well as alternating directions.

**Common Mistakes:** Favoring the dominant hand instead of doing both sides evenly

**Primary Muscle Groups:** Wrists, forearms

# Spine Roll

The Spine Roll is a gentle way to warm up your spine before more intense exercise. Begin in an all-fours position with your hands and knees on the ground. Your knees should be directly under your hips with your hands directly under your shoulders. Take a deep breath and compress your spine by lifting your tailbone and pushing your hips out to create an arch in your lower back. Look up and press your chest forward while squeezing your shoulder blades down and back. From here begin to exhale as you slowly suck your stomach in, round your spine and tuck your chin to your chest. Repeat for several repetitions.

**Common Mistakes:** Unnecessary elbow bending, inability to isolate the movement of the spine

**Primary Muscle Groups:** Hips, back, neck

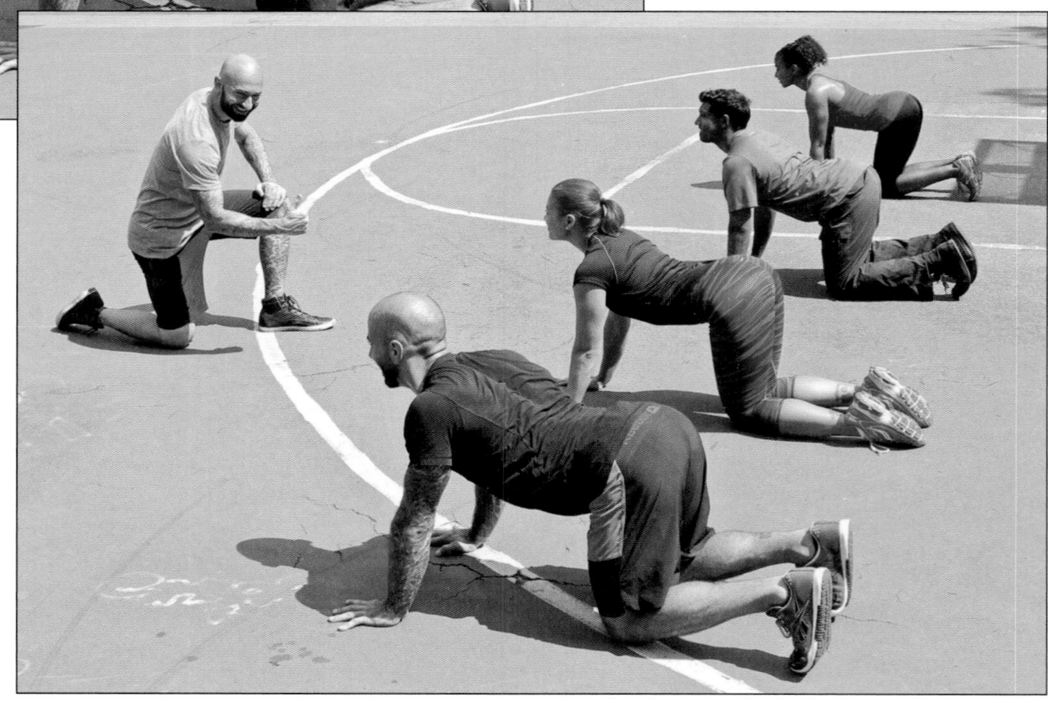

# Egg Beater

Egg Beaters are great for building active mobility in the hips. Lie on your back with your feet elevated and knees bent to approximately ninety degrees. Lay your arms on the ground next to your torso and begin rotating your feet around each other in a circle, keeping your knees pointed out to the sides. Practice this movement in both directions.

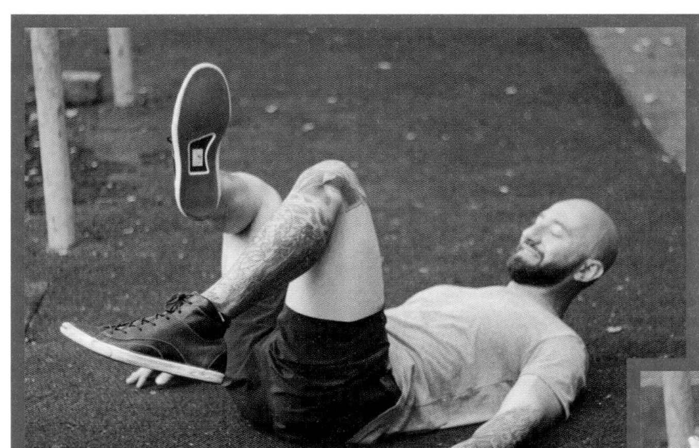

**Common Mistakes:** Moving too fast, excessive trunk movement

**Primary Muscle Groups:** Hips

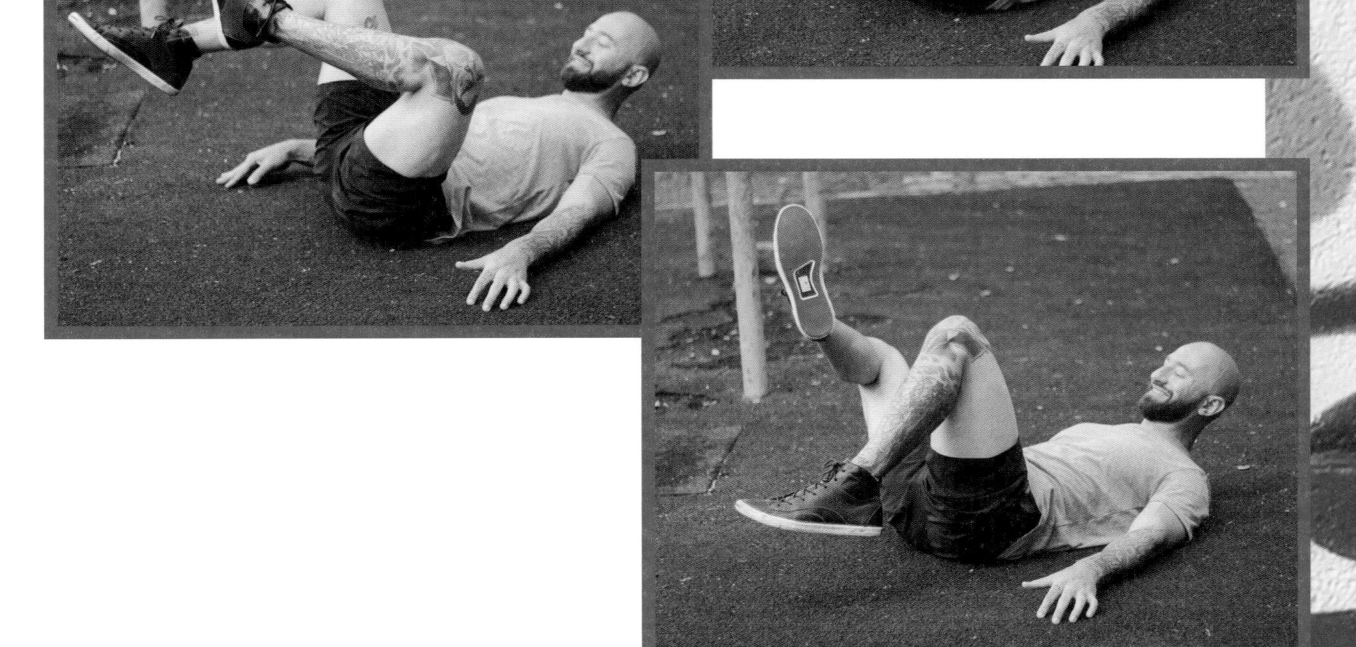

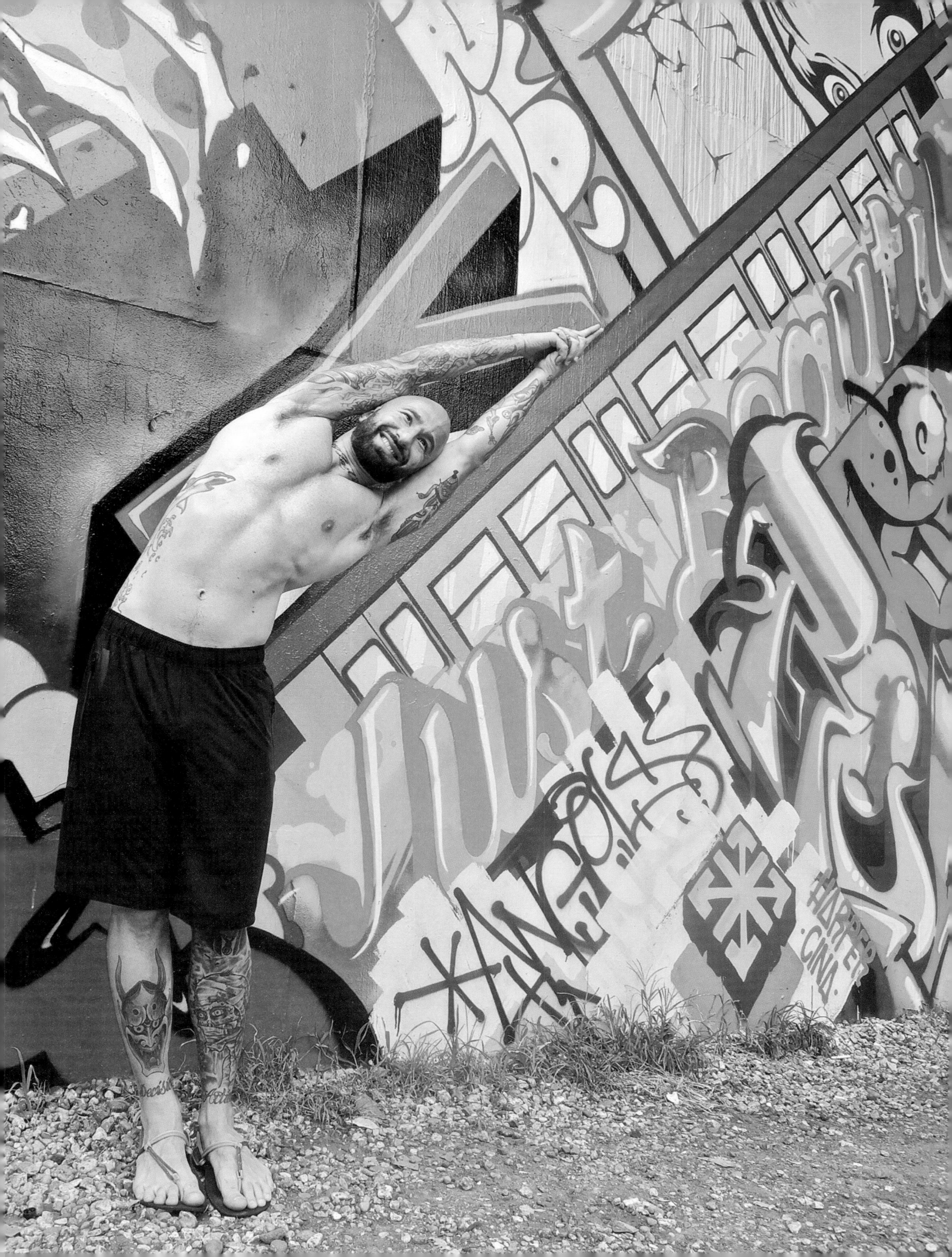

# STANDING STATICS

Though each posture in this section involves holding a static form, they are active exercises that involve strength, flexibility and alignment. The key to performing these moves is to utilize the breathing technique discussed in the last section along with the specific cues listed for each pose. You are going to be using the strength of certain muscles to stretch and activate others. Be patient with yourself and focus on the process. Respect your level and do not become short-sighted. Take your time working toward the full expression of each pose. Some will happen quicker than others. I'm still working on improving my form, too!

For these poses, I've included specific instructions to guide your breathing. I've also included "calisthenics counterparts" for each pose (when relevant), to demonstrate how improved mobility can have direct carryover into your strength training.

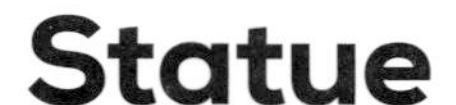

## Statue

On first sight, the Statue pose may look like you are just standing there. In a sense, this is correct. However, you are not "just" standing there. There are many subtle details to a proper Statue pose.

Begin in a narrow stance with your feet close together and toes touching (your heels should still be slightly apart). Squeeze your glutes and quads while spreading out your feet to grip the floor. Keep your weight equal throughout the front, back and sides of your feet. Breathe into your belly and feel your spine lengthen; visualize the top of your head reaching up toward the sky. Relax your shoulders and make your neck long. Let your arms hang down by your sides.

**Inhale:** Feel your belly fill up with air as your back straightens

**Exhale:** Contract your abdominals and reach the top of your head upward

**Common mistakes:** Shrugged or rounded shoulders, hyper-extended lower back

**Primary Muscle Groups:** Abs, glutes, low back, diaphragm

**Calisthenics Counterpart:** Push-up

The body's alignment in the Statue pose carries over directly to the alignment necessary for a proper Push-up.

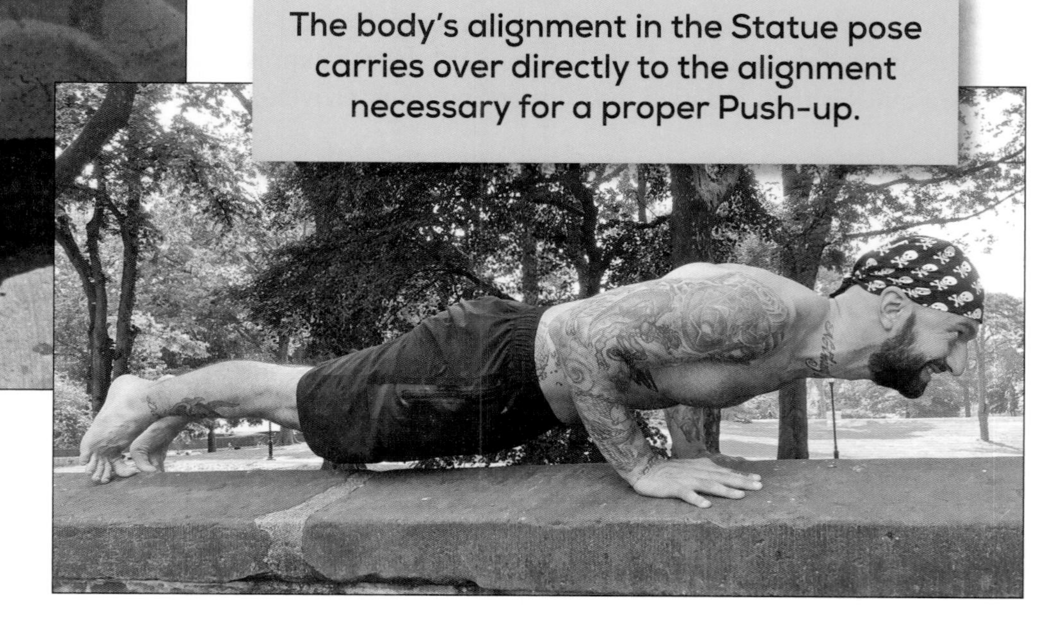

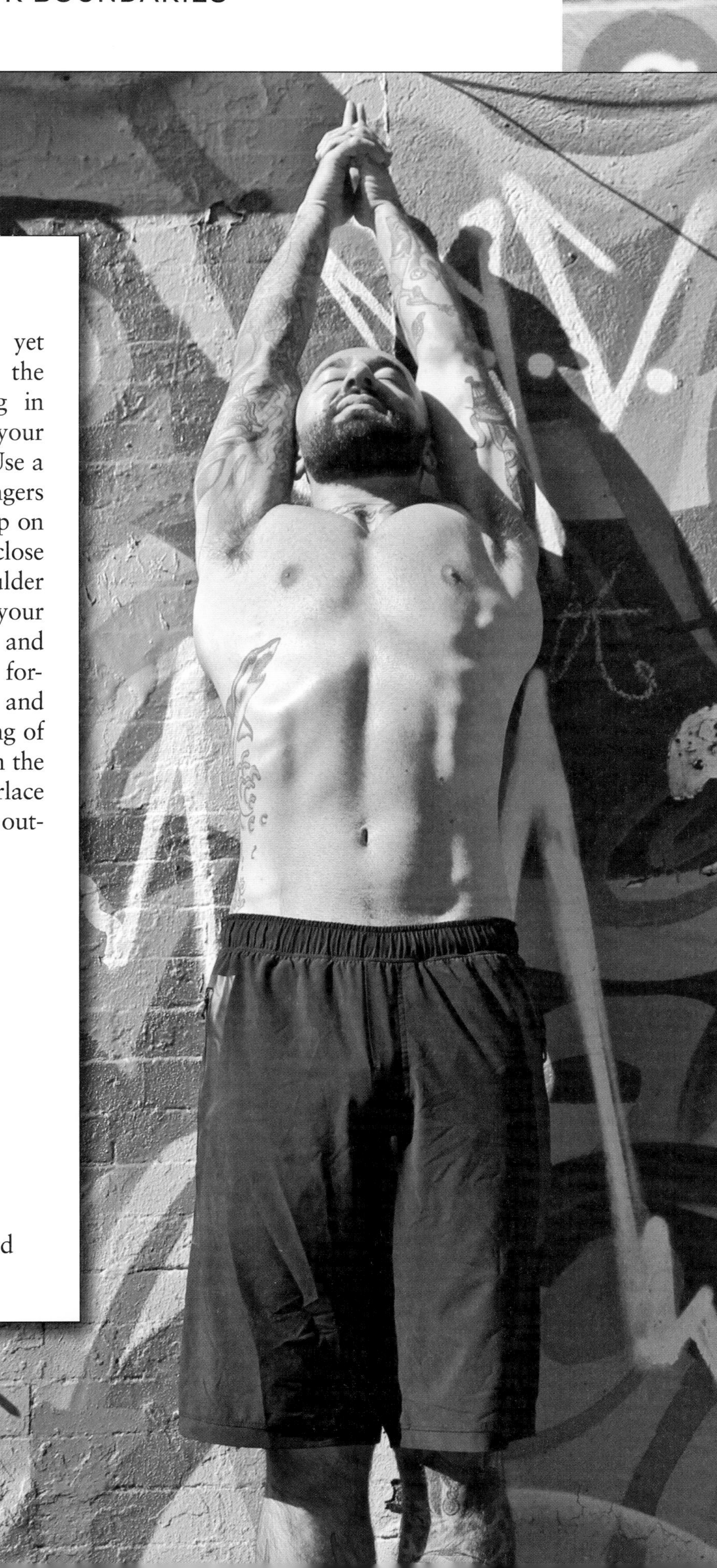

# Mountain

The Mountain pose is a simple, yet potentially challenging opener for the shoulders and upper back. Starting in Statue pose, reach your arms up over your head and clasp your hands together. Use a palm-to-palm grip, with your index fingers extended (switch which hand is on top on alternating efforts). Hug your biceps close to your head, allowing your shoulder blades to spread apart and slide up your back. Tilt your head back slightly and think about trying to press your chest forward while squeezing your glutes and hamstrings to prevent excessive arching of the lower back. For a deeper stretch in the wrists and forearms, you can interlace your fingers and rotate your palms outward.

**Inhale:** Reach your arms upward, lengthening the body

**Exhale:** Squeeze your glutes and abs

**Common mistakes:** Overly arched lower-back, bent arms

**Primary Muscle Groups:** Shoulders, glutes, abs

**Calisthenics Counterpart:** Handstand

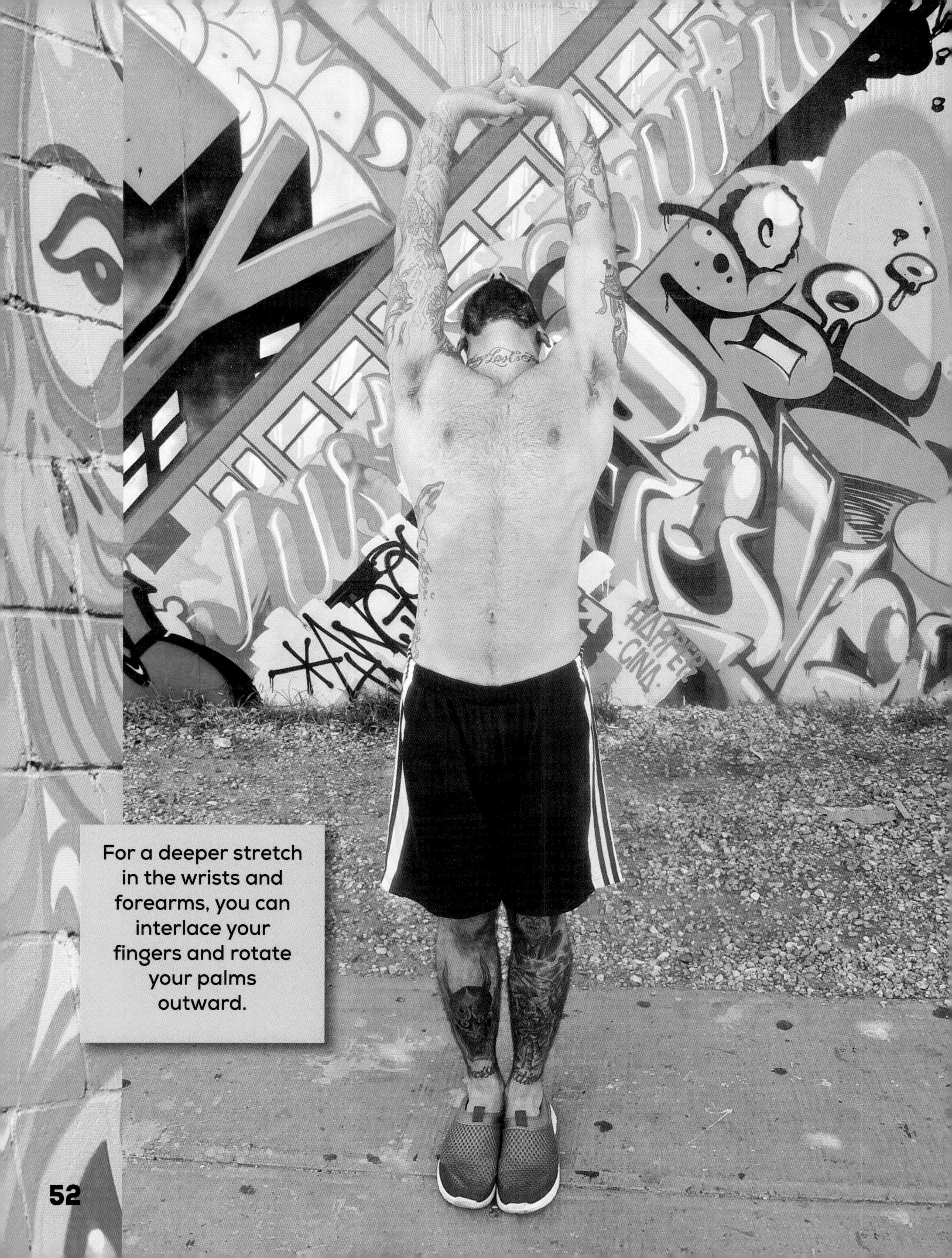


For a deeper stretch in the wrists and forearms, you can interlace your fingers and rotate your palms outward.

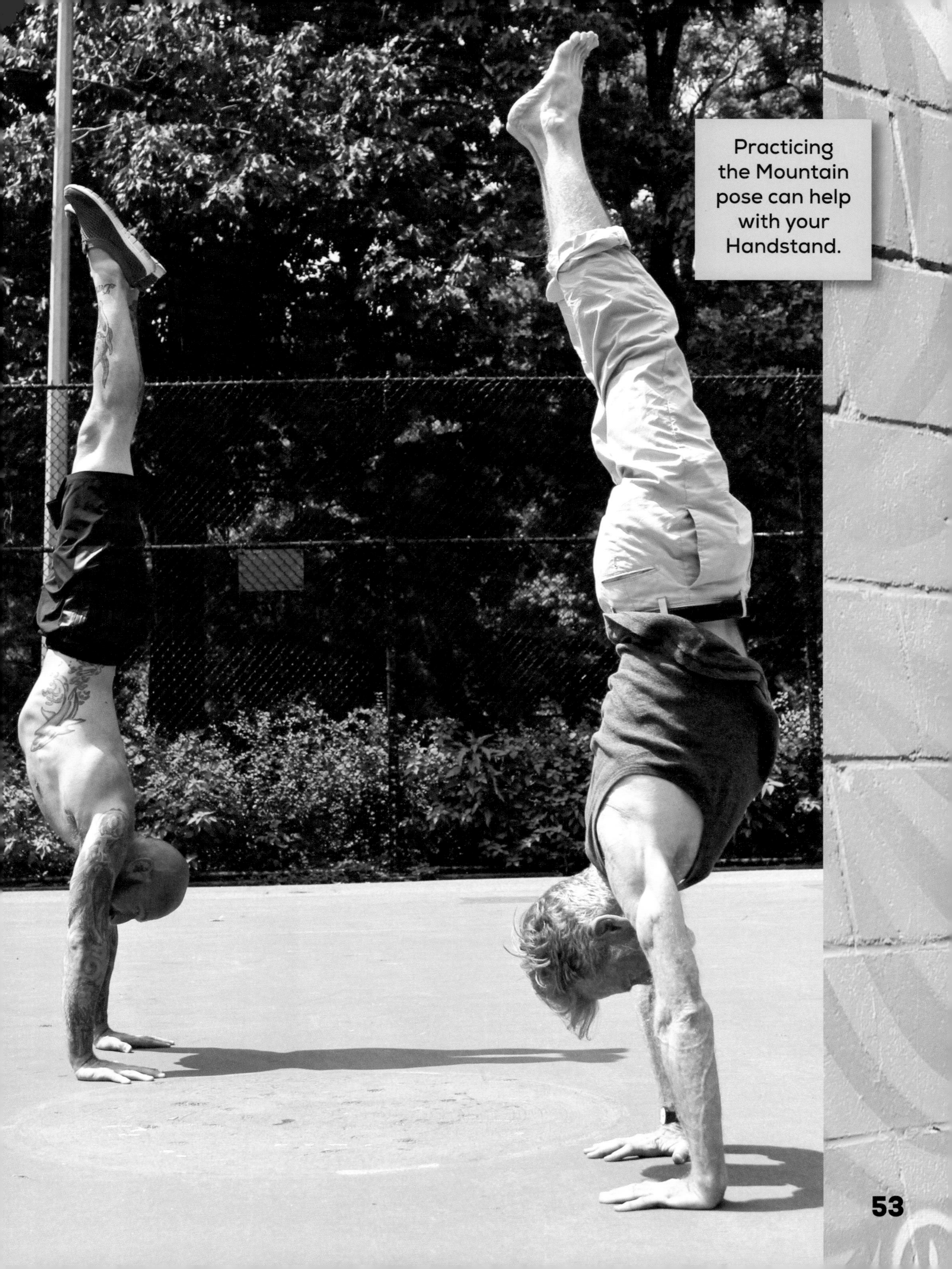

Practicing the Mountain pose can help with your Handstand.

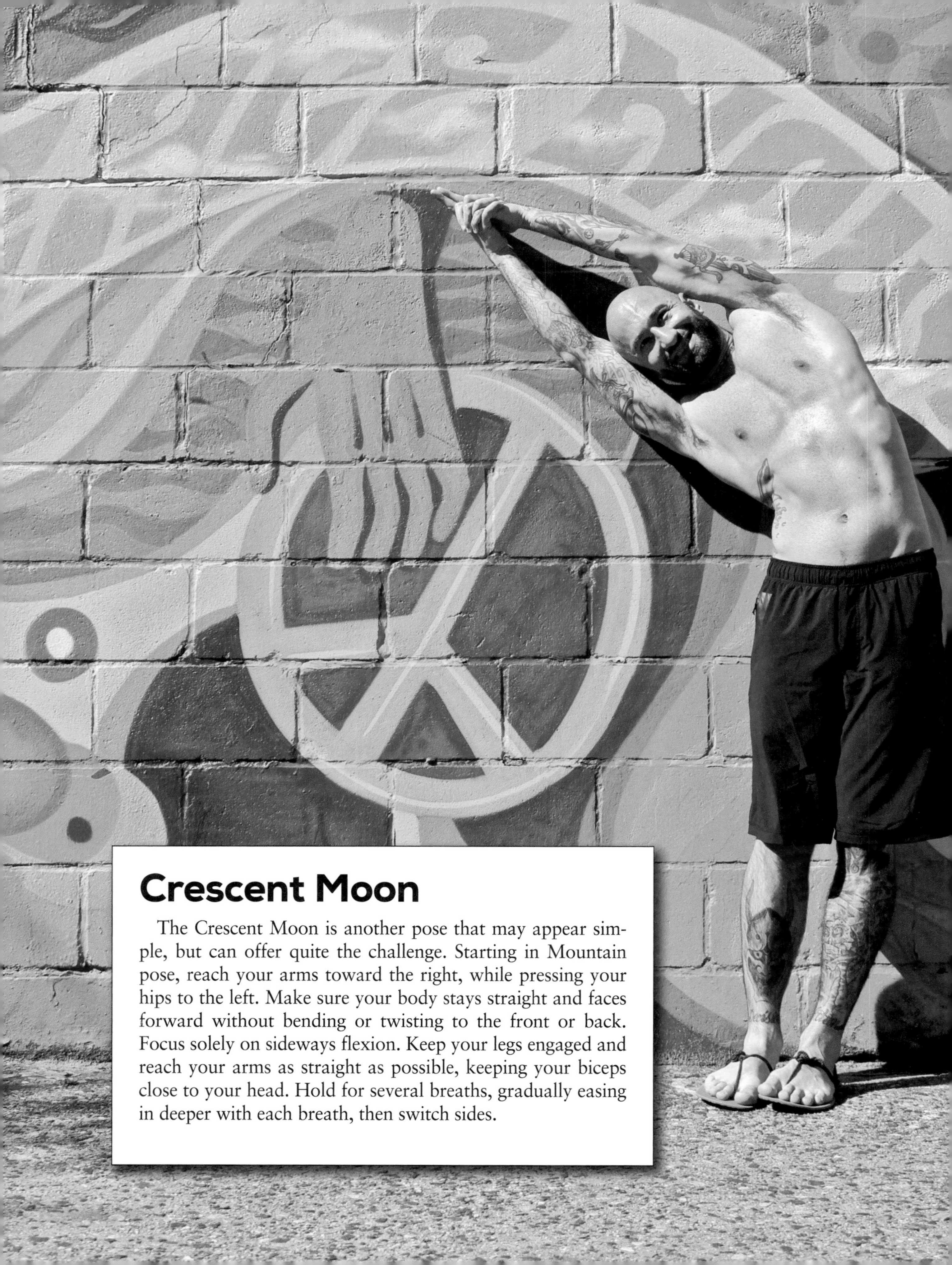

## Crescent Moon

The Crescent Moon is another pose that may appear simple, but can offer quite the challenge. Starting in Mountain pose, reach your arms toward the right, while pressing your hips to the left. Make sure your body stays straight and faces forward without bending or twisting to the front or back. Focus solely on sideways flexion. Keep your legs engaged and reach your arms as straight as possible, keeping your biceps close to your head. Hold for several breaths, gradually easing in deeper with each breath, then switch sides.

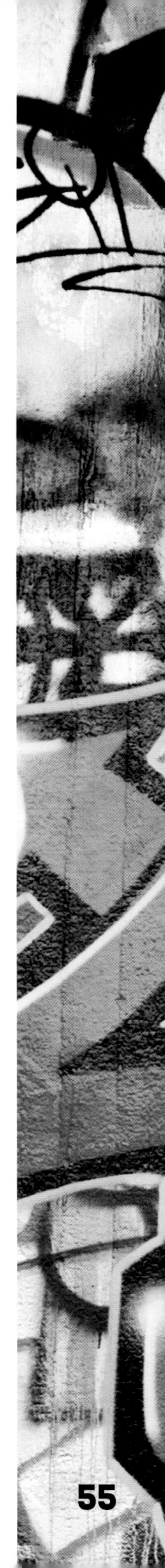

**Inhale:** Reach your arms up and away from your body

**Exhale:** Push your hips in the opposite direction of your arms

**Common Mistakes:** Rotating the trunk instead of bending to the side, letting the arms come too far in front of the rest of the body

**Primary Muscle Groups:** Obliques, lats, triceps, hips

**Calisthenics Counterpart:** Flag Hang

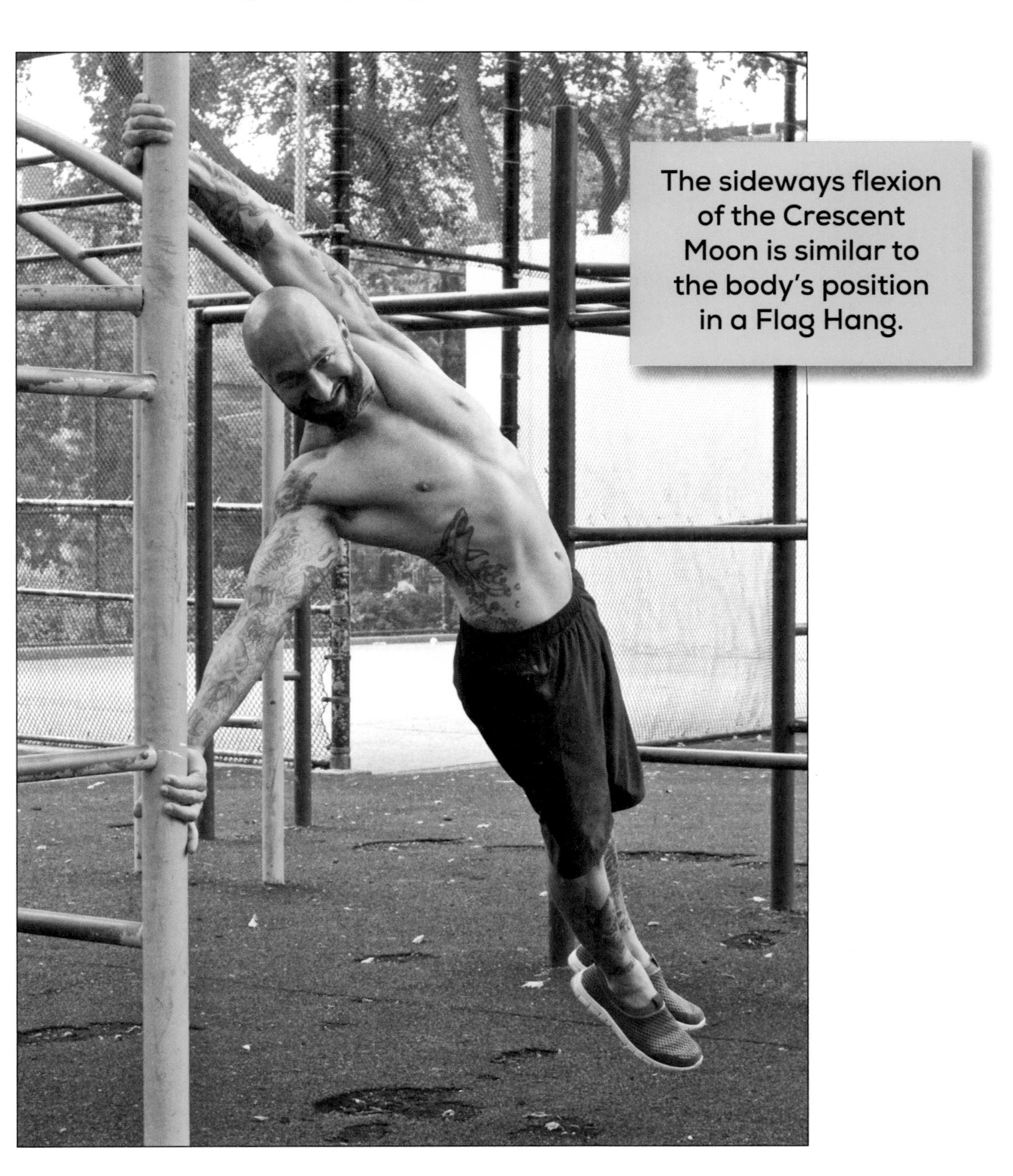

The sideways flexion of the Crescent Moon is similar to the body's position in a Flag Hang.

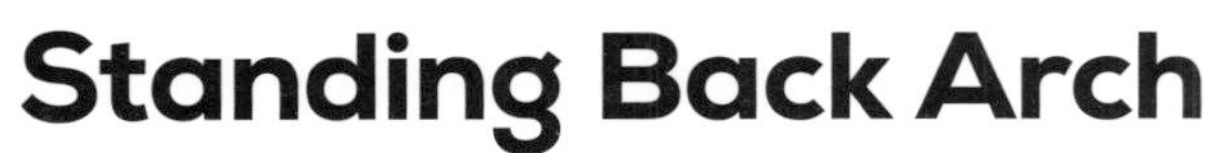

# Standing Back Arch

The Standing Back Arch is a great primer for spinal mobility. Start in Statue pose and clasp your hands behind your back with your fingers interlaced. Press your chest out while squeezing down and back through your shoulder blades. Look up and gradually let your head drop back while slowly shifting your gaze back behind you. Squeeze your glutes and continue to open your chest. For an added stretch, try rotating your palms outward while keeping your fingers clasped. Try to avoid bending your knees.

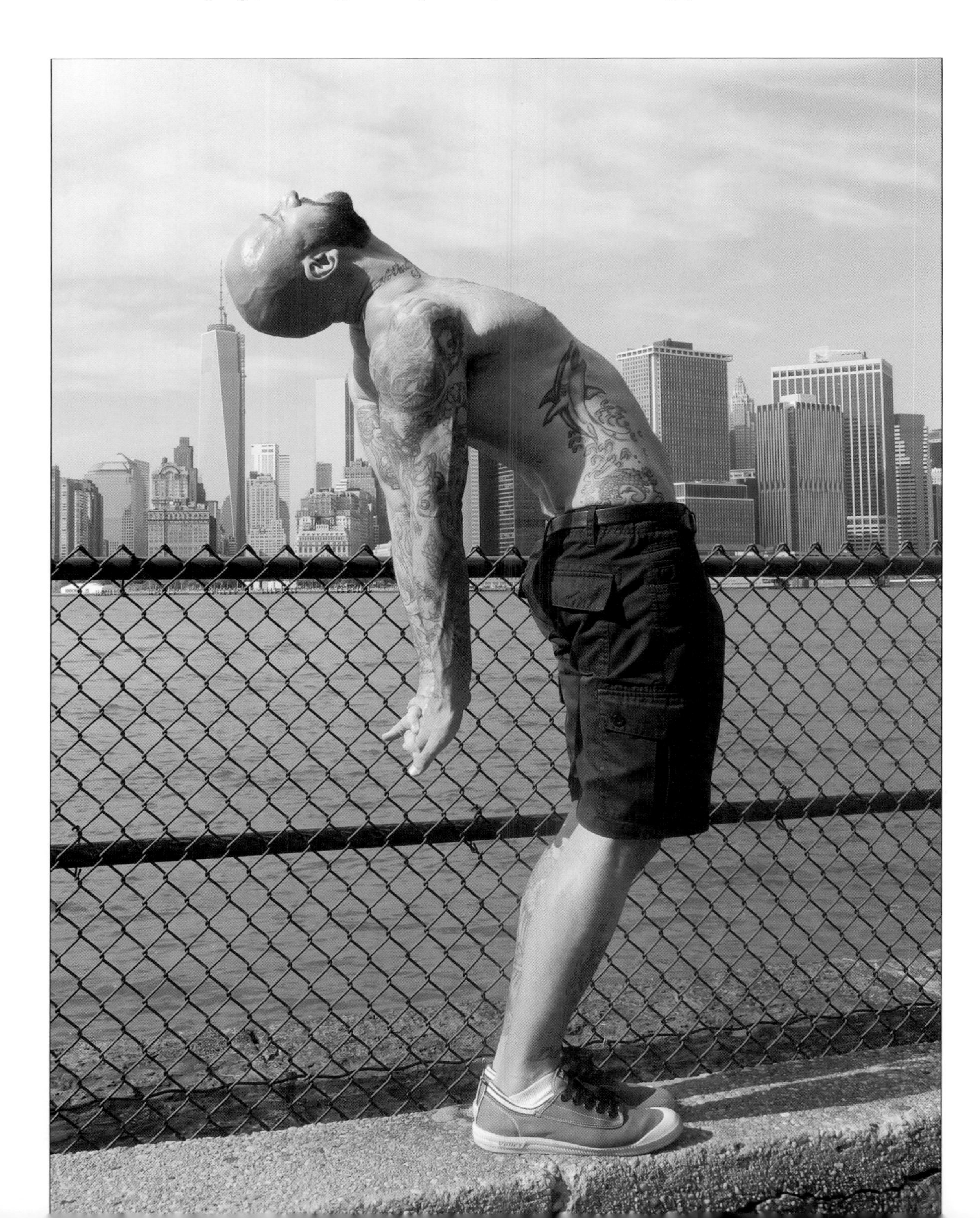

**Inhale:** Lengthen your spine

**Exhale:** Squeeze down and back through your shoulder blades while looking farther and farther behind your back

**Common Mistakes:** Shrugged shoulders, excessive knee flexion

**Primary Muscle Groups:** Chest, shoulders, abs

**Calisthenics Counterpart:** Short Bridge

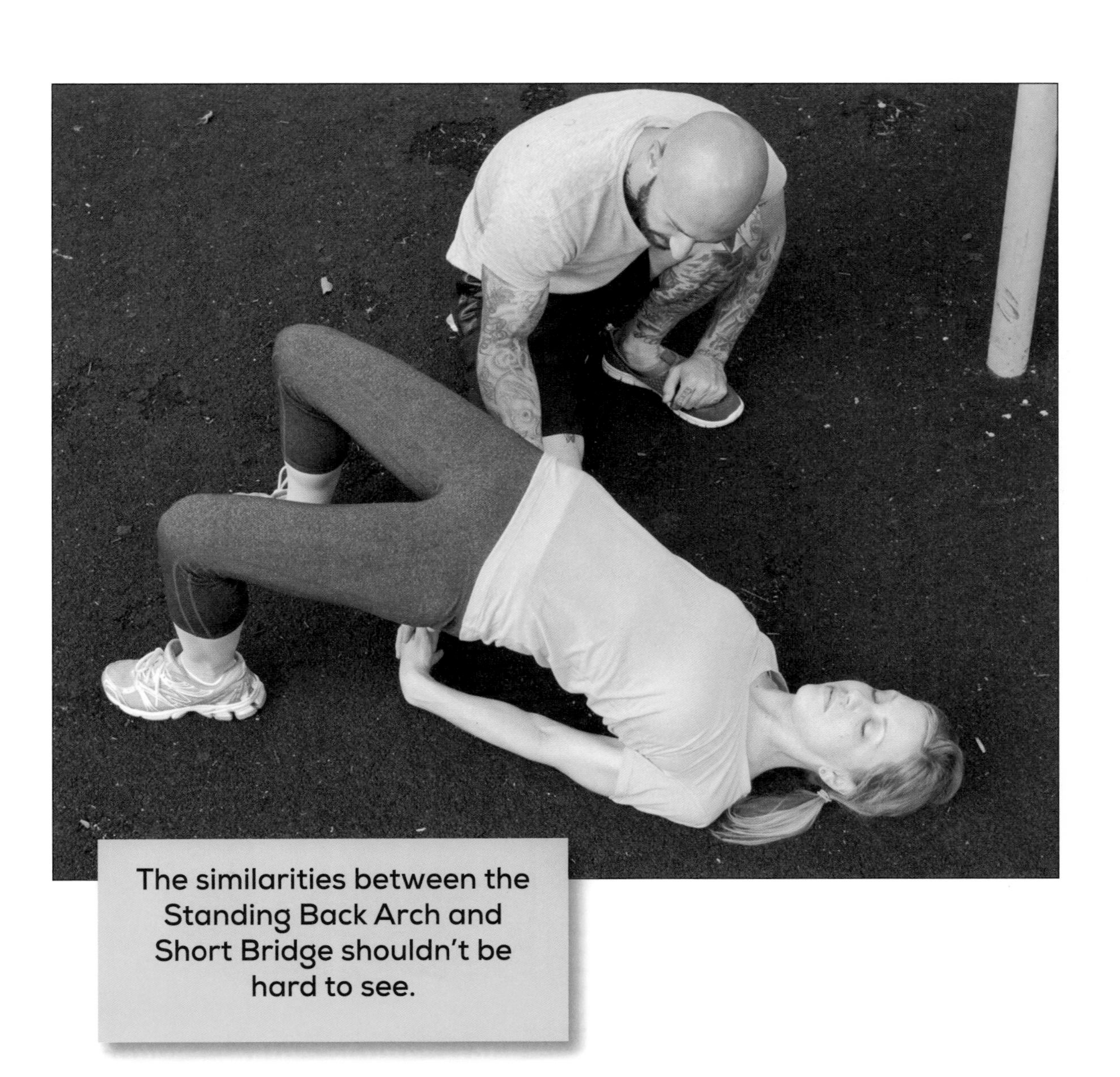

The similarities between the Standing Back Arch and Short Bridge shouldn't be hard to see.

# Half Forward Bend

The Half Forward Bend is a gentle hamstring stretch that's great for beginners. Starting in Statue pose, lean forward from your hips with a flat back and place your hands palms-down on your thighs. Slowly start pushing your hands against your legs while bending further forward from the waist. Focus on keeping your back as straight as you can while pitching your chest forward as your reach your hips back. Your legs and torso will wind up looking like the number 7. Bend your knees slightly if you need to in order to keep from rounding your back.

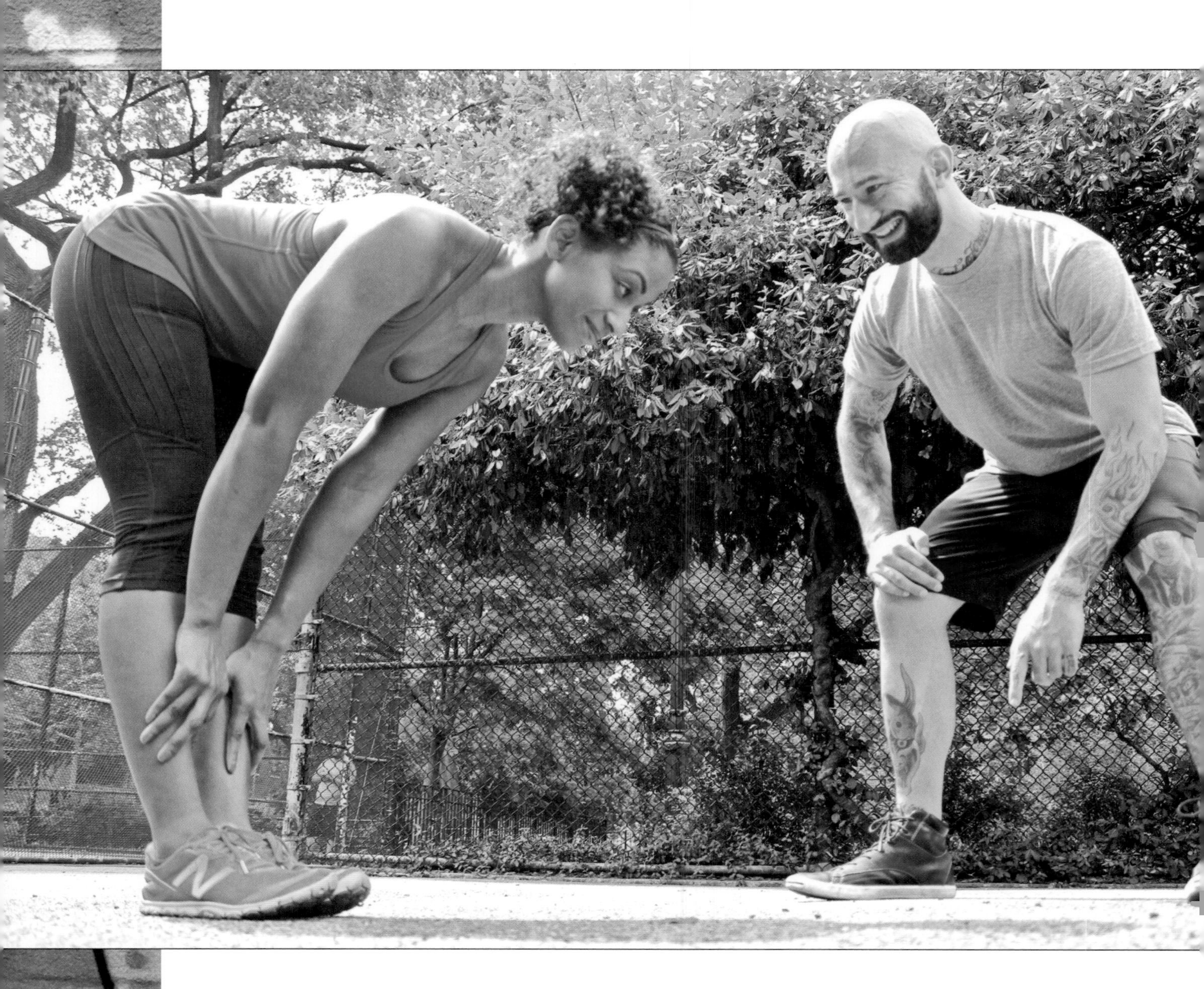

**Inhale:** Lengthen your spine and lift your head

**Exhale:** Hinge from the hips, gradually increasing the stretch in your hamstrings

**Common Mistakes:** Excessive rounding of the spine, shrugged shoulders

**Primary Muscle Groups:** Hamstrings, calves

**Calisthenics Counterpart:** Hanging Leg Raise

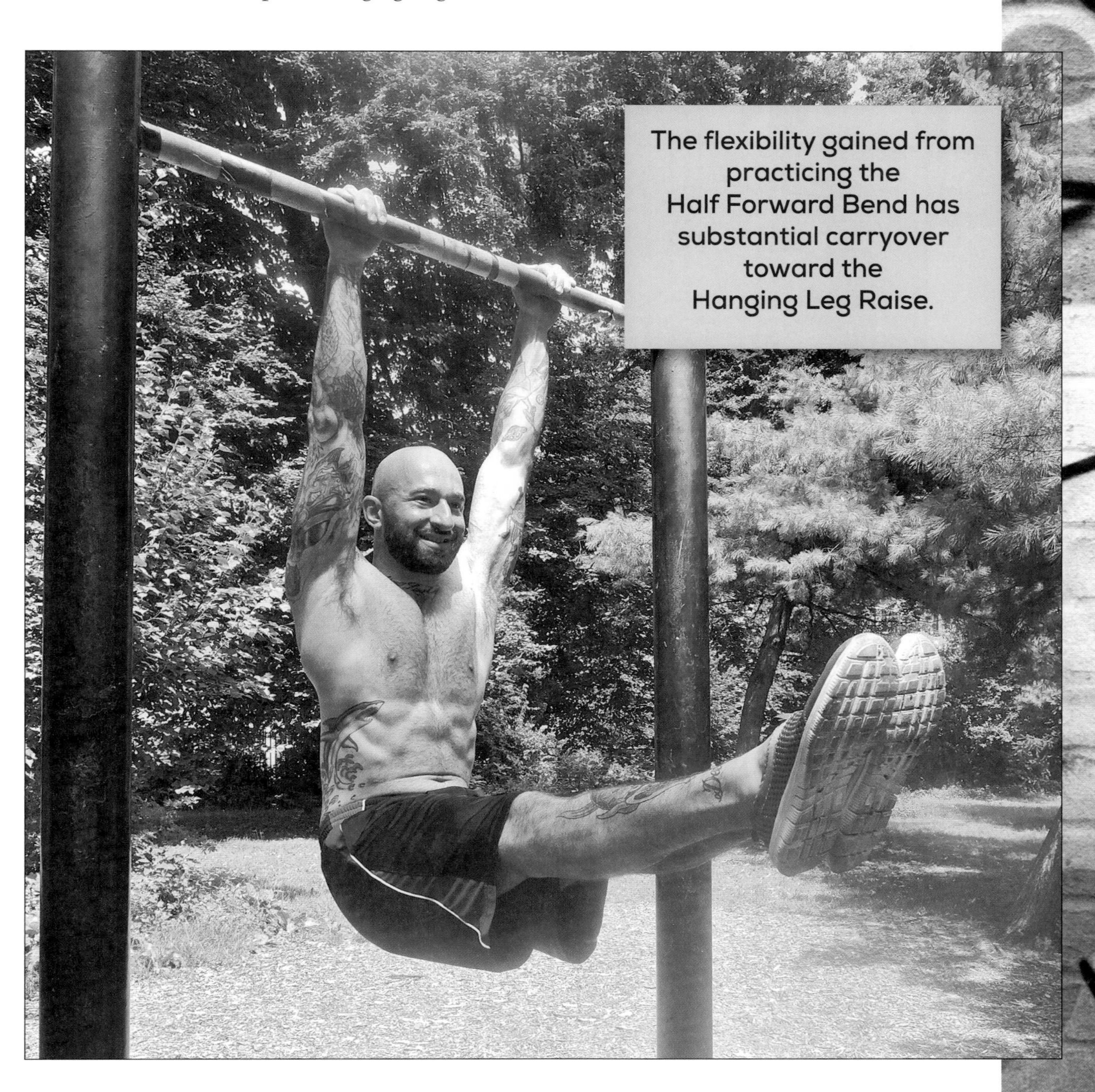

The flexibility gained from practicing the Half Forward Bend has substantial carryover toward the Hanging Leg Raise.

## Full Forward Bend

The Full Forward Bend offers a deep stretch for the hamstrings, lower back and calves. From the Half Forward Bend position, slowly relax your head, neck and spine to let your upper body hang down. Reach your hands toward the floor or to your heels. If you're able to grab your heels, you can gently use them for added leverage to bring yourself deeper into the stretch. You may keep a slight bend in the knees if you lack the flexibility to perform the pose with them straight.

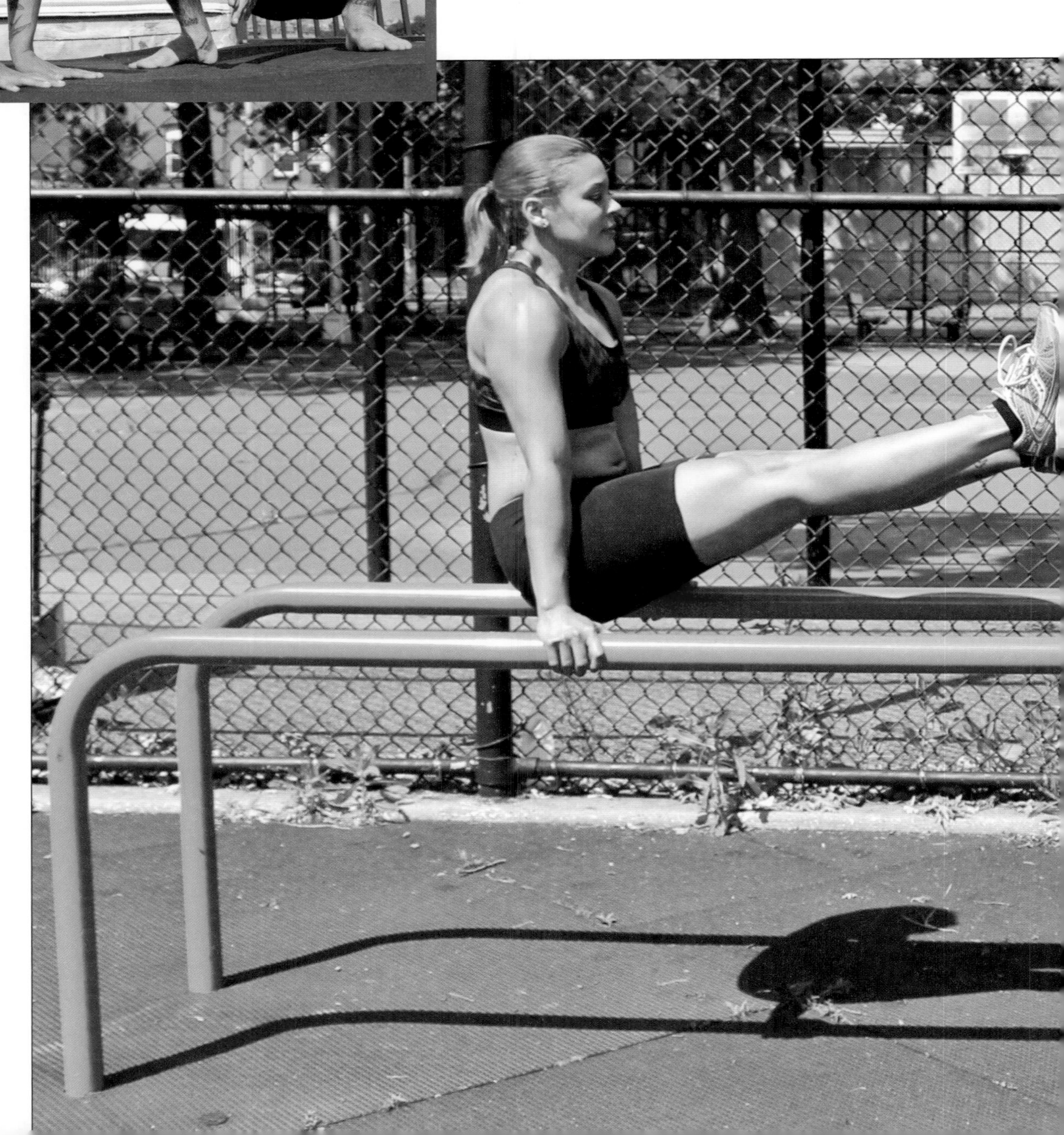

**Inhale:** Fill your belly with air, lengthening the spine

**Exhale:** Relax deeper toward the floor

**Common Mistakes:** Excessive upper-body tension

**Primary Muscle Groups:** Hamstrings, lower back, calves

**Calisthenics Counterpart:** L-Sit

Hamstring flexibility is crucial for performing an L-Sit.

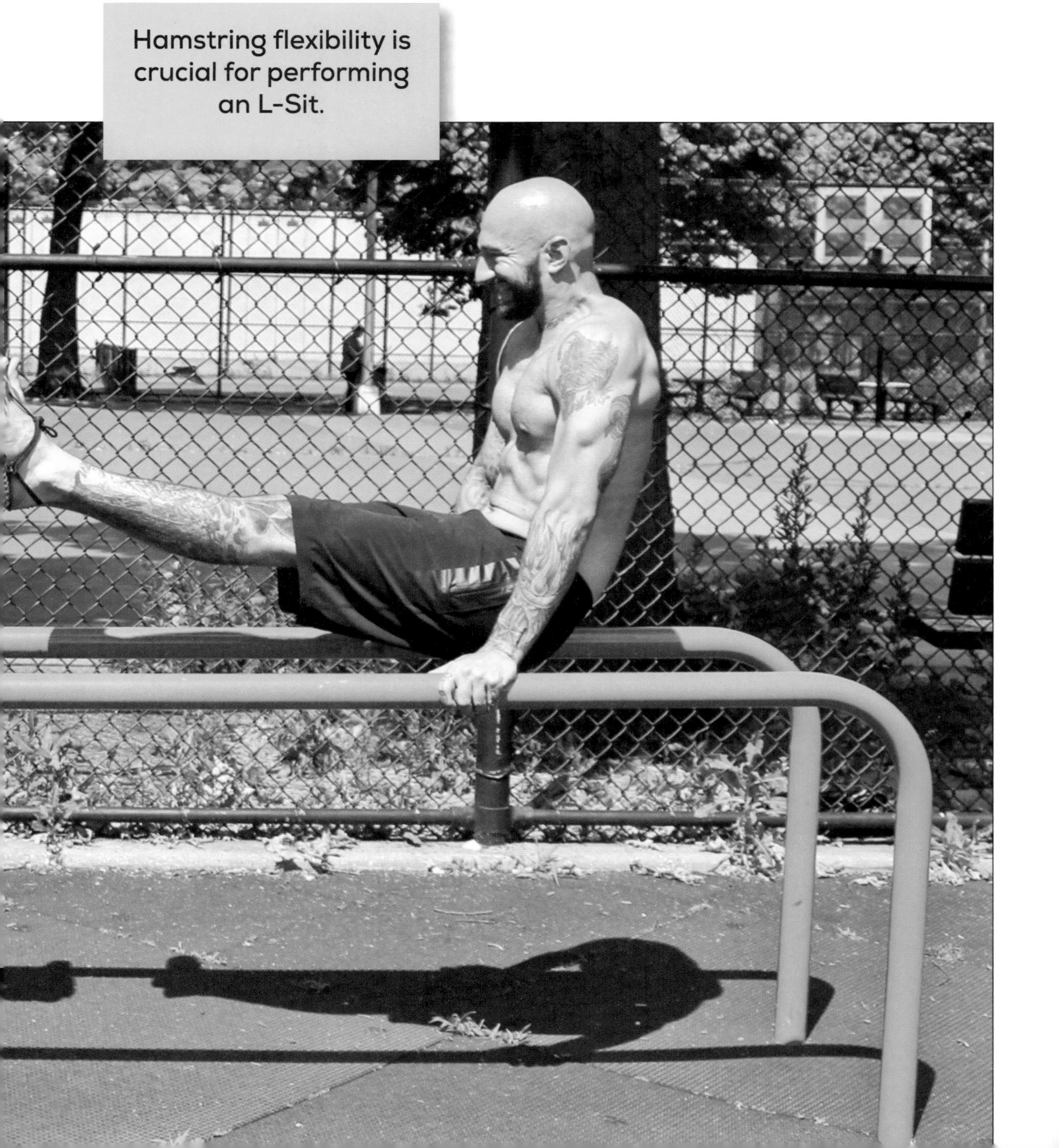

# Standing Plow

Beginning in the Standing Back Arch position, bend forward from the waist while rotating your arms away from your body to facilitate a deep opening of the chest and shoulders, while simultaneously stretching the hamstrings and calves. Let your head drop and reach your arms as far from your body as you can. Though some degree of flexion may be unavoidable, do your best to keep your elbows and knees straight when performing this posture.

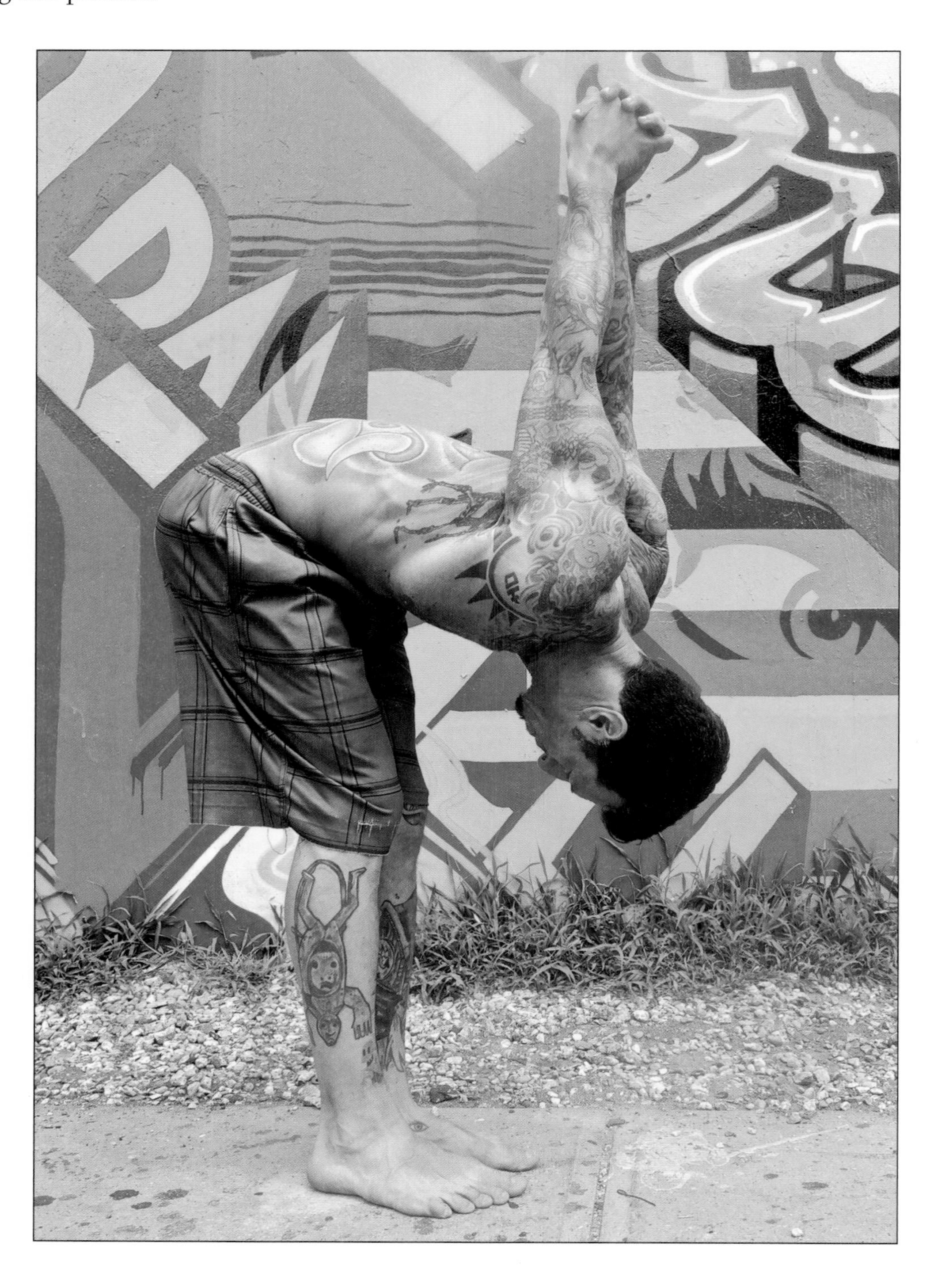

**Inhale:** Lengthen your spine and lift your arms farther up your back

**Exhale:** Gradually push deeper into your forward bend

**Common Mistakes:** Excessive knee and/or elbow bending

**Primary Muscle Groups:** Shoulders, pecs, forearms, low back, hamstrings, calves

**Calisthenics Counterpart:** Skin the Cat

The shoulder flexibility required to Skin the Cat can be achieved through practicing the Standing Plow.

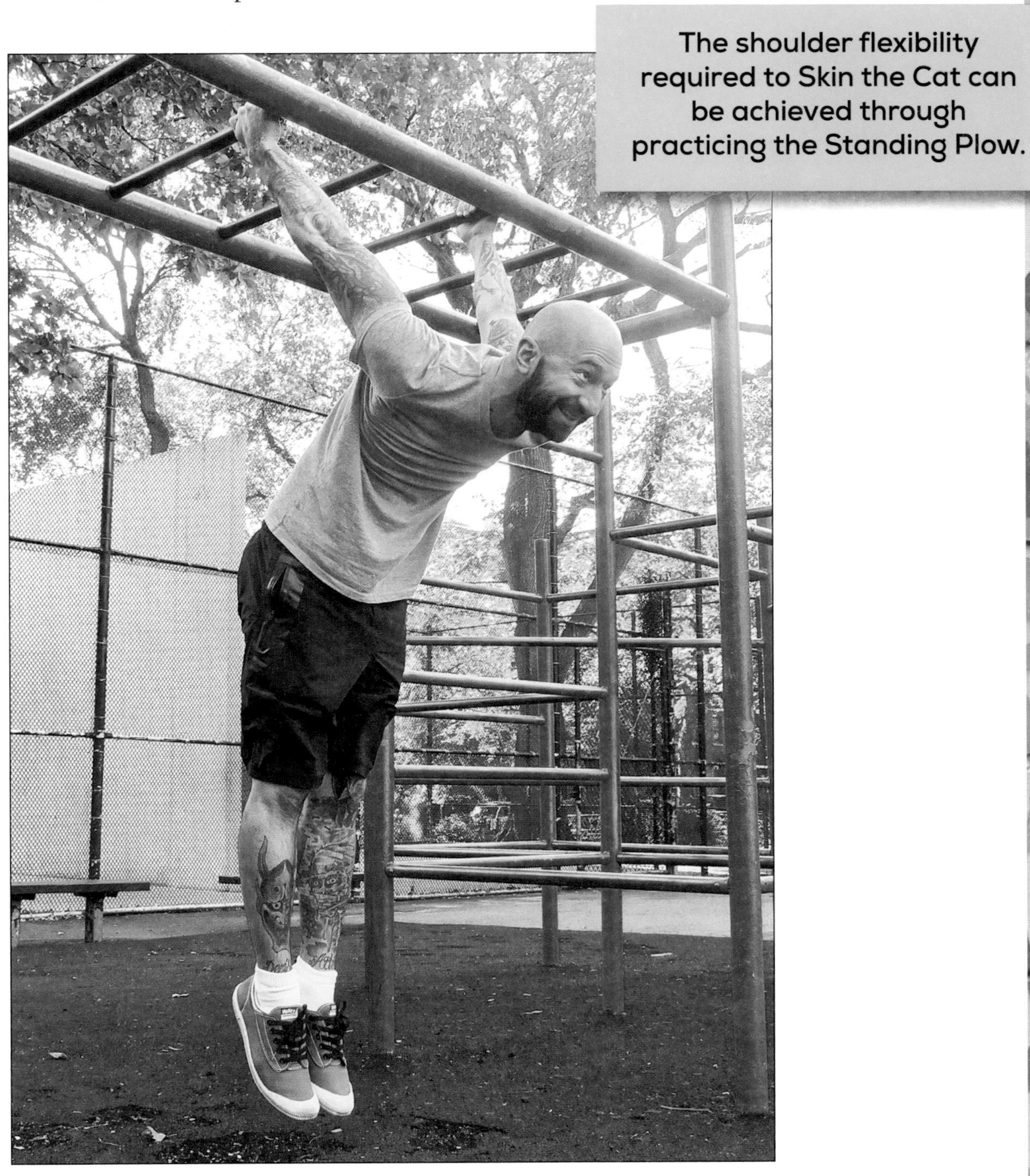

# Standing Straight Arm Wall Stretch

The Standing Straight Arm Wall Stretch is a great way to open up tight shoulders and pecs. Stand facing a wall or other sturdy object and reach your right arm all the way out to the side. Press the entire inside of your arm against the wall from your fingertips to the top of your biceps. Step your right leg in front of your left and begin twisting away from the wall while looking over your left shoulder. Repeat on the opposite side.

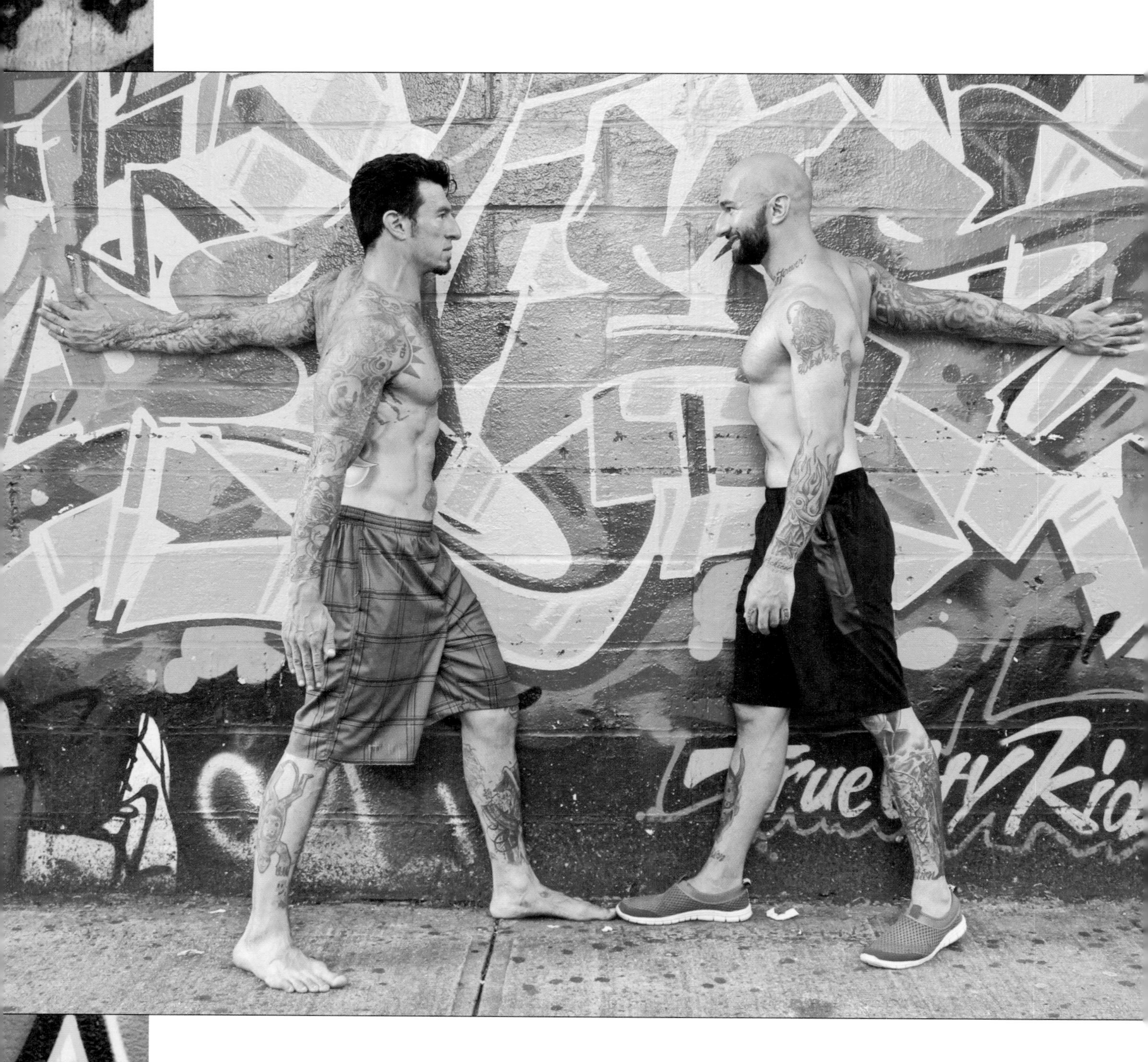

**Inhale:** Lengthen your spine and drop your shoulders

**Exhale:** Twist away from the wall while pressing your hips forward and looking over the opposite shoulder

**Common Mistakes:** Excessively shrugged shoulders, wrong leg in front

**Primary Muscle Groups:** Front delts, pecs, biceps, forearms

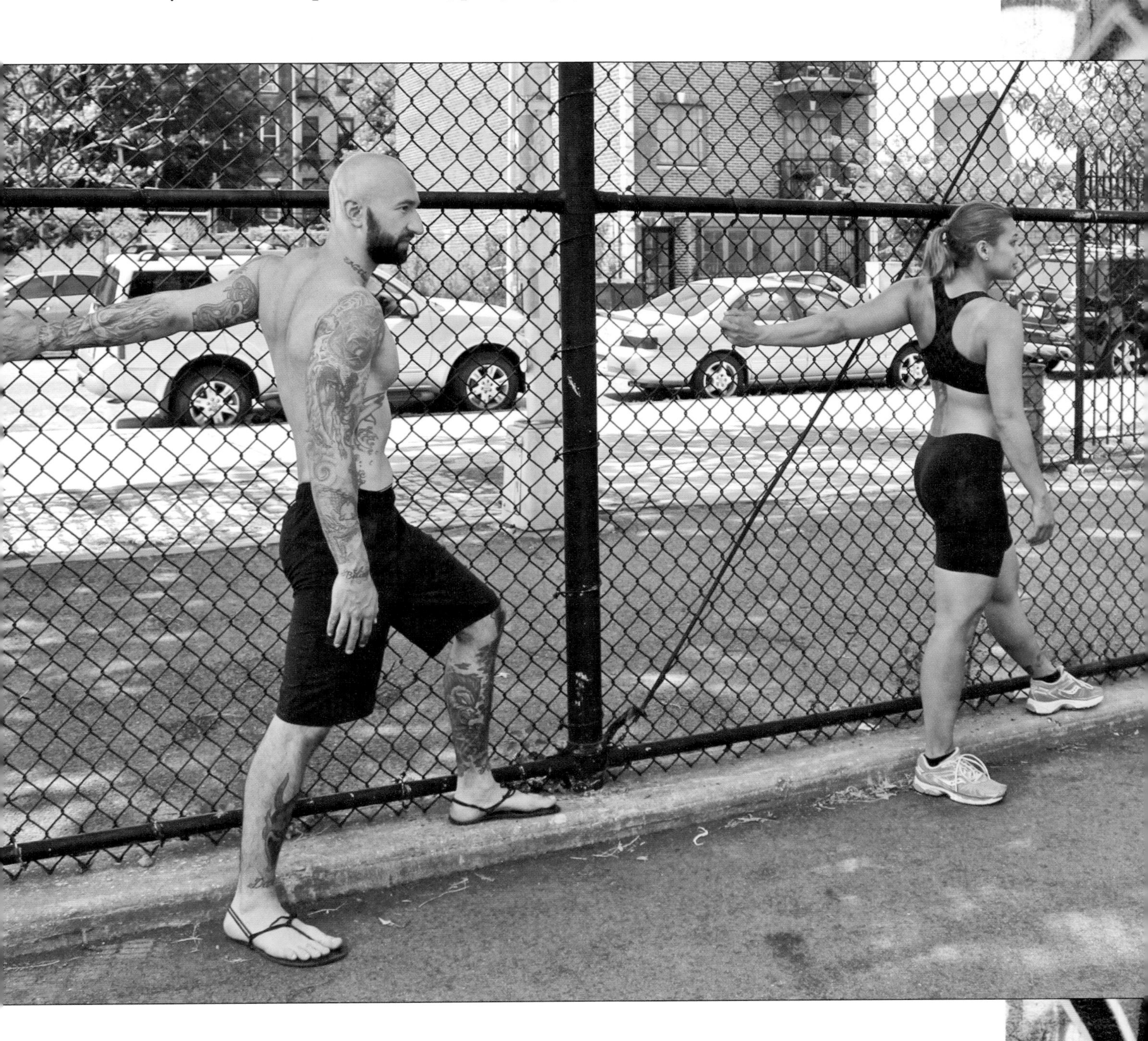

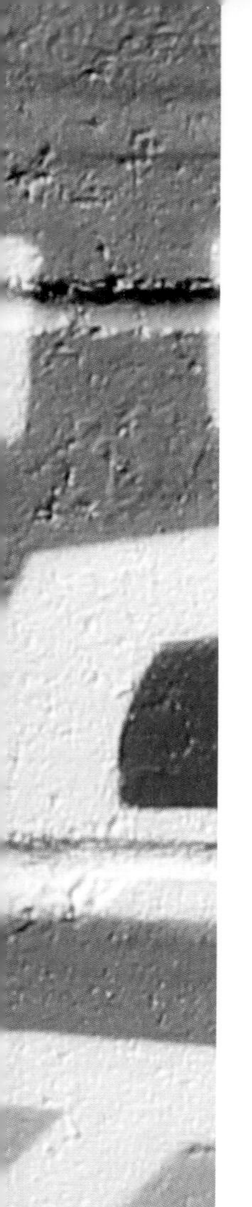

# Standing Bent Arm Wall Stretch

This pose is the same as the Standing Straight Arm Wall Stretch except the arm being stretched is bent to 90 degrees at the elbow (fingers pointed up). This changes the angle of the stretch, putting more emphasis on the chest while deemphasizing the biceps, forearms and shoulders.

**Inhale:** Lengthen your spine and press your arm to the wall

**Exhale:** Twist your trunk away from the wall and look over your shoulder

**Common Mistakes:** Excessively shrugged shoulders, wrong leg in front

**Primary Muscle Groups:** Pecs, front delts

**Calisthenics Counterpart:** Elevated Push-up

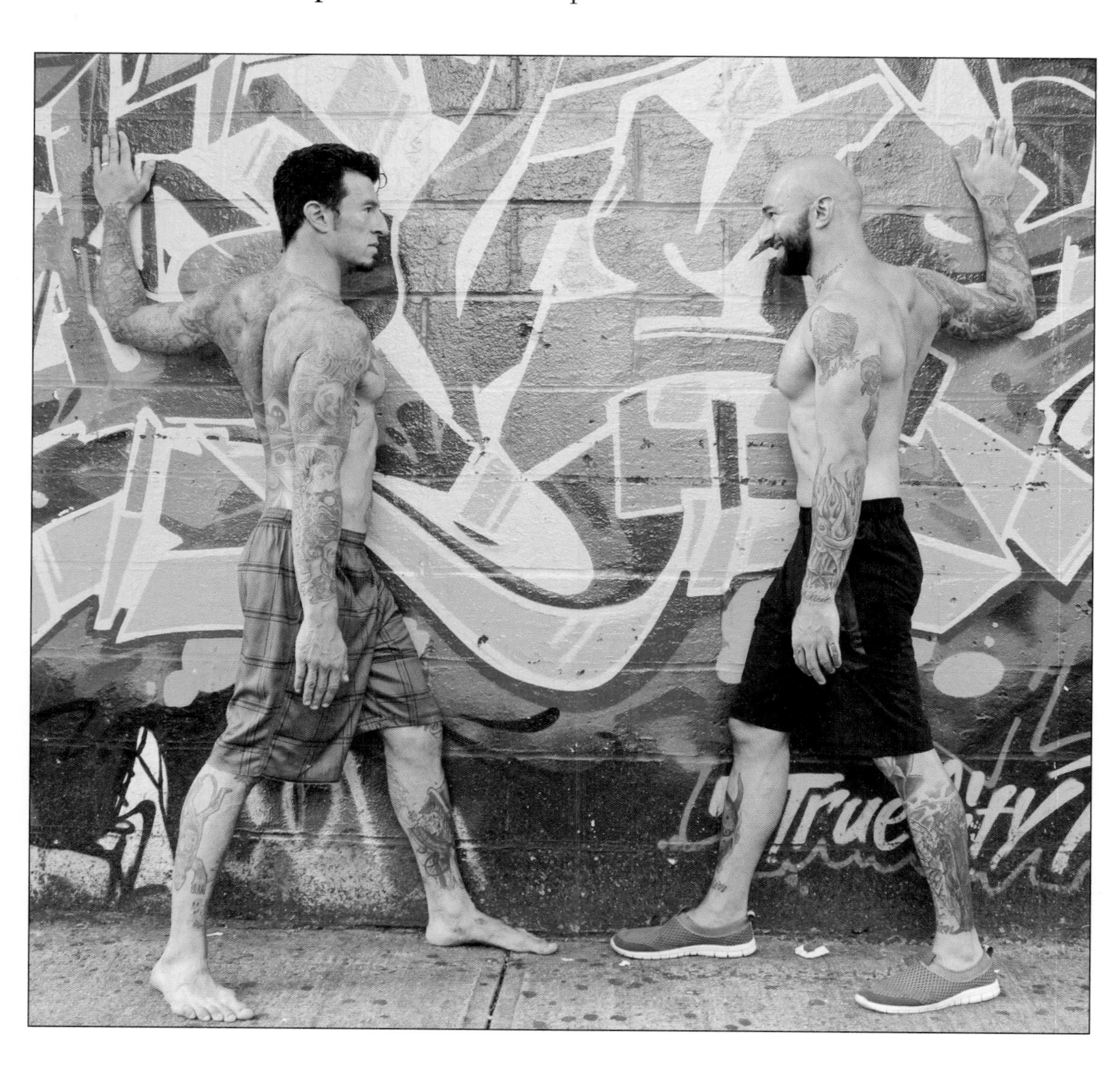

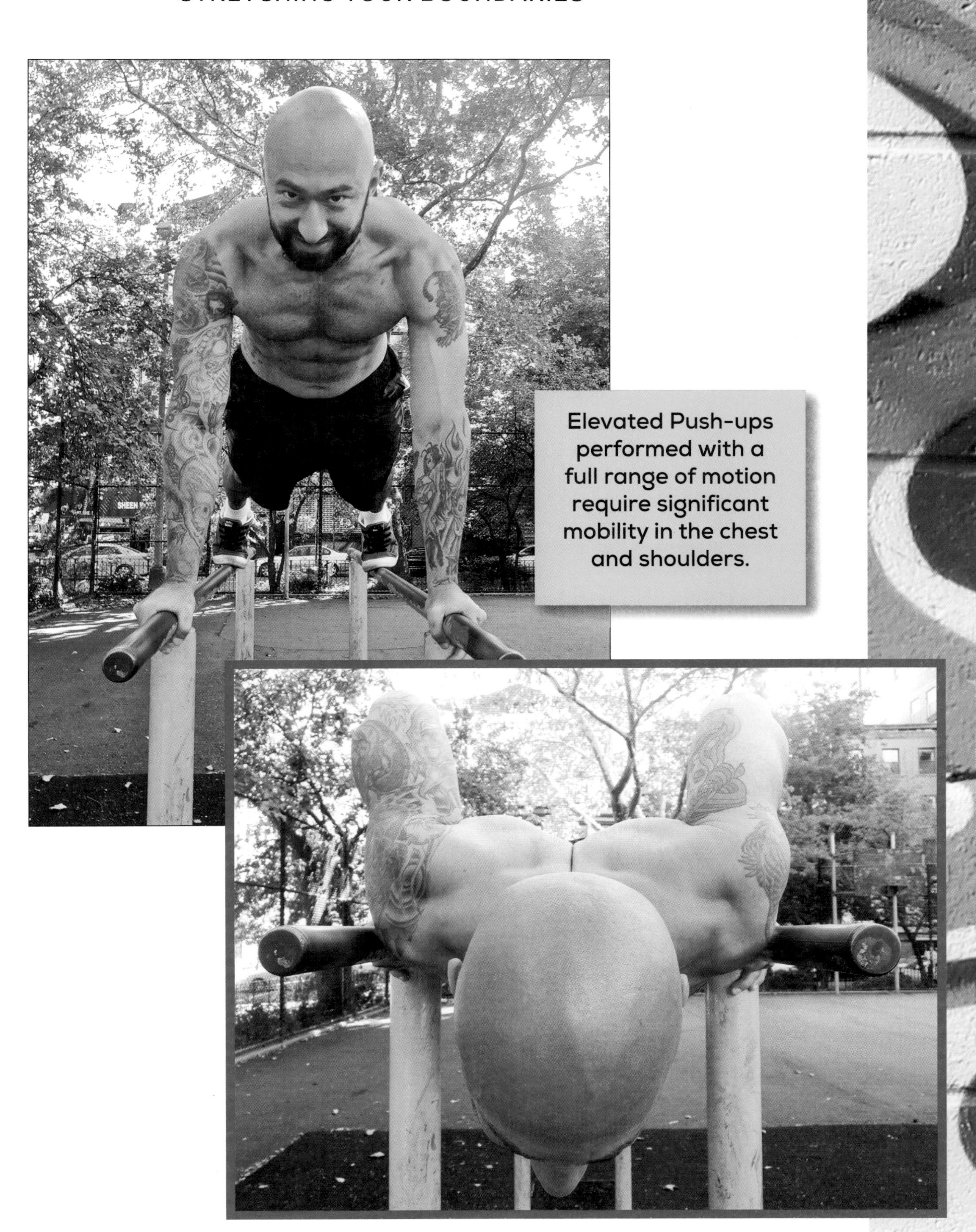

Elevated Push-ups performed with a full range of motion require significant mobility in the chest and shoulders.

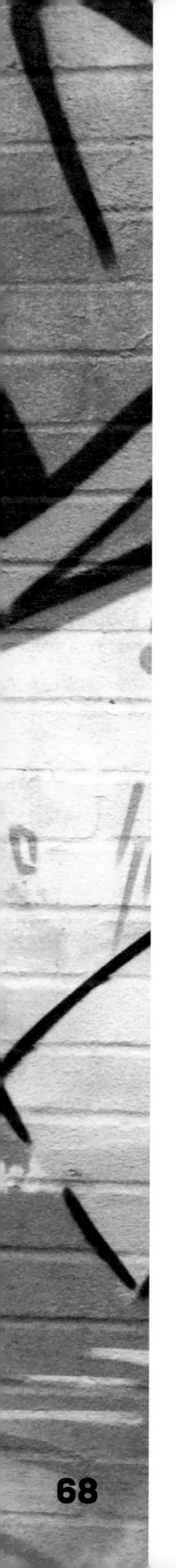

# Standing Rear Delt Stretch

The Standing Rear Delt Stretch targets the back of the shoulder. From a standing position, reach one arm across the front of your body while grabbing along the triceps with your opposite hand. Keep your chest up and your shoulders down in their sockets as you pull the arm straight across your body. Try to get your extended arm parallel to the ground without shrugging your shoulder or bending your elbow. Make sure to stretch both sides evenly.

**Inhale:** Lift your head and lengthen your spine

**Exhale:** Pull your elbow down and in toward your body, squeeze your shoulder blades down

**Common Mistakes:** Shrugged shoulders, particularly on the side being stretched

**Primary Muscle Groups:** Rear delts

**Calisthenics Counterpart:** Meathook

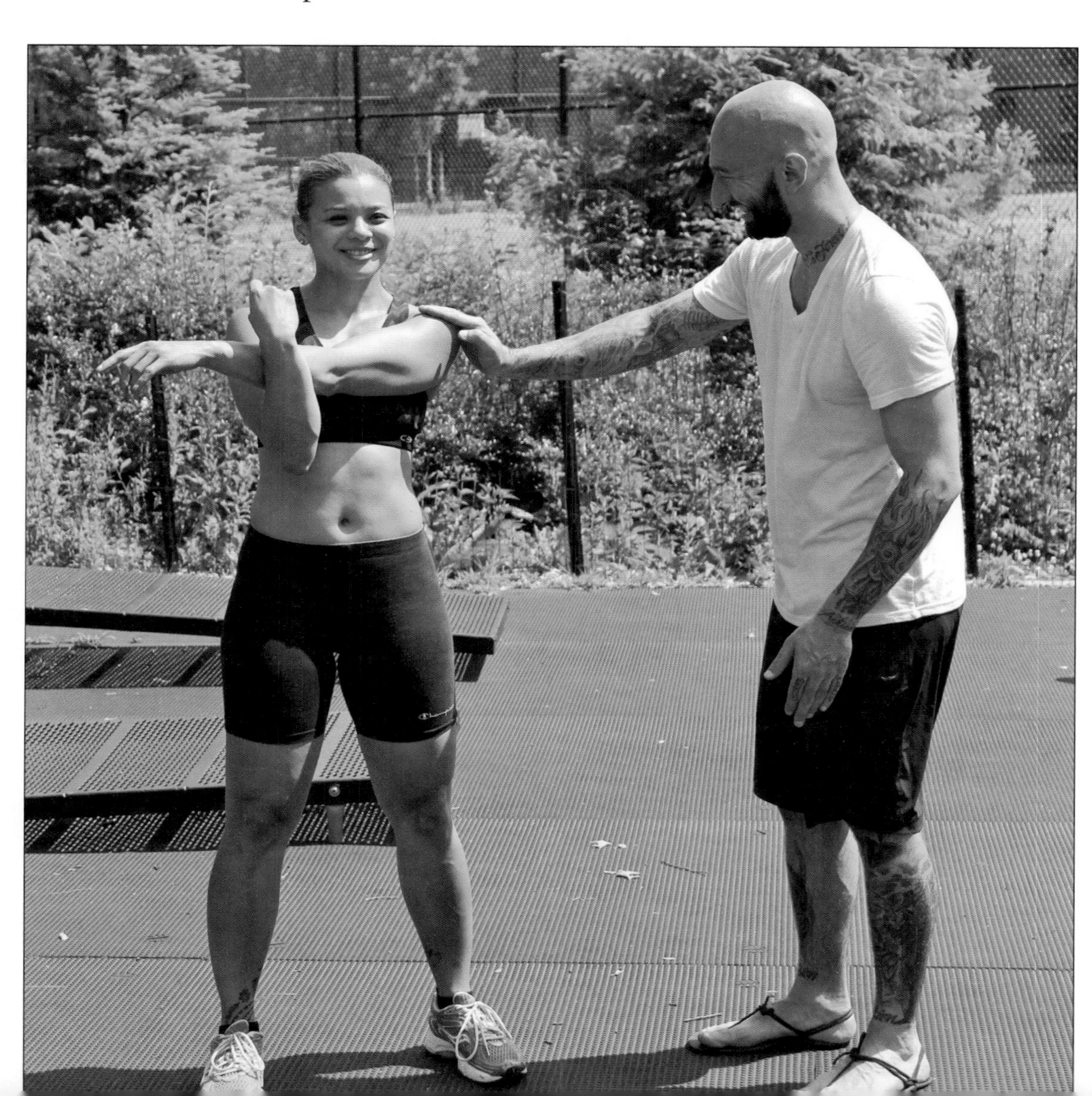

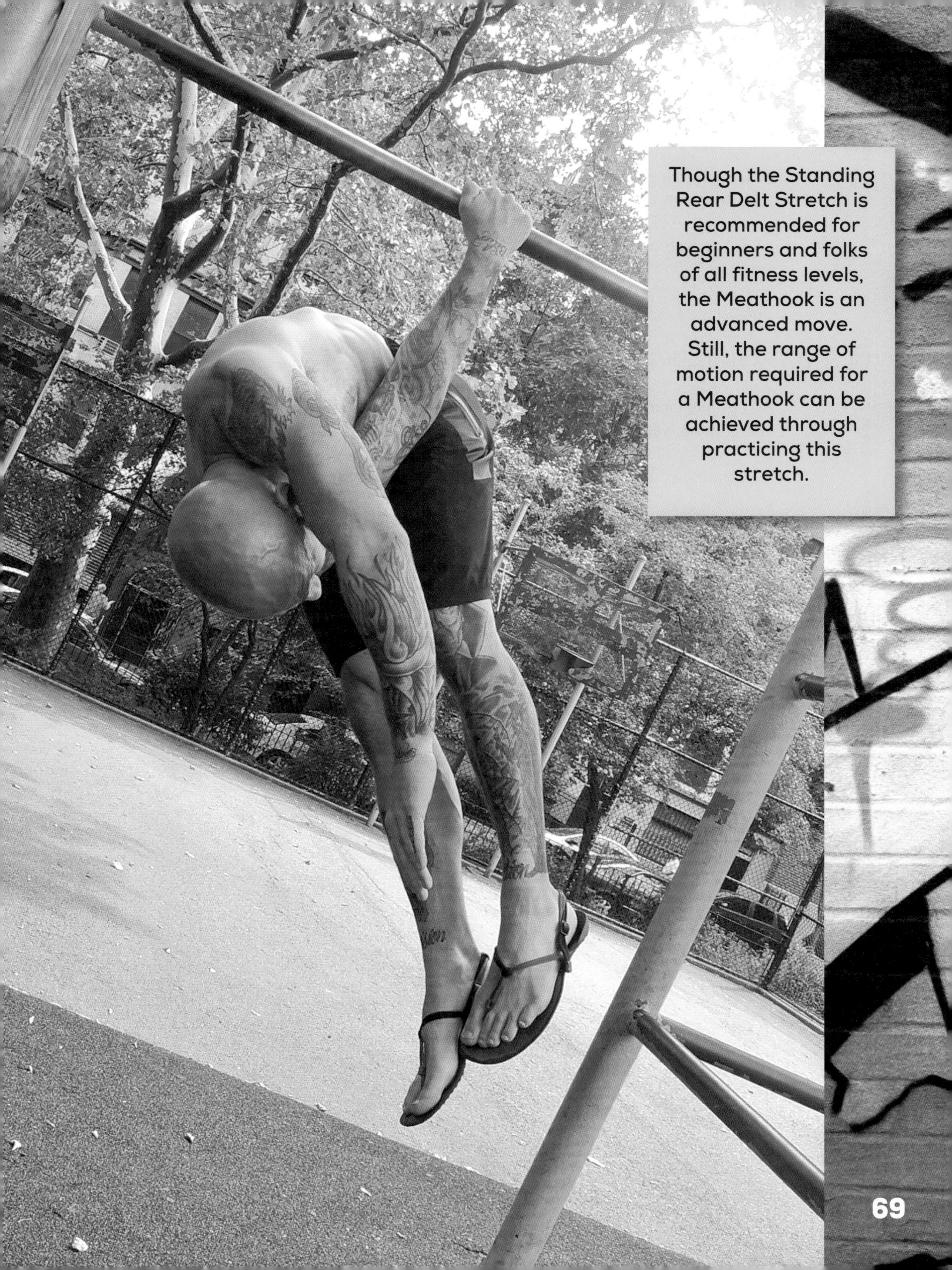

Though the Standing Rear Delt Stretch is recommended for beginners and folks of all fitness levels, the Meathook is an advanced move. Still, the range of motion required for a Meathook can be achieved through practicing this stretch.

# Standing Triceps Stretch

The Standing Triceps Stretch is a great opener for the entire upper-arm region, including the chest, shoulders and back. From Statue pose, raise one arm in the air then bend it back at the elbow, reaching in between your shoulder blades. Now use your opposite hand to grab your elbow and pull the arm farther back. Stand tall, engaging your abdominals to prevent hyperextending your lower back. Try to avoid letting your chin get pushed down to your chest. You may find it helpful to use the back of your head for added leverage to press into your arm to deepen the stretch. Repeat on both sides.

**Inhale:** Lift your head and lengthen your spine

**Exhale:** Gently pull down on your elbow with your assisting arm and reach your free hand in between your shoulder blades

**Common Mistakes:** Shrugged shoulders, tucked chin

**Primary Muscle Groups:** Triceps, shoulders, chest, back

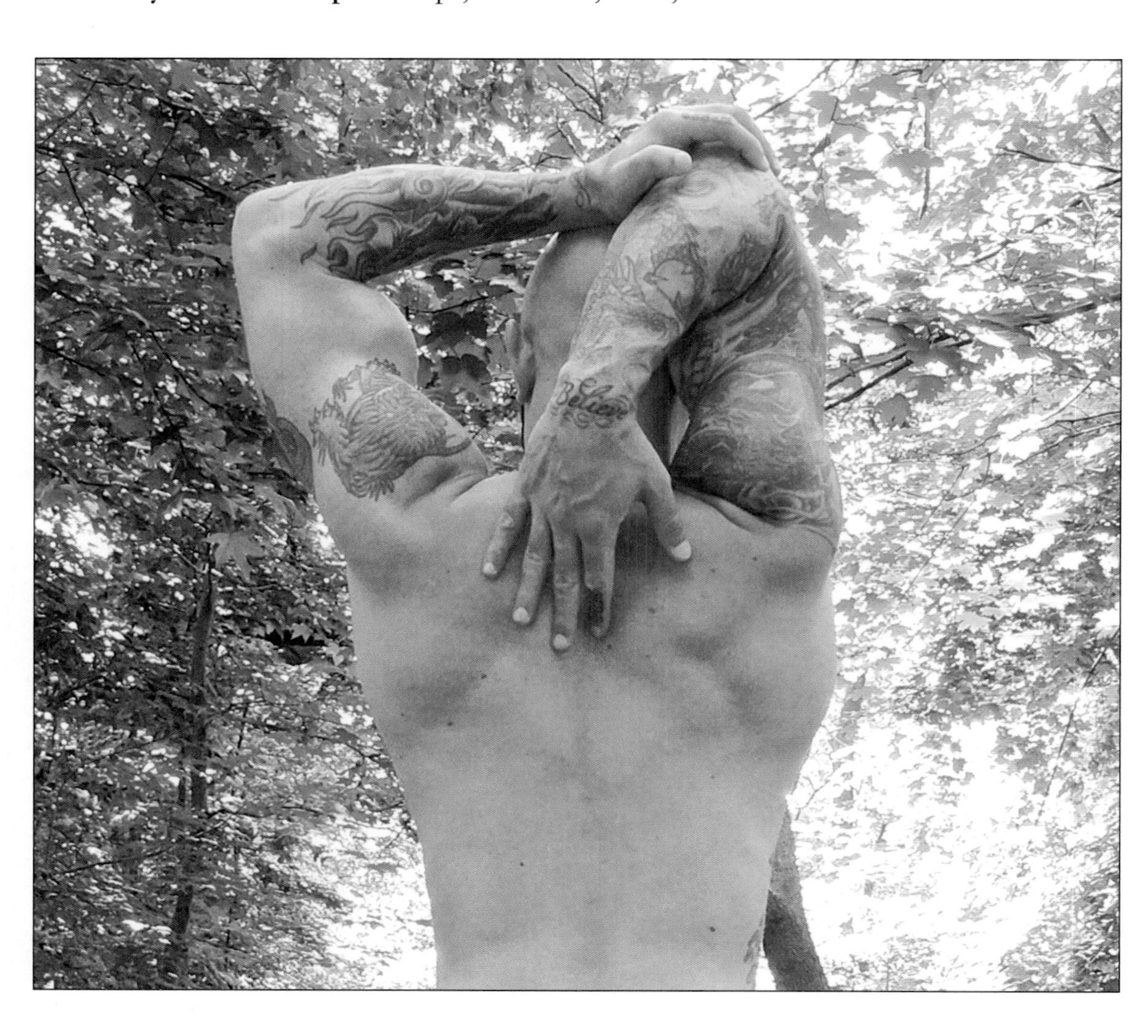

# Standing Triceps Stretch with Bind

From the Standing Triceps Stretch position, remove the assisting arm and reach it behind your back from the bottom up. The objective is to clasp your fingers together behind your back, with your bottom hand positioned palm-out and top hand facing the body. Remember to keep your chin up and back straight. Beginners should start by holding a cloth in both hands, which will allow them to remain farther apart, gradually working toward bringing the hands closer together (and eventually into a full bind) over time. Repeat on both sides, bearing in mind that it is very common for one side to be tighter than the other.

**Inhale:** Lift your head and lengthen your spine

**Exhale:** Gently squeeze your hands closer together

**Common Mistakes:** Shrugged shoulders, tucked chin

**Primary Muscle Groups:** Triceps, shoulders, chest, back

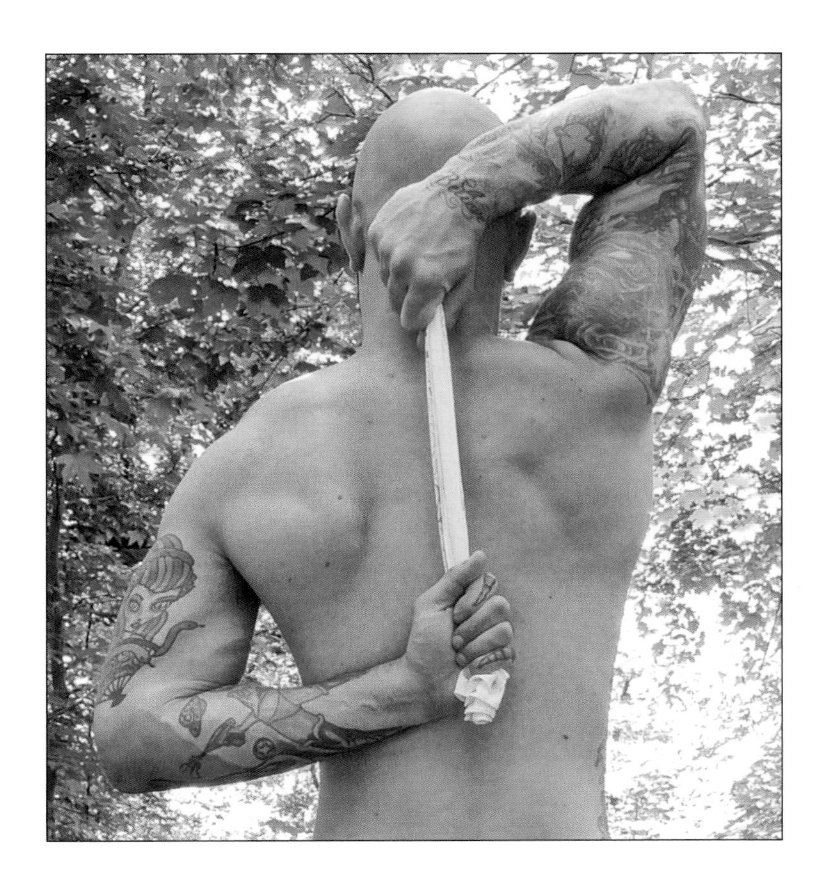

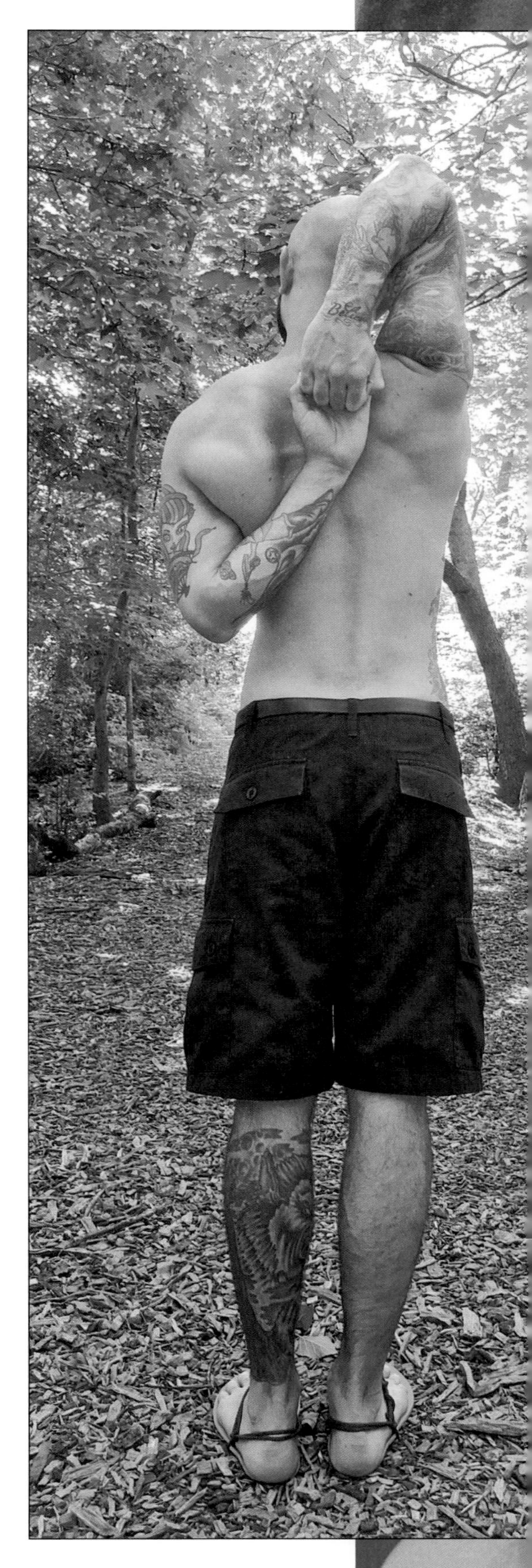

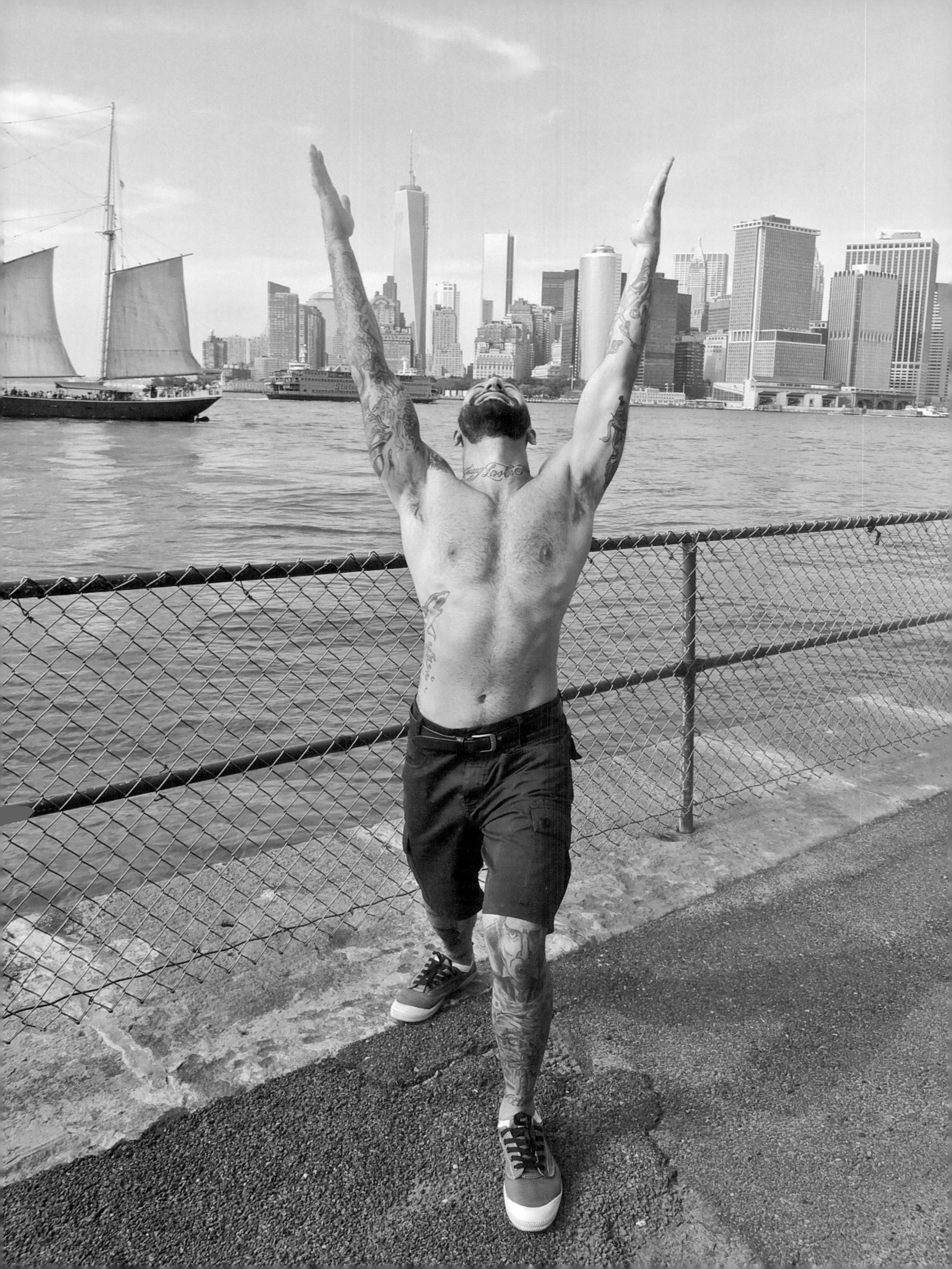

# Warrior One

Warrior One is a fantastic pose with many subtle challenges. From Statue pose, take a big step forward with your left leg, then bring your right foot to a forty-five degree angle so the heel of your front foot lines up with the instep of your back foot. Keep your hips facing forward and bend your front knee. If you're tight in the hips, adjust your right leg slightly out to the right side, maintaining the forty-five degree angle of the foot. You should feel a stretch in your calf and your hip flexor on the right side. Reach your arms up overhead, but be careful not to shrug your shoulders. Lift your chest tall, but keep your shoulder blades depressed. Repeat on both sides.

**Inhale:** Lengthen your spine and reach up with your arms

**Exhale:** Press your back heel into the ground, while pushing your hips forward

**Common Mistakes:** Shrugged shoulders, twisted hips

**Primary Muscle Groups:** Hip flexors, calves, chest, back

**Calisthenics Counterpart:** Pull-up (bottom position)

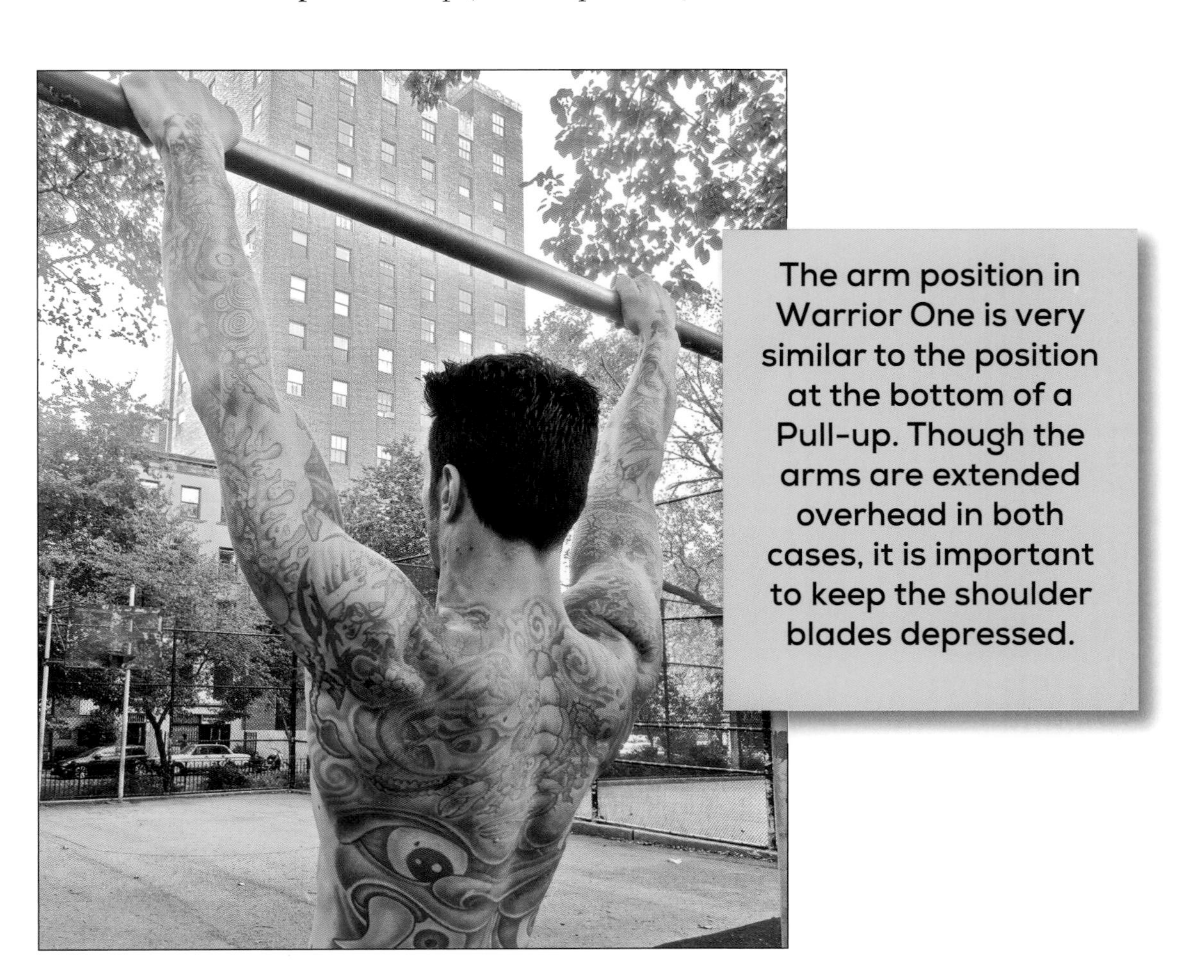

The arm position in Warrior One is very similar to the position at the bottom of a Pull-up. Though the arms are extended overhead in both cases, it is important to keep the shoulder blades depressed.

# Warrior Two

Beginning in Warrior One, rotate your hips to the side, as though you were attempting to slide between a vary narrow passageway. Reach your arms straight out to the sides so they are parallel to the floor, again being mindful to avoid shrugging your shoulders. Suck in your stomach, tuck your hips under and squeeze your glutes. Do your best to keep your front knee from bowing inward as you bend your leg until the top of your thigh is parallel to the ground. Turn your head to the side and look over your front hand. You may need to widen your stance from the Warrior One position. Repeat on both sides.

**Inhale:** Lift your chest and tuck your hips under

**Exhale:** Sink into your front knee, drop your shoulders and reach your arms all the way out to the sides

**Common Mistakes:** Excessive inward bowing of the front knee, shrugged shoulders

**Primary Muscle Groups:** Hips, hamstrings

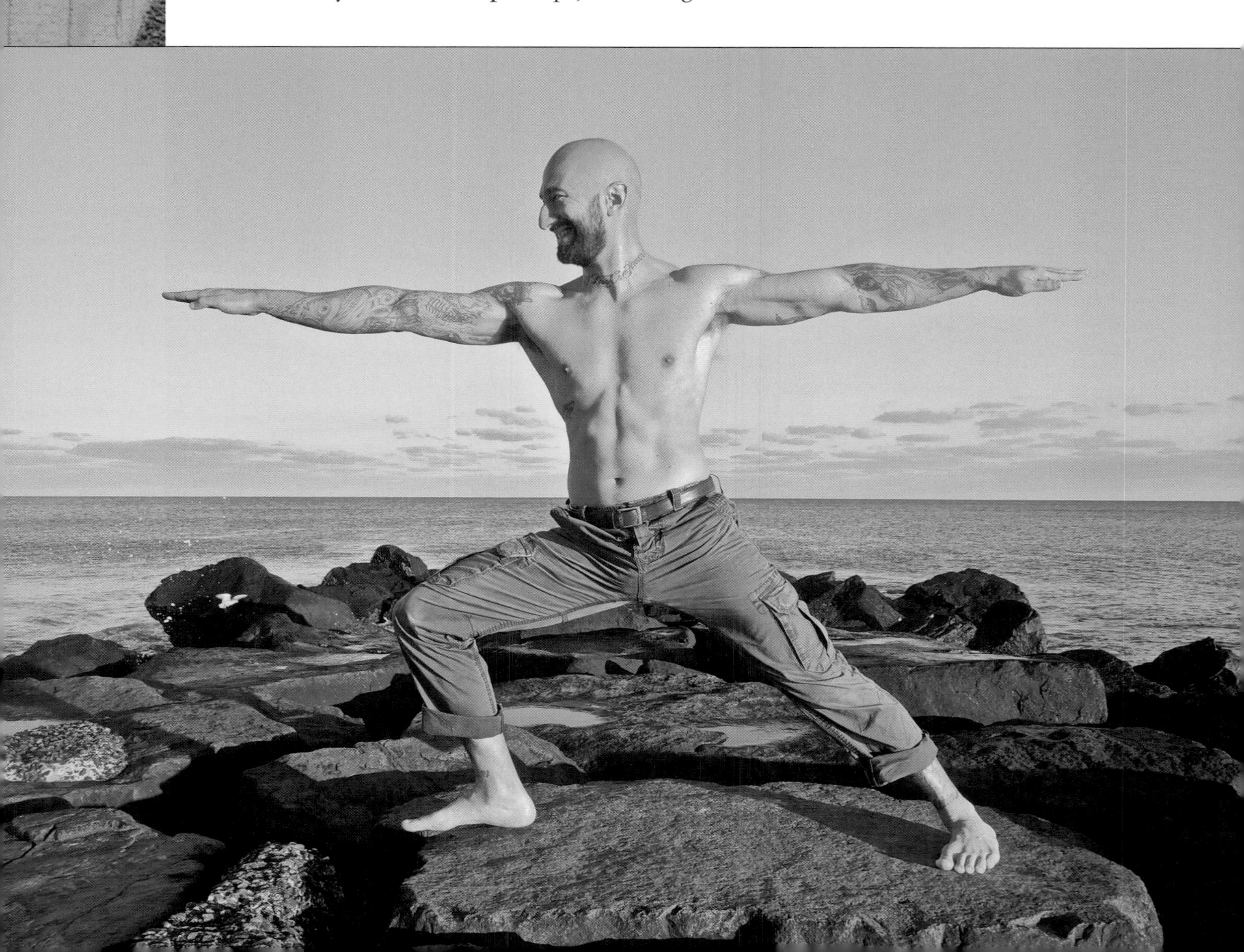

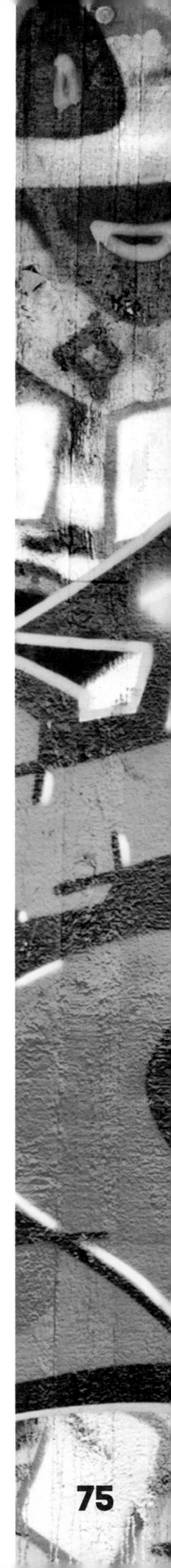

# Triangle

From the Warrior Two position, bend at the waist so your trunk moves closer toward your front leg, reaching your front hand all the way out to the side. Continue flexing your trunk to bring your front hand to your ankle. Your opposite arm should be reaching straight up into the air. Though you may need to rotate your trunk a bit to get low enough, the eventual goal should be to perform this move as pure sideways flexion with your trunk staying in line with your legs. Imagine yourself between two panes of glass. You may need to bend your front leg a bit to get down low enough. Though I recommend working toward extending that leg over time, a bent front knee is perfectly acceptable when starting out.

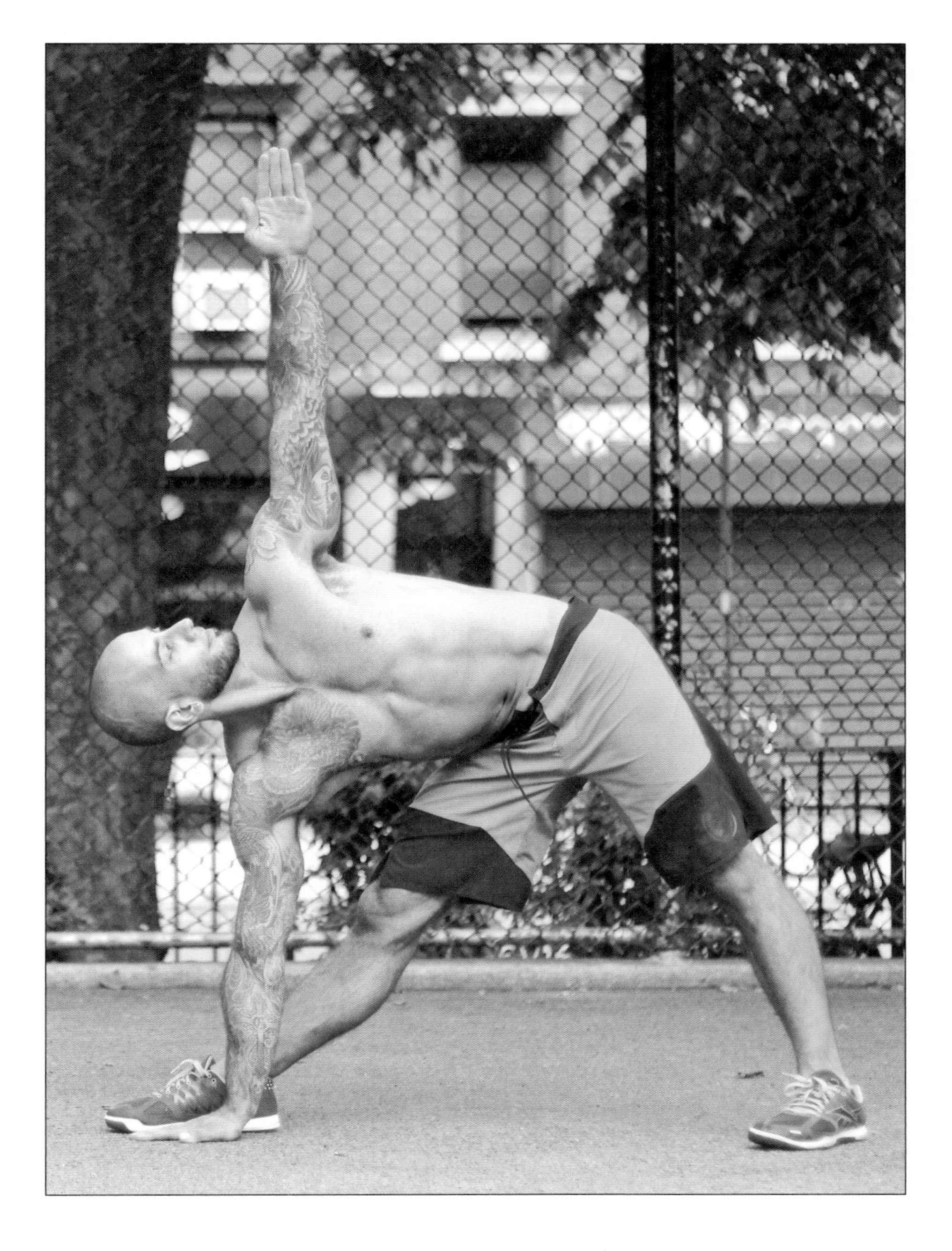

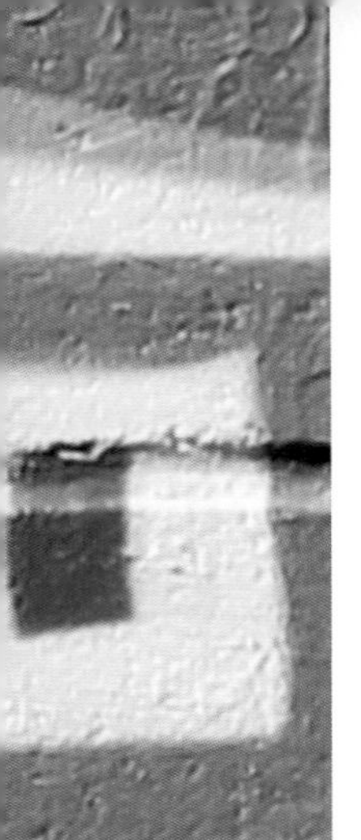

**Inhale:** Lengthen your spine and reach your arms as long as you can

**Exhale:** Gradually push further into sideways trunk flexion

**Common Mistakes:** Trunk rotation in place of sideways flexion, excessive forward spinal flexion

**Primary Muscle Groups:** Lats, obliques, hamstrings, hips

It's okay to bend your front leg a bit when starting out with Triangle.

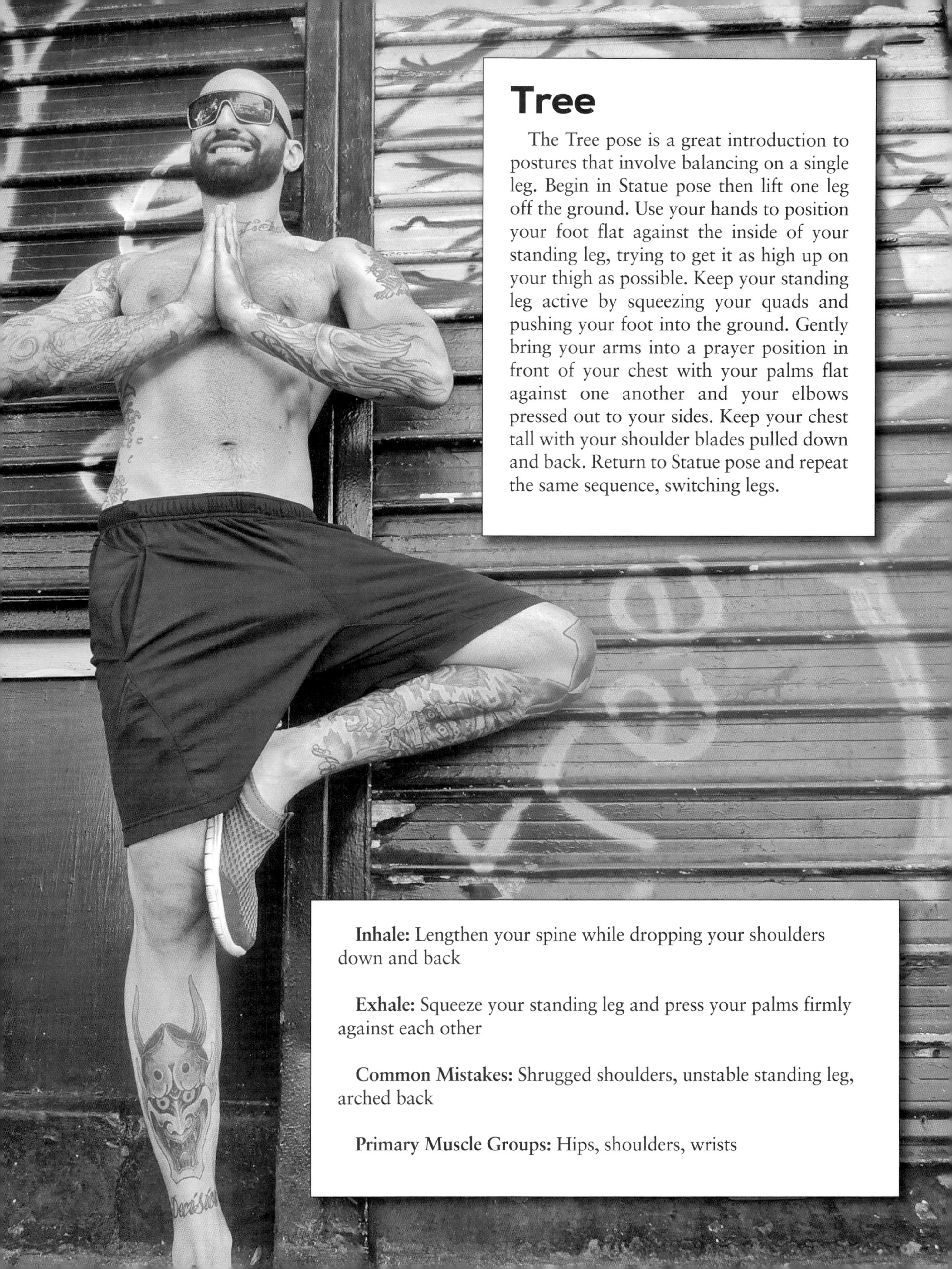

# Tree

The Tree pose is a great introduction to postures that involve balancing on a single leg. Begin in Statue pose then lift one leg off the ground. Use your hands to position your foot flat against the inside of your standing leg, trying to get it as high up on your thigh as possible. Keep your standing leg active by squeezing your quads and pushing your foot into the ground. Gently bring your arms into a prayer position in front of your chest with your palms flat against one another and your elbows pressed out to your sides. Keep your chest tall with your shoulder blades pulled down and back. Return to Statue pose and repeat the same sequence, switching legs.

**Inhale:** Lengthen your spine while dropping your shoulders down and back

**Exhale:** Squeeze your standing leg and press your palms firmly against each other

**Common Mistakes:** Shrugged shoulders, unstable standing leg, arched back

**Primary Muscle Groups:** Hips, shoulders, wrists

# Standing Quad Stretch

The Standing Quad Stretch is another great single leg posture for beginners. Begin in Statue pose then lift your right leg, bend your knee and reach your right arm behind you to grab your ankle. Squeeze your knees together and bring your heel all the way to your backside, keeping your back straight. You may hold onto an object for support or keep a slight bend in your standing leg if you need to.

**Inhale:** Lengthen your spine and tighten your glutes

**Exhale:** Squeeze your heel toward your backside

**Common Mistakes:** Knee flaring out to the side, creasing at the hips

**Primary Muscle Groups:** Quads, hip flexors

**Calisthenics Counterpart:** Shrimp Squat

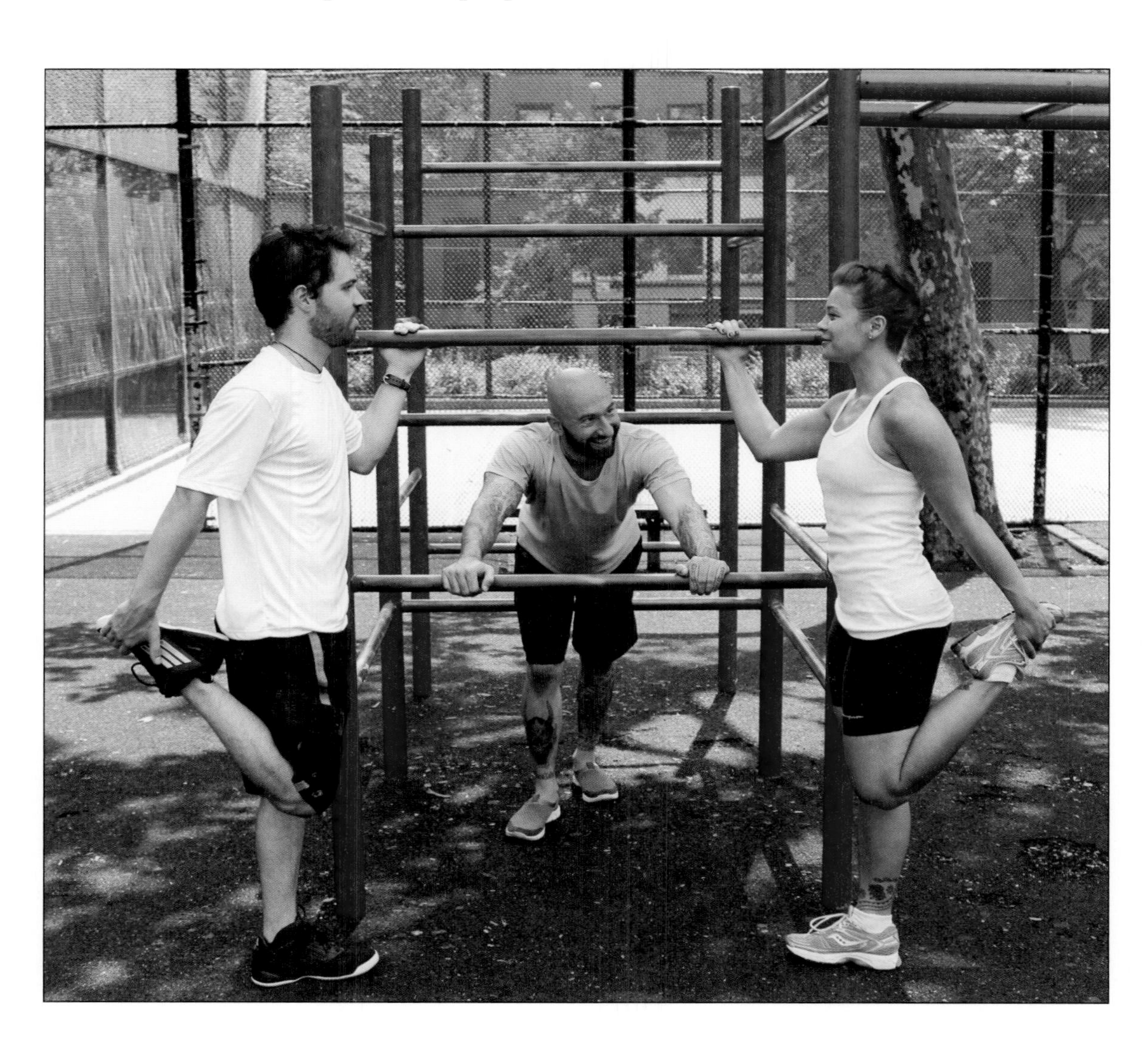

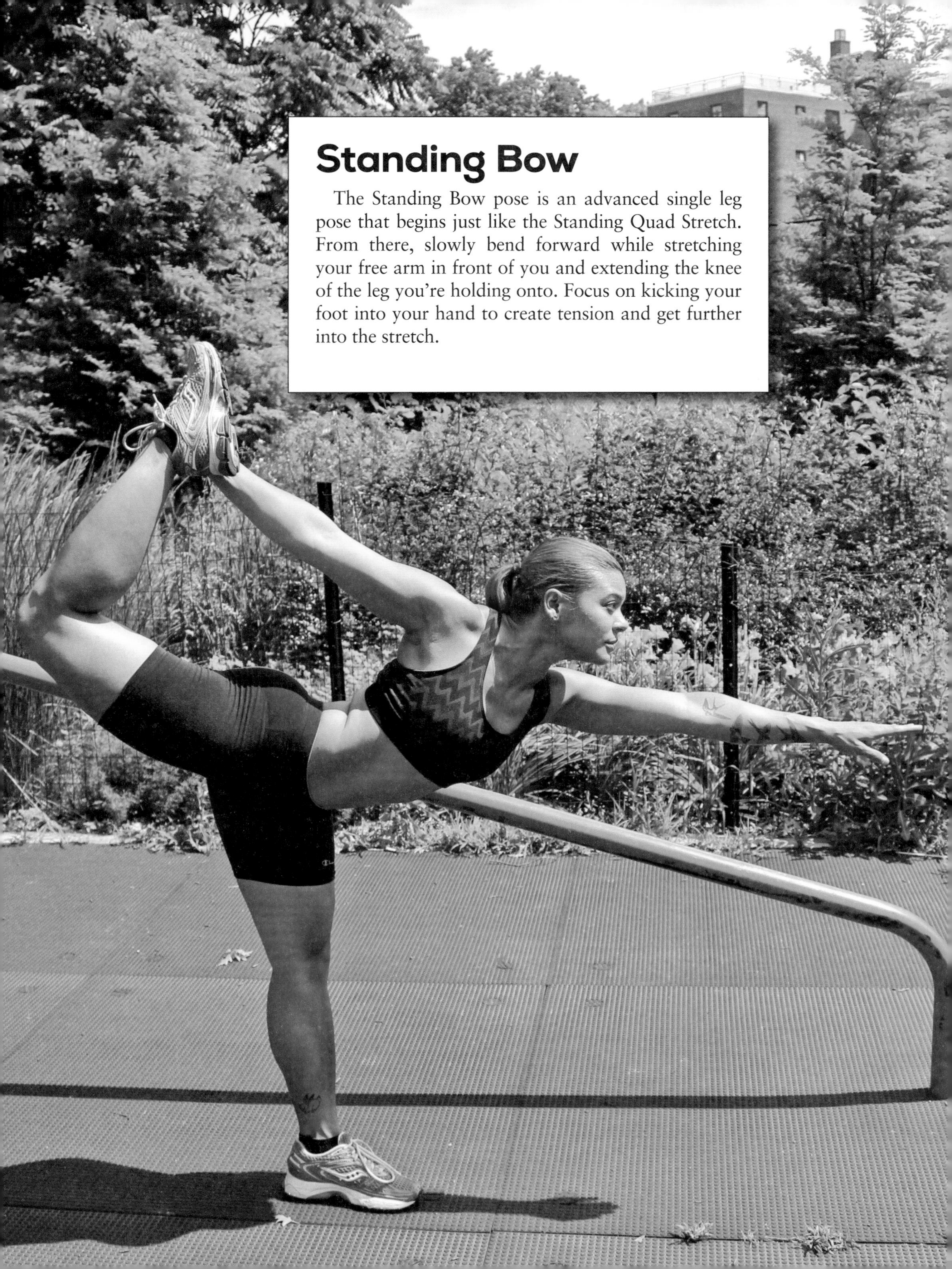

## Standing Bow

The Standing Bow pose is an advanced single leg pose that begins just like the Standing Quad Stretch. From there, slowly bend forward while stretching your free arm in front of you and extending the knee of the leg you're holding onto. Focus on kicking your foot into your hand to create tension and get further into the stretch.

Just like the Standing Quad Stretch, feel free to begin with a wall or other object for support, eventually working toward performing the move freestanding. As this is an advanced pose, it may take years of practice to achieve in it's fullest expression.

**Inhale:** Lift your chest and reach your front arm forward

**Exhale:** Lean forward and kick your back leg into your hand

**Common Mistakes:** Rotating the hips sideways

**Primary Muscle Groups:** Hip flexors, quads, chest and shoulders

**Calisthenics Counterpart:** Shrimp Squat

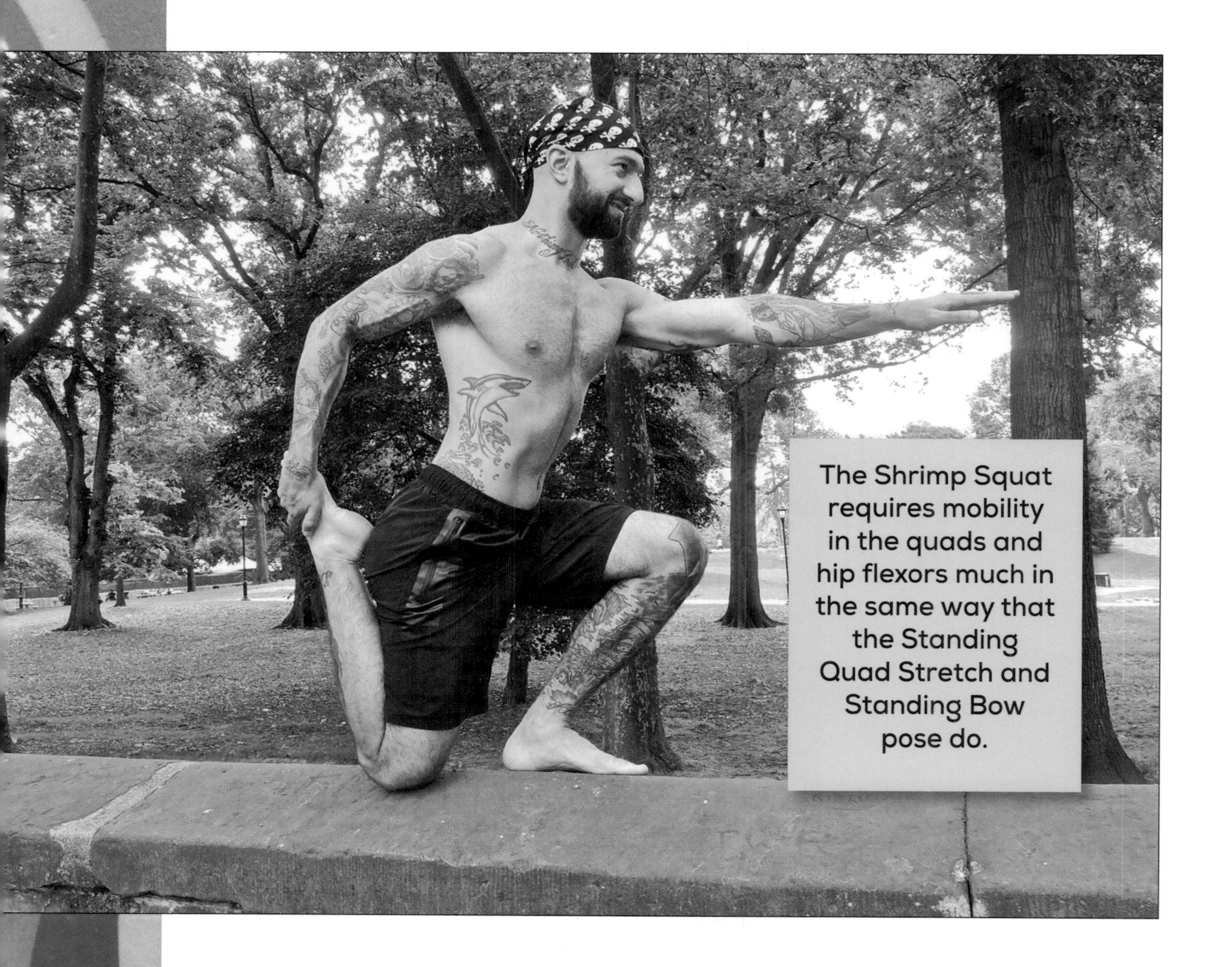

The Shrimp Squat requires mobility in the quads and hip flexors much in the same way that the Standing Quad Stretch and Standing Bow pose do.

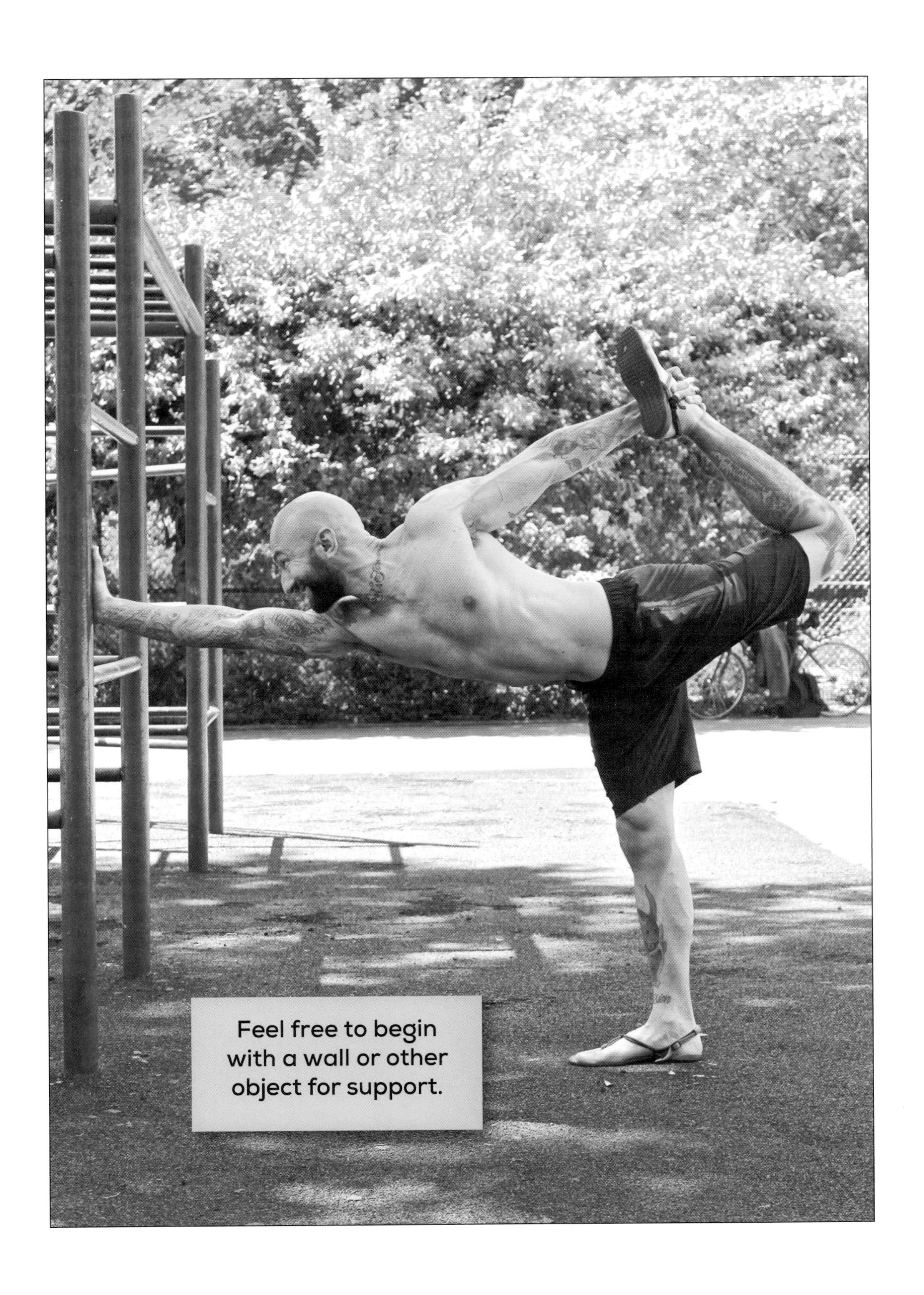

Feel free to begin with a wall or other object for support.

# Bound Eagle

The Bound Eagle pose involves wrapping your arms and legs around each other to stretch the shoulders and hips. Start in Statue pose and reach one arm under the other, criss-crossing at the elbows in front of your chest. Try to bend your arms far enough back to get your palms against one another. The bottom of one palm should line up with the top of the other. Now bend your knees and cross your legs in the same fashion, wrapping your foot behind your opposite ankle, if possible. Make sure to switch arms and legs during alternating efforts in order to get both sides of your body evenly.

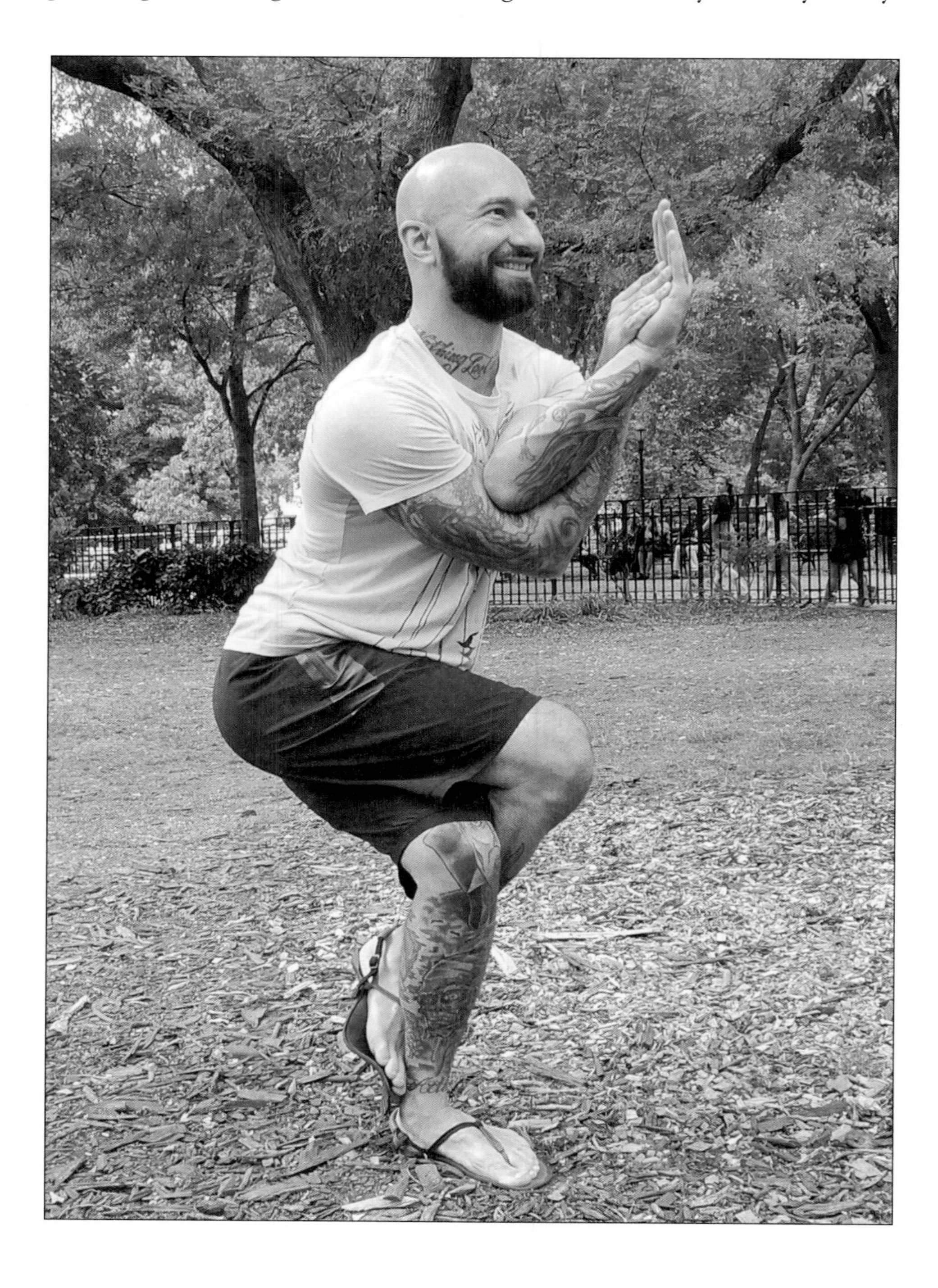

**Inhale:** Lengthen your back and breathe into your belly

**Exhale:** Constrict your arms and legs, wrapping yourself up tightly

**Common Mistakes:** Hunched back, shrugged shoulders, excessive knee torque

**Primary Muscle Groups:** Rear delts, rotator cuff, hips

**Calisthenics Counterpart:** Elbow Lever

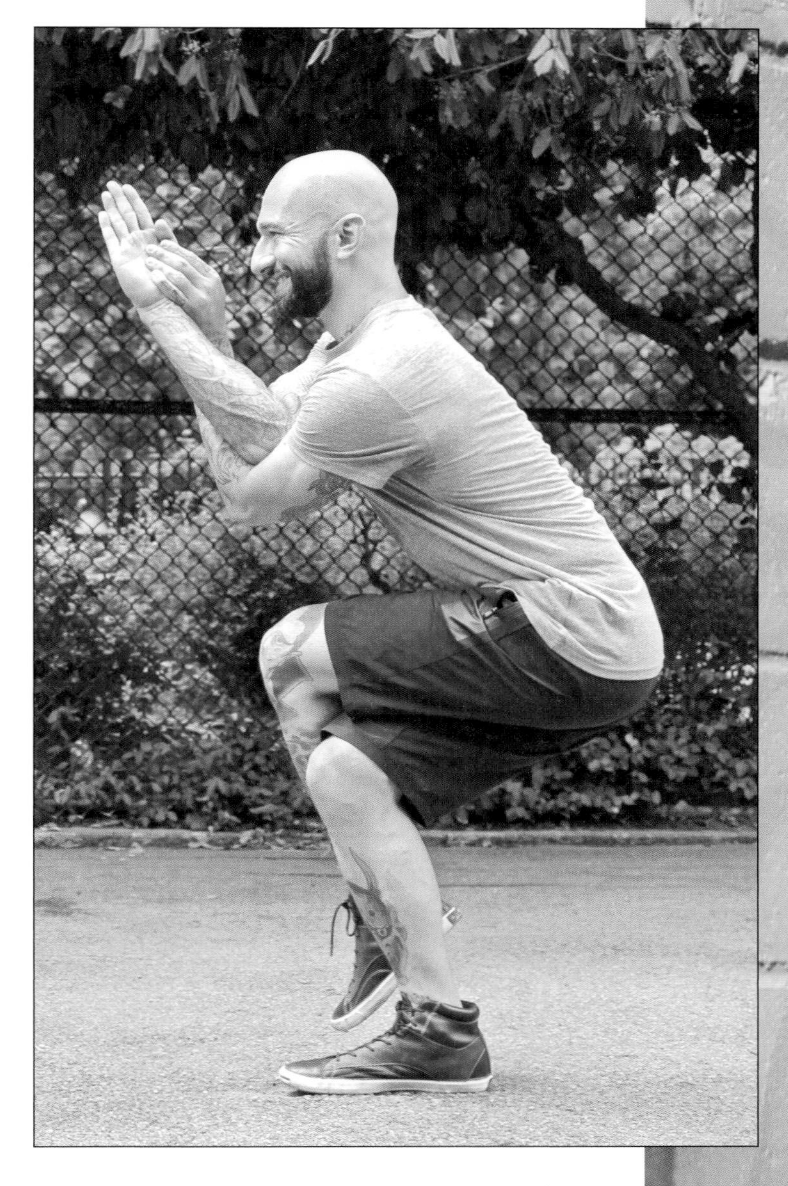

The ability to rotate the elbow far enough inside the hip is often a limiting factor for learning the Elbow Lever. The Bound Eagle pose can be very helpful for facilitating a greater range of motion in this area.

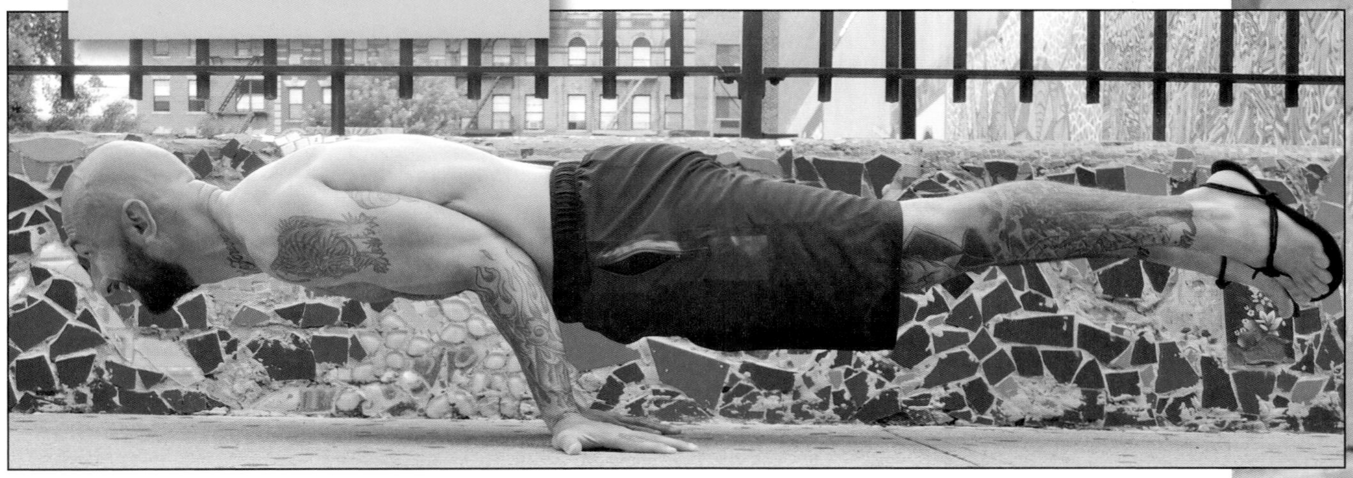

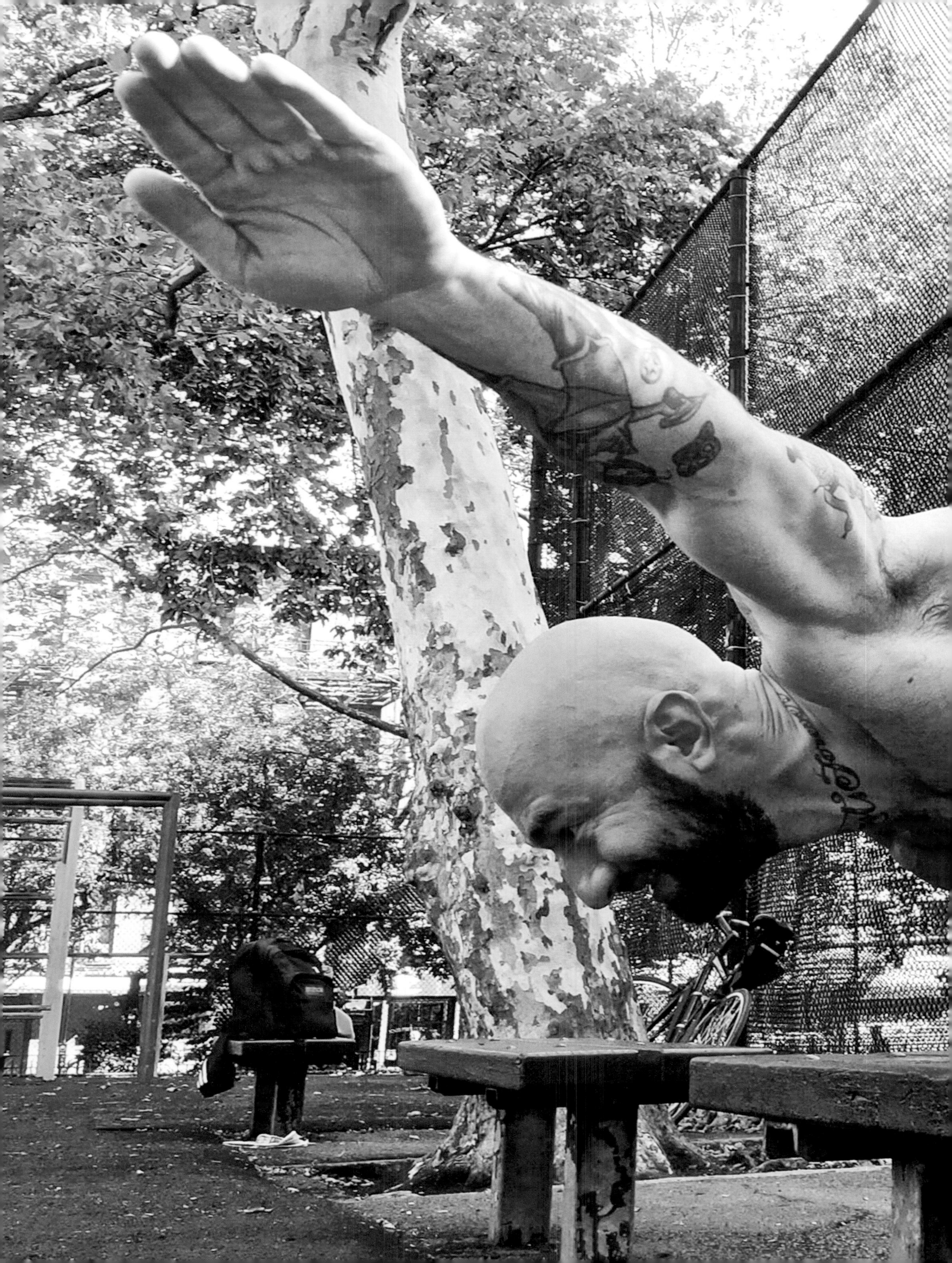

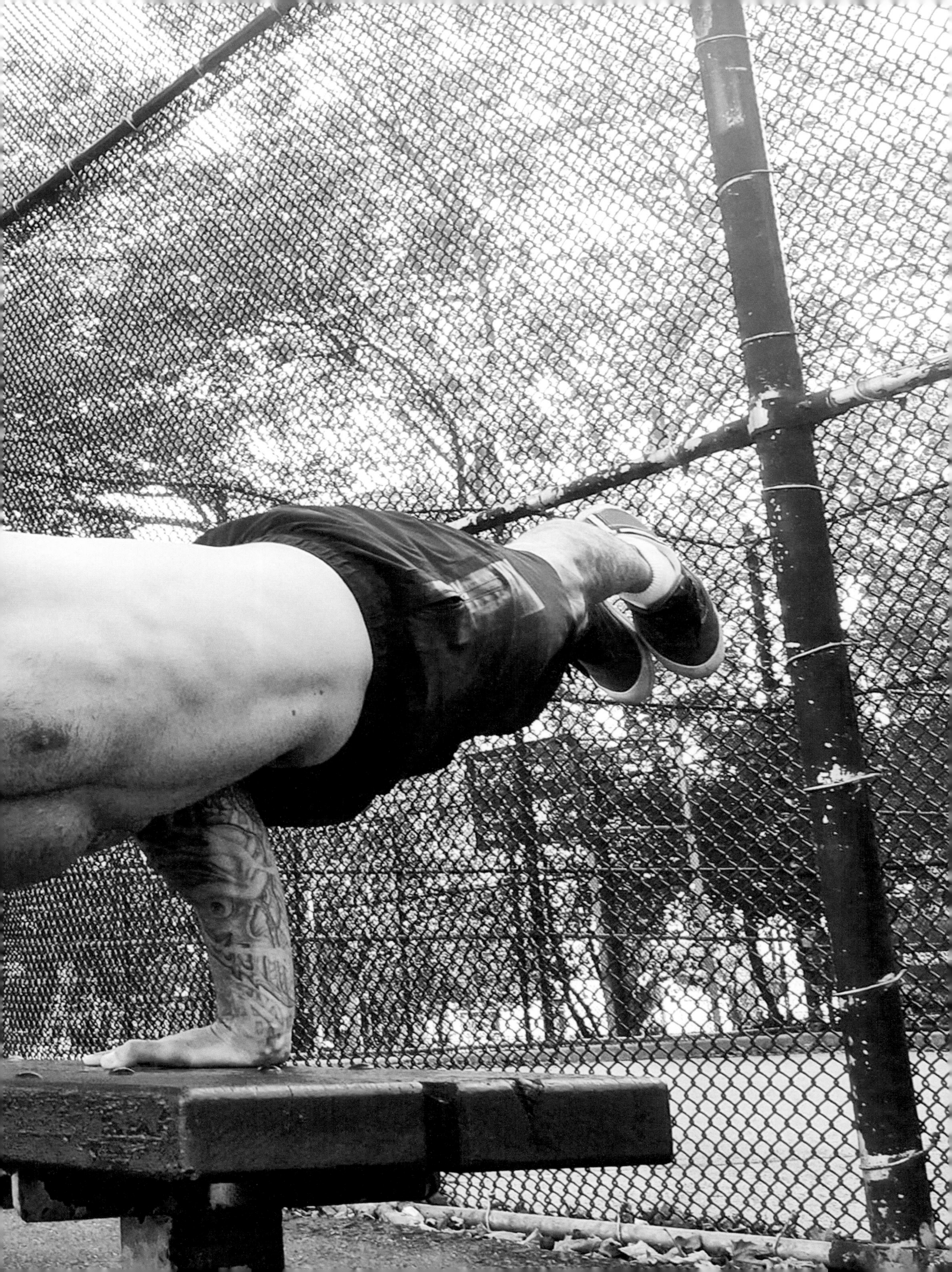

# Drinking Bird

Also known as Warrior Three, the Drinking Bird is another challenging single-leg posture. From Statue pose, reach your arms straight up in the air over your shoulders. Lift one foot off the floor and slowly tip forward on your standing leg by bending from your hip. The idea is to reach your back leg all the way behind you with your back flat and arms extended straight overhead. Be careful to avoid rotating to the side on the way down. The position resembles that of a drinking bird toy. Slowly return to Statue pose and repeat on the other side. Beginners may find it helpful to hold onto an object for balance and/or maintain a slight bend in the standing leg.

**Inhale:** Reach your arms up and lengthen your spine.

**Exhale:** Hinge deeper into your hips, reach your free leg all the way back and press into the ground with your standing leg

**Common Mistakes:** Externally rotating at the hip (twisting to the side)

**Primary Muscle Groups:** Hamstrings, calves

**Calisthenics Counterpart:** Single Leg Deadlift

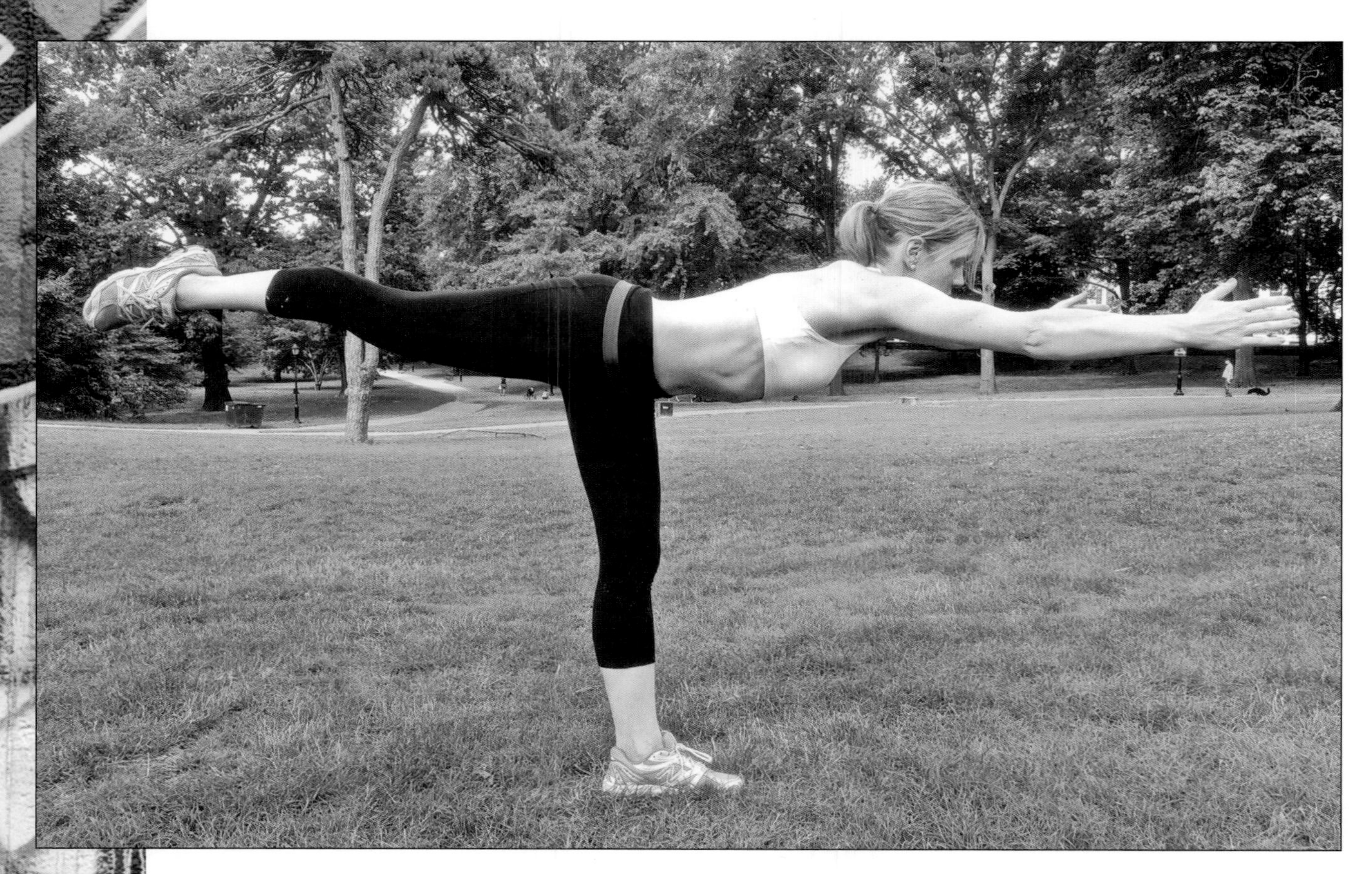

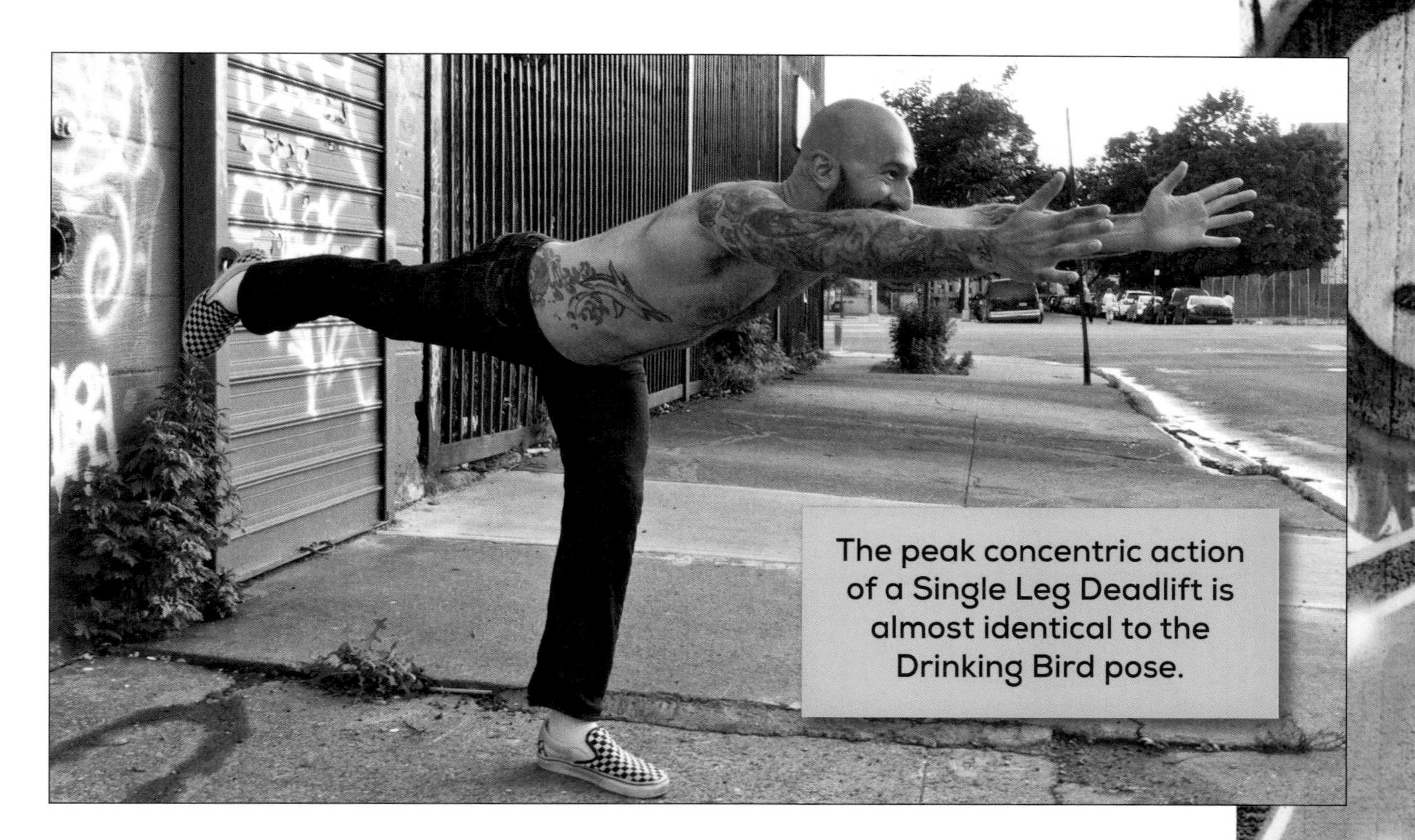

The peak concentric action of a Single Leg Deadlift is almost identical to the Drinking Bird pose.

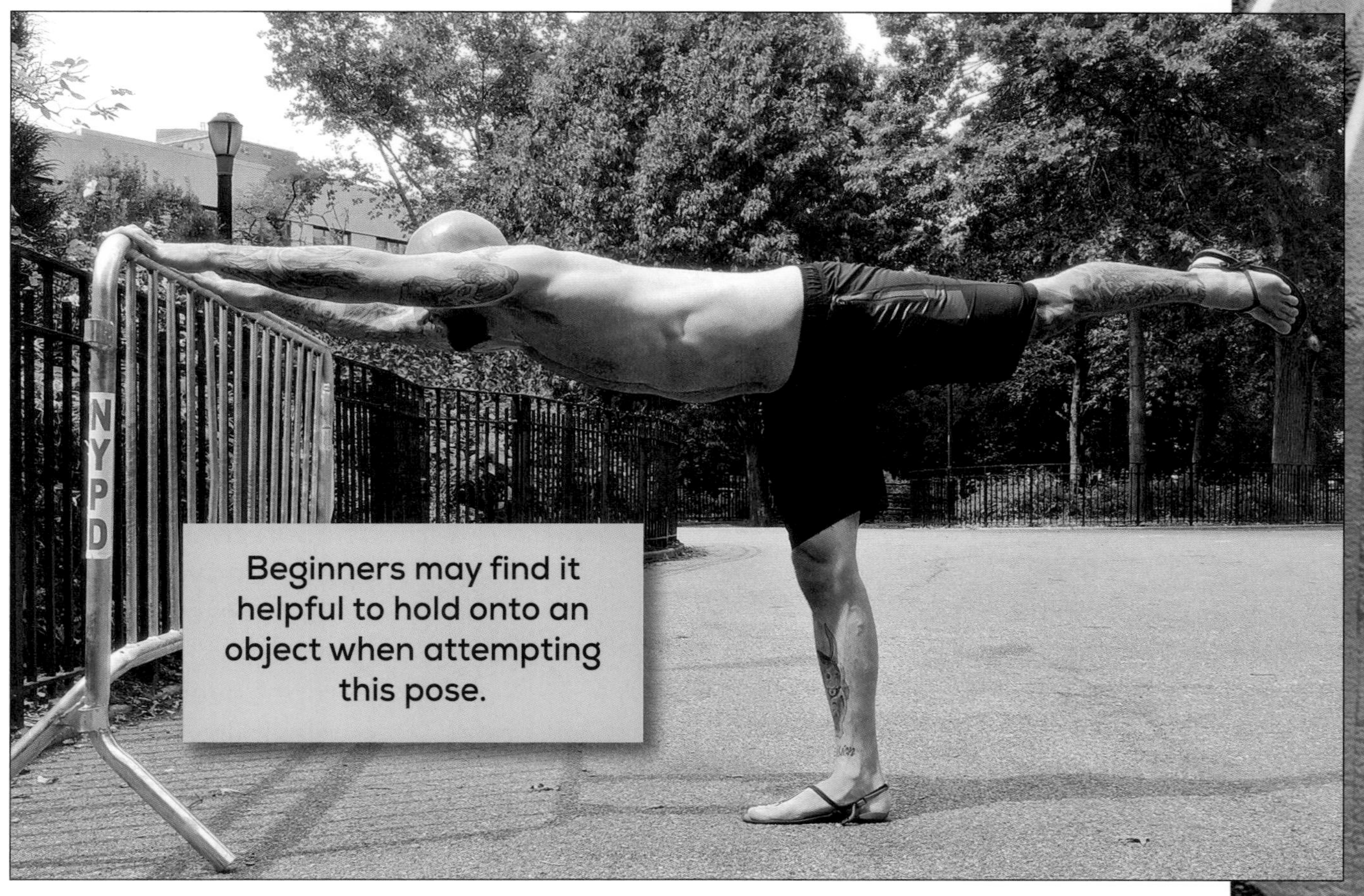


Beginners may find it helpful to hold onto an object when attempting this pose.

# Standing Single Leg Foot Hold

The Standing Single Leg Foot Hold can be a balance challenge as well as a great stretch. Begin in Statue pose and lift one foot off the floor, bringing your knee as high as you can toward your chest. Slowly reach over and grab beneath your foot with both hands. Your fingers should be interlaced. Keep your standing leg locked with your trunk as upright as possible.

**Inhale:** Lengthen your spine and drop your shoulder blades

**Exhale:** Squeeze your standing leg and press your heel into the floor

**Common Mistakes:** Bending the standing leg

**Primary Muscle Groups:** Hamstrings, hip flexors

**Calisthenics Counterpart:** Half Tuck Front Lever

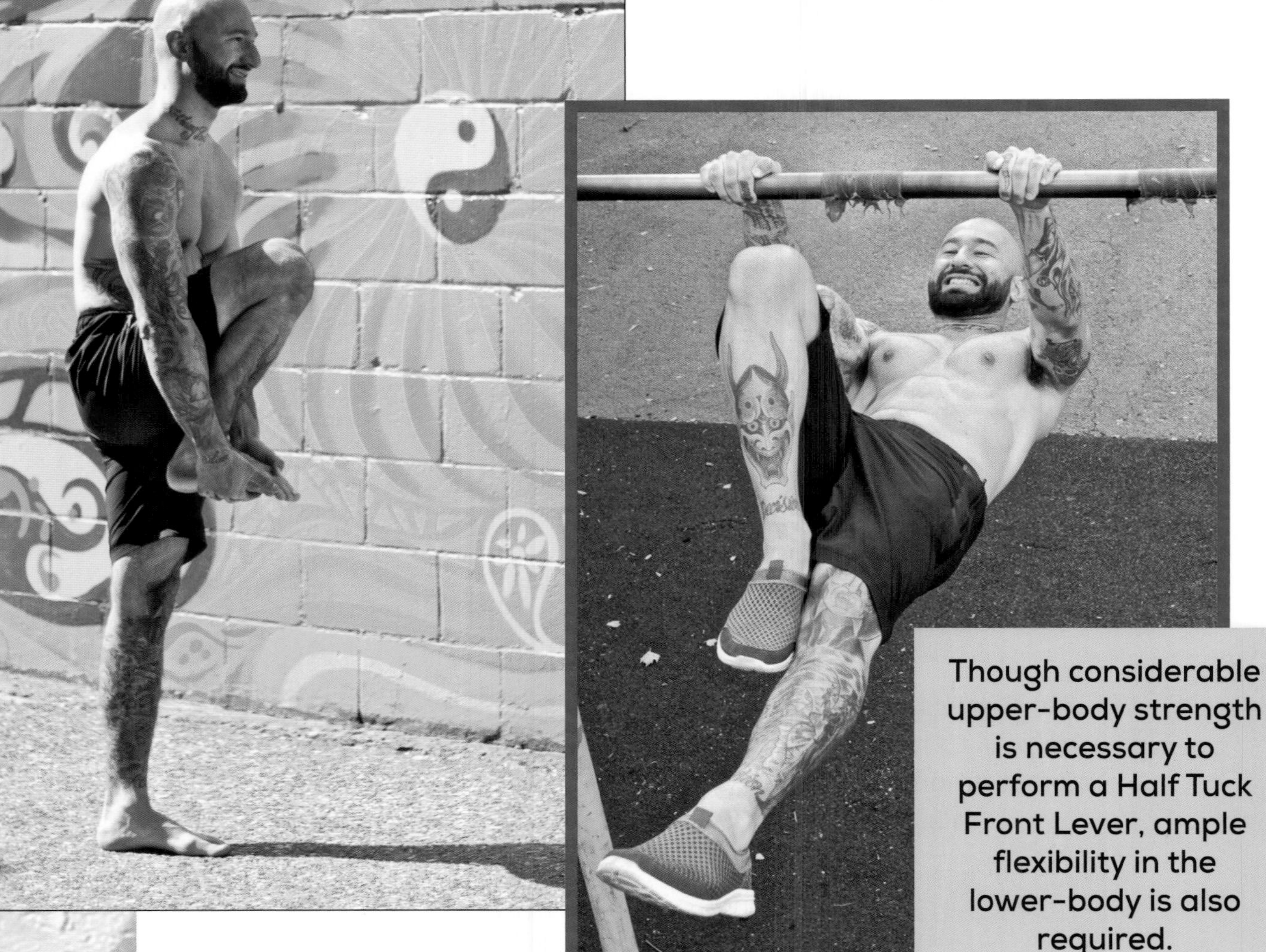

Though considerable upper-body strength is necessary to perform a Half Tuck Front Lever, ample flexibility in the lower-body is also required.

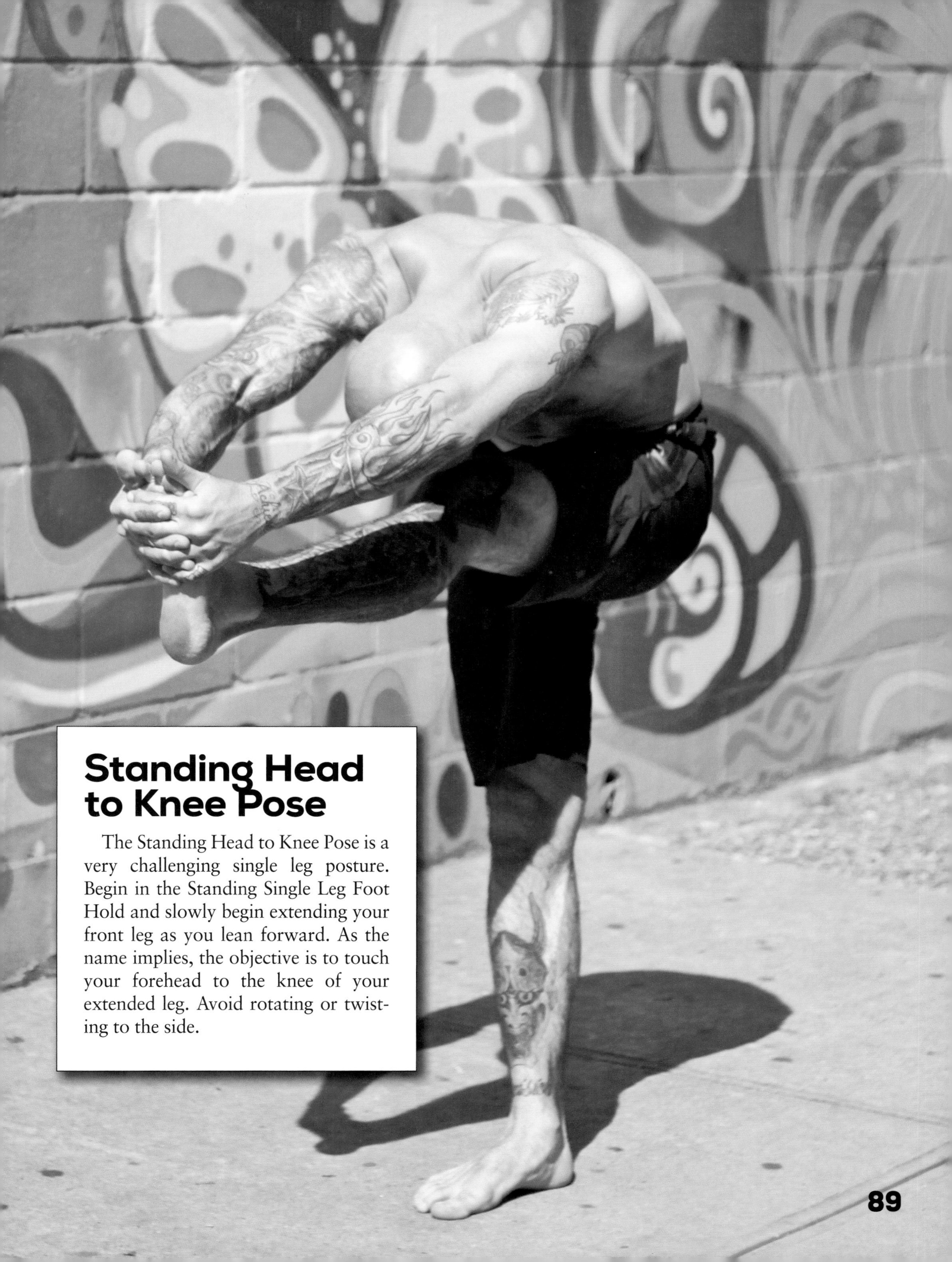

## Standing Head to Knee Pose

The Standing Head to Knee Pose is a very challenging single leg posture. Begin in the Standing Single Leg Foot Hold and slowly begin extending your front leg as you lean forward. As the name implies, the objective is to touch your forehead to the knee of your extended leg. Avoid rotating or twisting to the side.

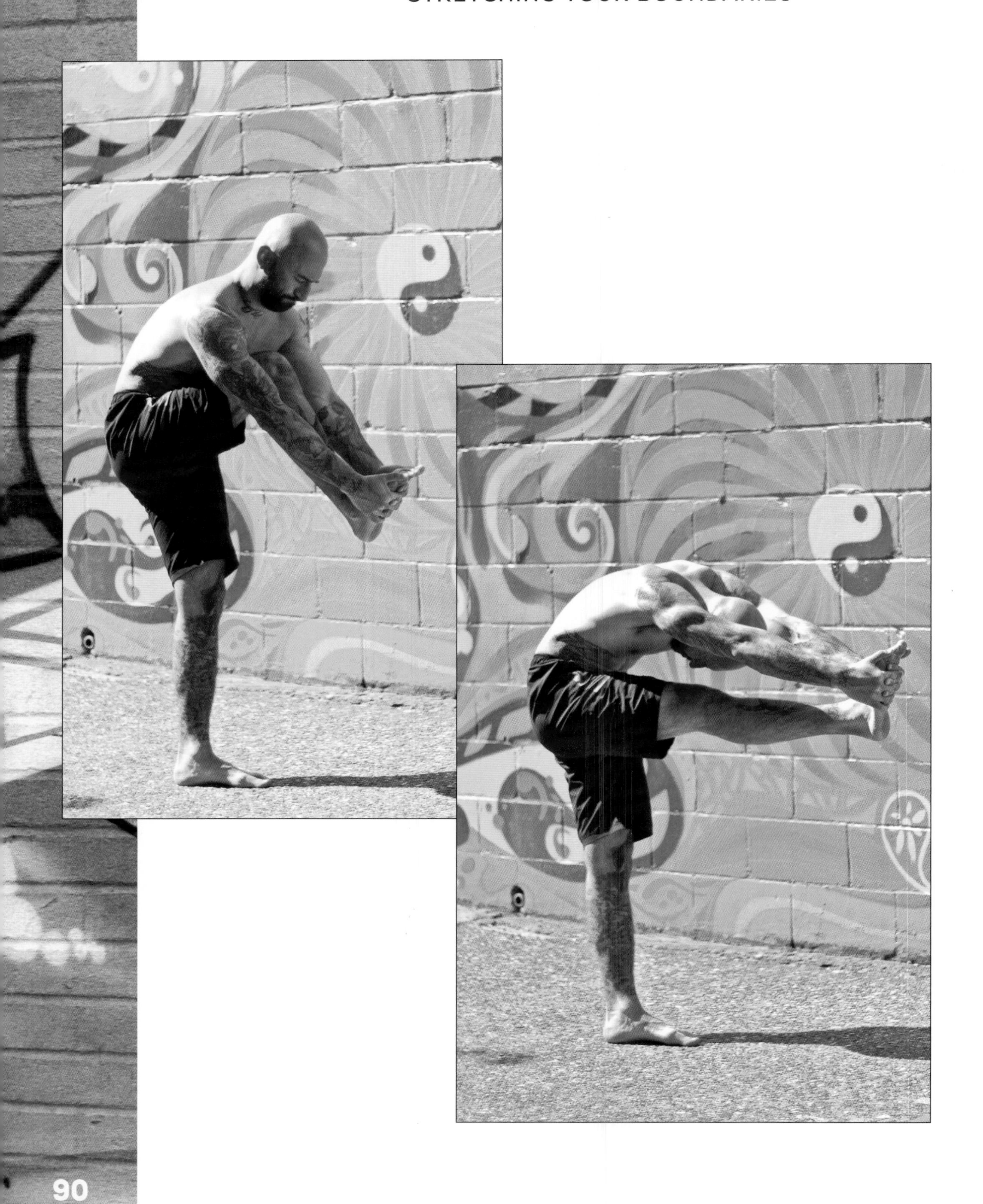

**Inhale:** Press your foot into the palms of your hands while creating tension through your arms

**Exhale:** Lean forward from your hips, aiming your head for your knee

**Common Mistakes:** Overextending the hamstrings by attempting to straighten the leg too quickly

**Primary Muscle Groups:** Hamstrings, calves, lower back

**Calisthenics Counterpart:** Pistol Squat

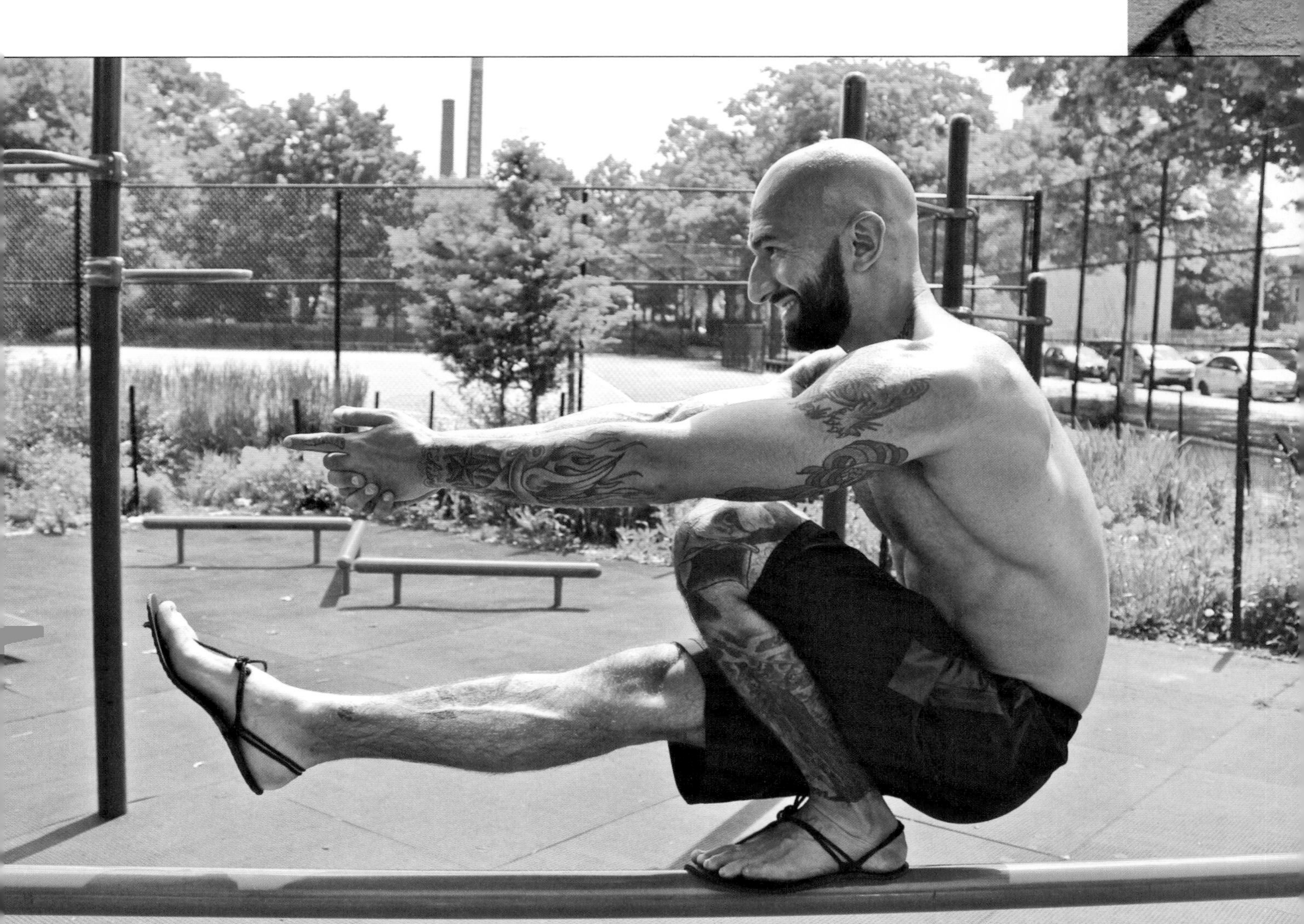

Practicing the Standing Head to Knee Pose helps your ability to hold one leg extended straight in front of your body while balancing on the other as you would in a Pistol Squat.

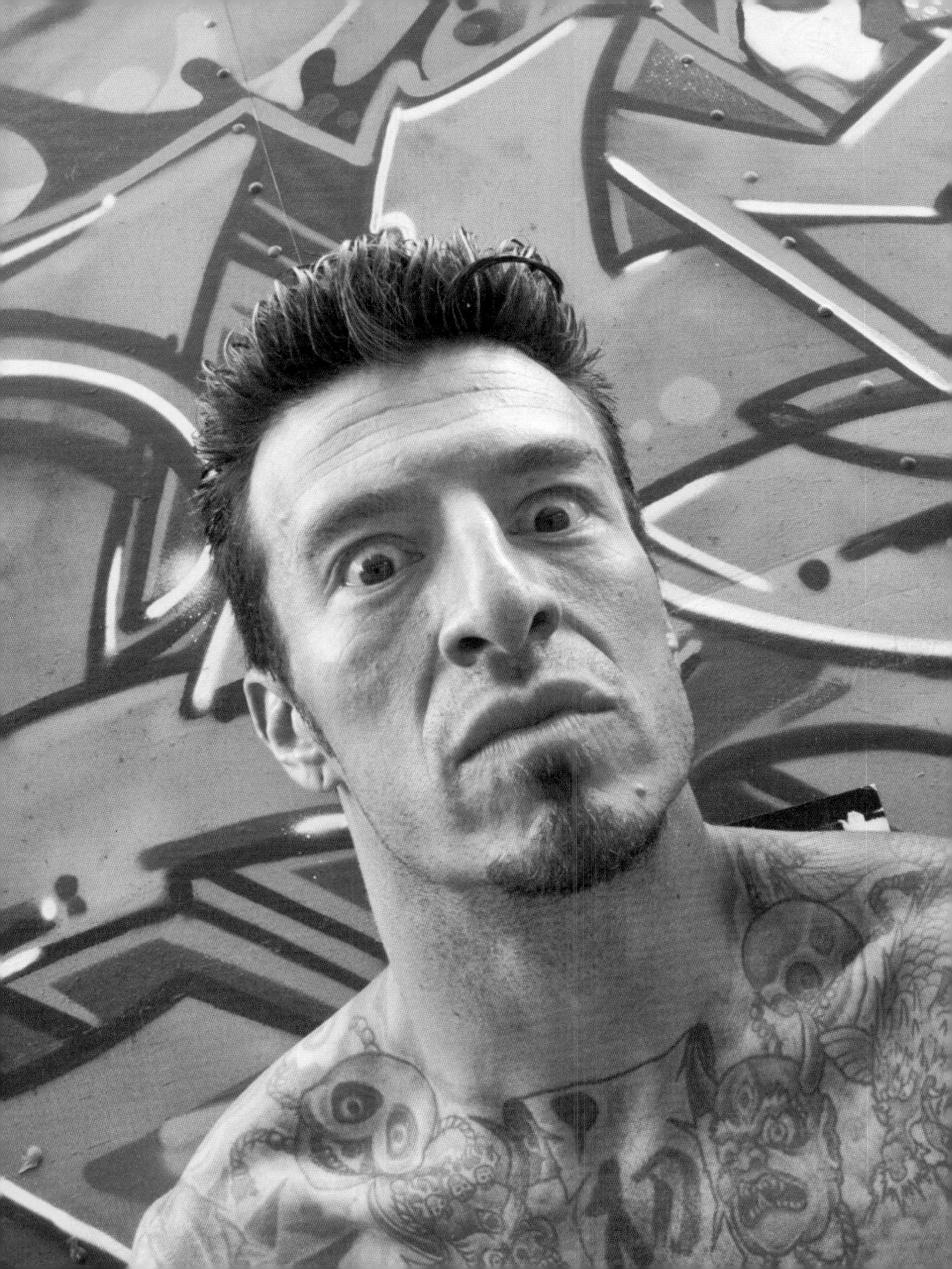

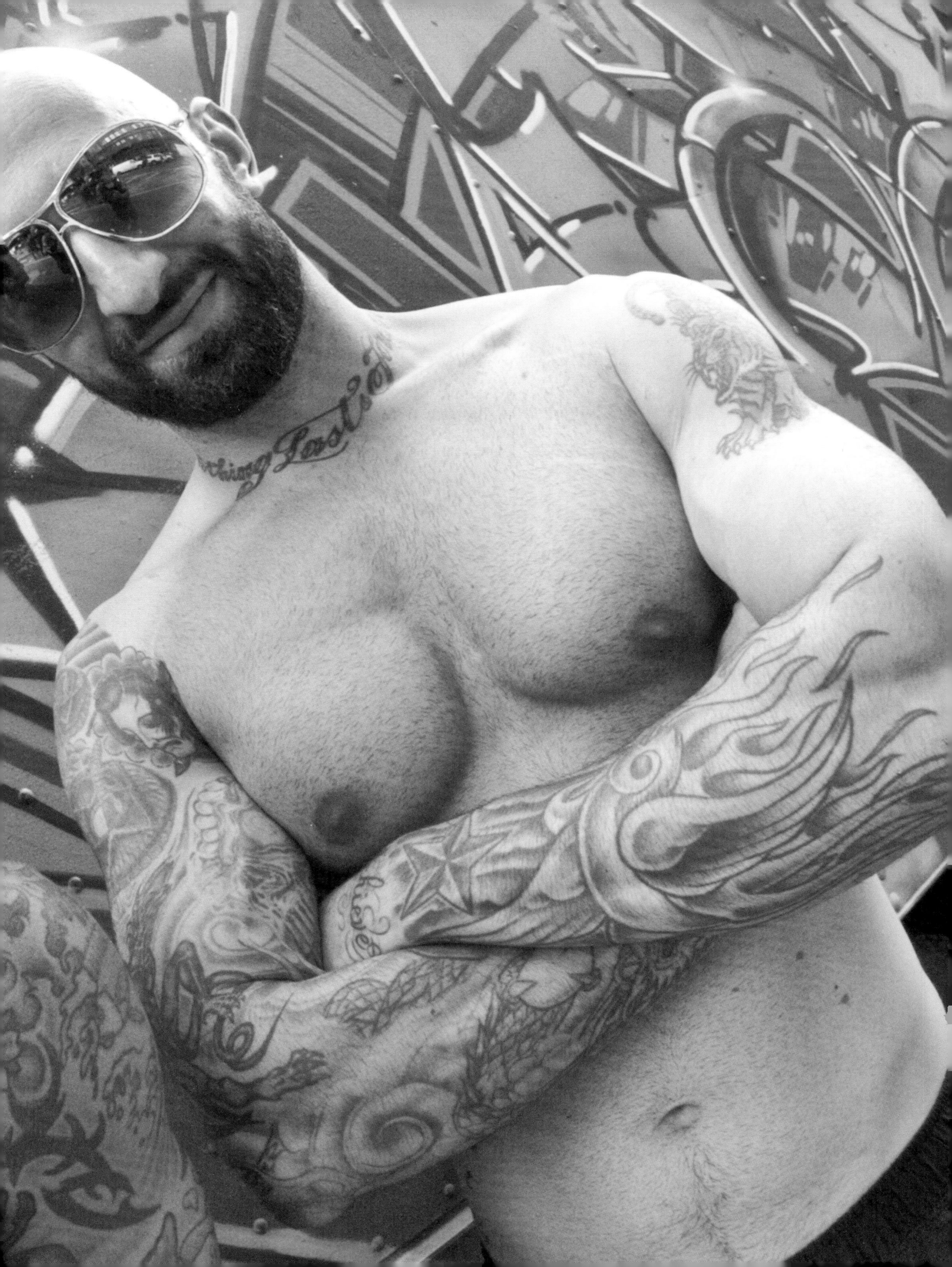

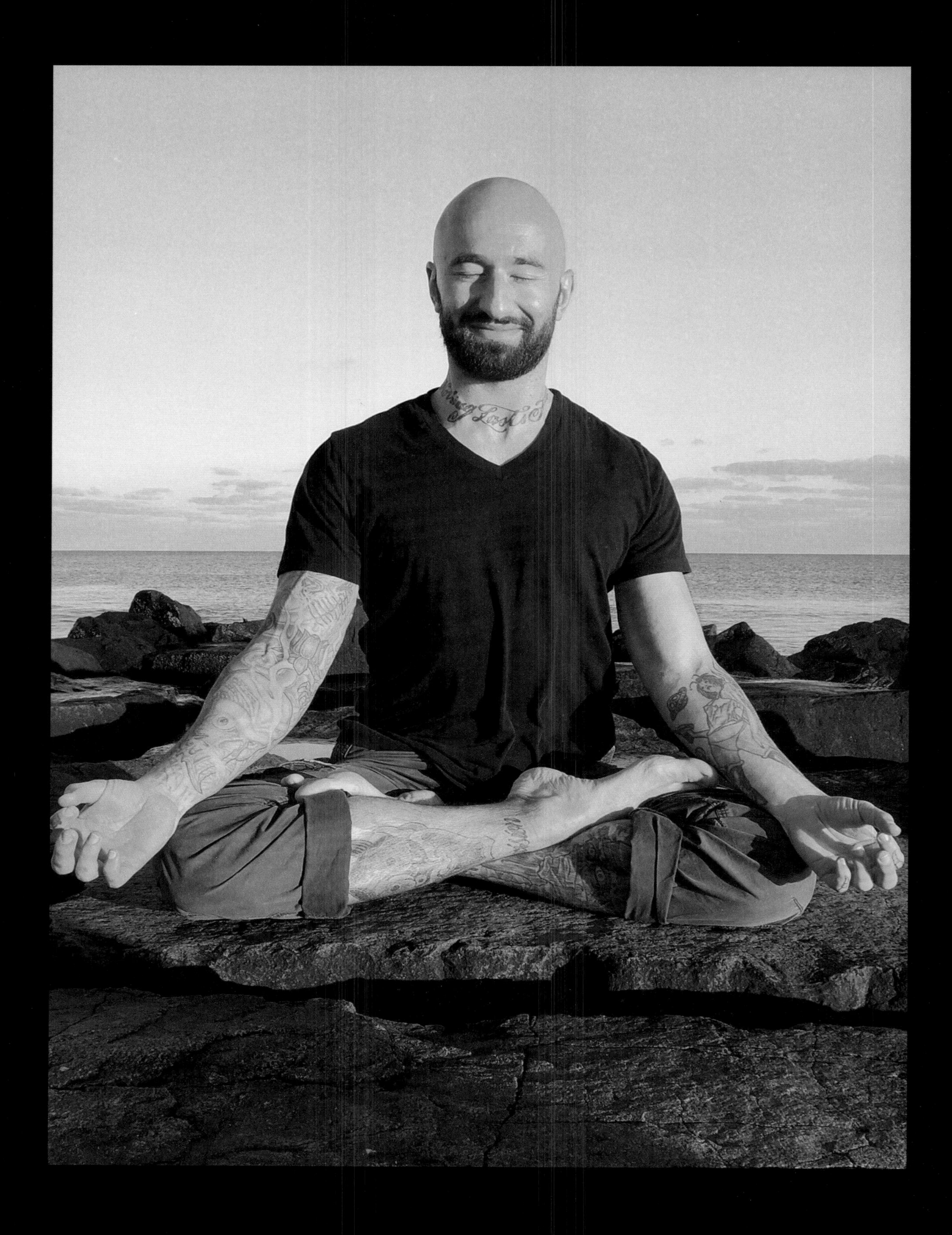

# GROUNDED STATICS

This final grouping of stretches is made up of static postures that involve squatting, kneeling, sitting and lying down. Many of these poses share similarities to certain standing poses presented in the last section. Though you will find some of these exercises less demanding than those in the previous sections, they may challenge you in their own unique ways. I again implore you to experiment with these various postures firsthand, being mindful to respect your body's current capabilities. Stay focused, train hard and have fun!

## Deep Squat Hold

Holding the bottom position of a Squat as a stretch can help increase your active range of motion when performing Squats in your strength workouts. Start by squatting down as low as you can with your feet flat on the floor. Keep your back as straight as possible, focusing on bending from your hips instead of your spine. From here, slowly slide your elbows inside of your knees and bring your palms together into a prayer position. Use your elbows for leverage against your inner thighs to get deeper into the stretch. Be careful to keep your knees in alignment with your toes.

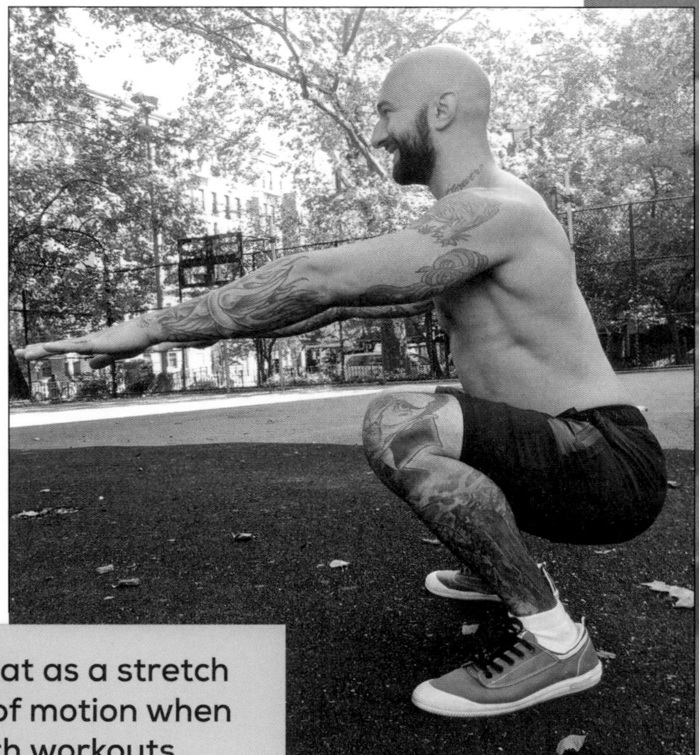

**Holding the bottom position of a Squat as a stretch can help increase your active range of motion when performing squats in your strength workouts.**

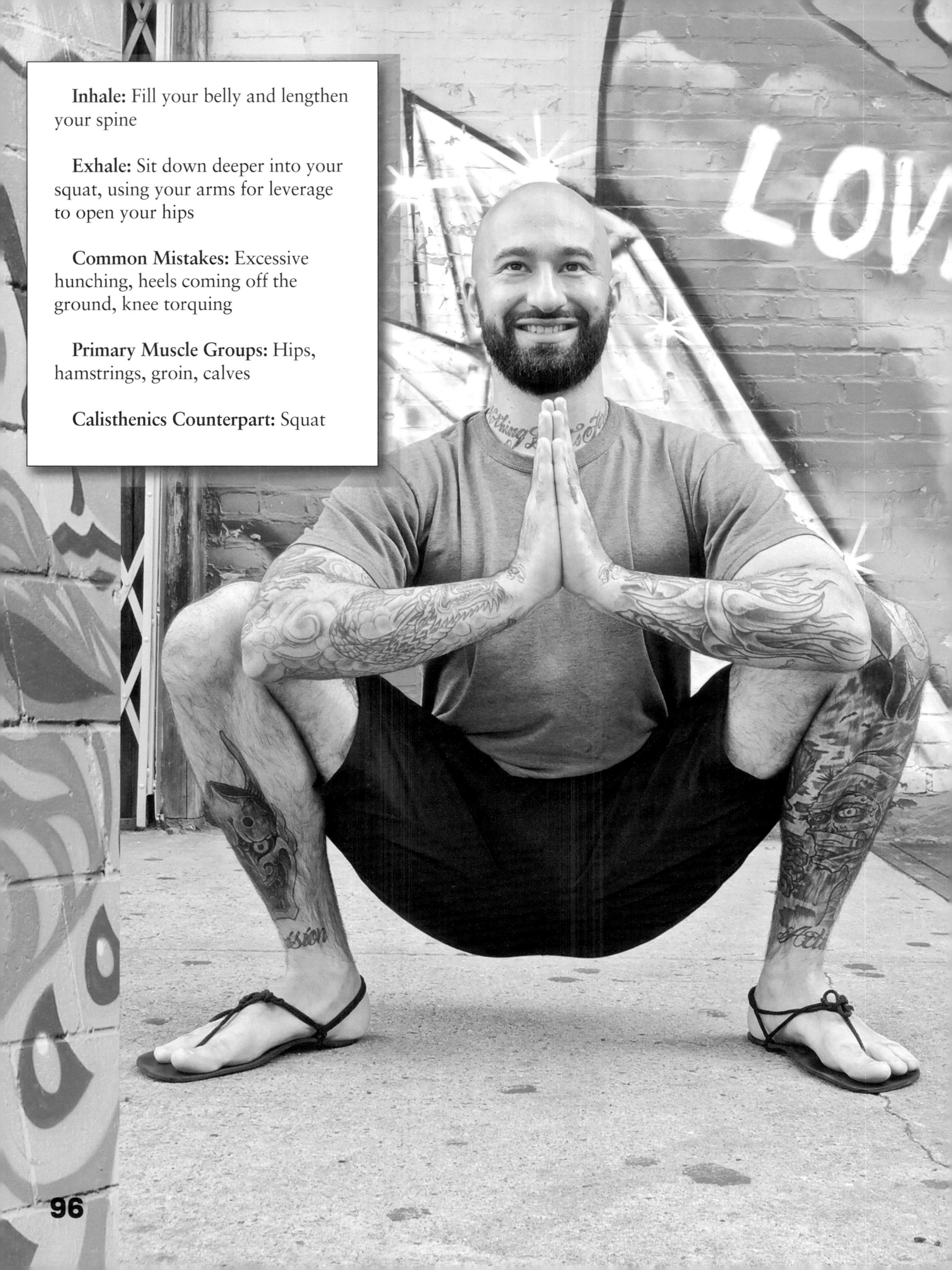

**Inhale:** Fill your belly and lengthen your spine

**Exhale:** Sit down deeper into your squat, using your arms for leverage to open your hips

**Common Mistakes:** Excessive hunching, heels coming off the ground, knee torquing

**Primary Muscle Groups:** Hips, hamstrings, groin, calves

**Calisthenics Counterpart:** Squat

# Deep Squat with Internal Shoulder Rotation

The Deep Squat with Internal Shoulder Rotation is a great combination stretch for your upper and lower body. Begin in a Deep Squat Hold and reach your left hand behind you, like you were reaching for your left back pocket. The back of your left wrist will rest on the outside of your left hip. Slowly bring your left elbow inside of your left knee, using the leverage of your leg to gently squeeze the elbow closer to your body. Repeat on your right side, doing each arm separately.

**Inhale:** Sit back into your squat and lengthen your spine

**Exhale:** Use your leg to gently squeeze your arm in toward your body

**Common Mistakes:** Overly hunched back, knee torquing

**Primary Muscle Groups:** Rear delts, hips, hamstrings

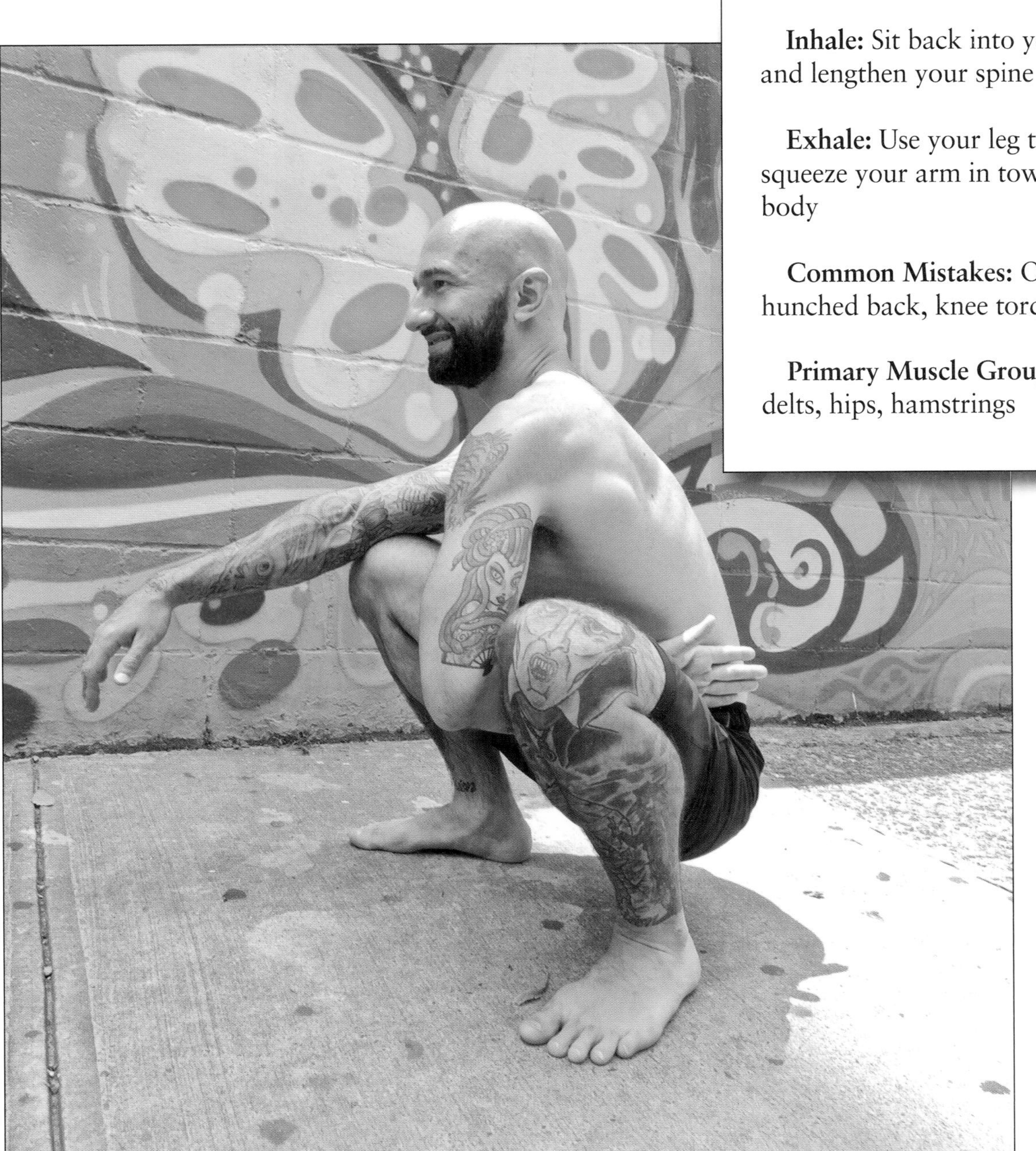

# Noose

The Noose pose takes the Deep Squat With Internal Shoulder Rotation a bit farther while adding a degree of trunk rotation to the picture. From the previous position, release your hand from behind your hip, instead reaching it around your shin and knee. Look over your opposite shoulder and begin twisting your trunk while bringing your free arm behind your back to bind your hands. As with all binds, you may need to start by holding a cloth in your hands before you will be ready to clasp them together.

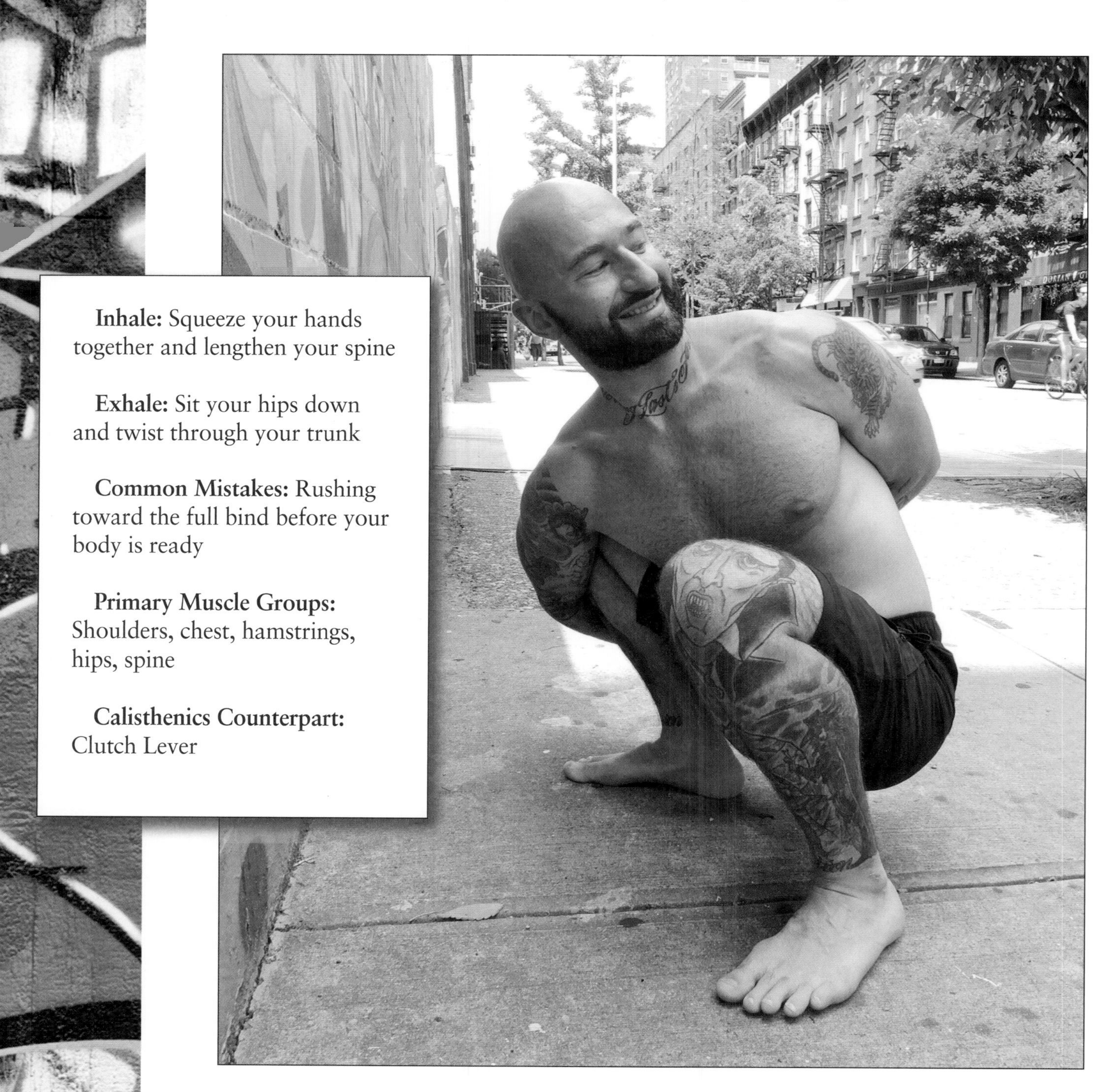

**Inhale:** Squeeze your hands together and lengthen your spine

**Exhale:** Sit your hips down and twist through your trunk

**Common Mistakes:** Rushing toward the full bind before your body is ready

**Primary Muscle Groups:** Shoulders, chest, hamstrings, hips, spine

**Calisthenics Counterpart:** Clutch Lever

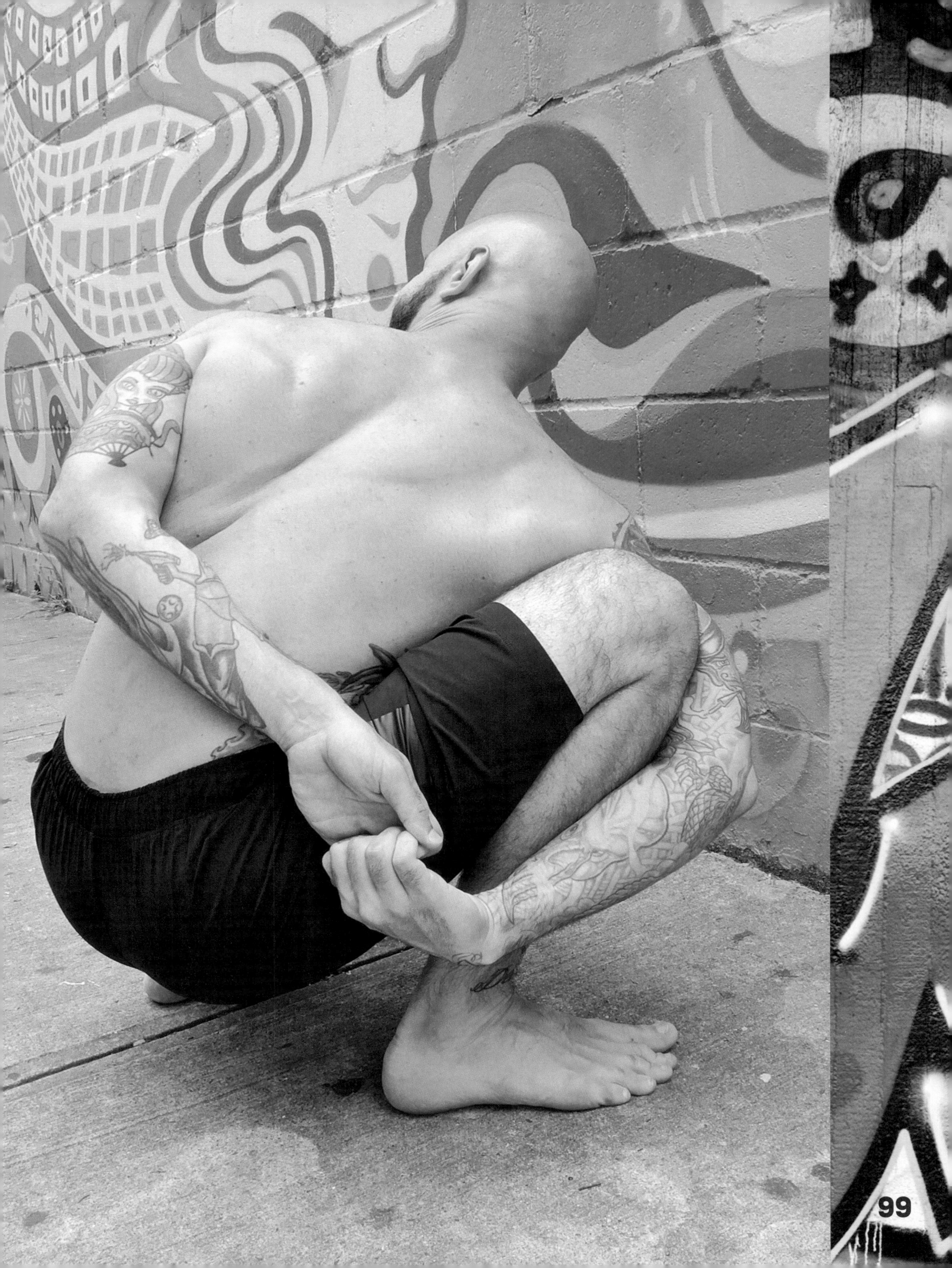

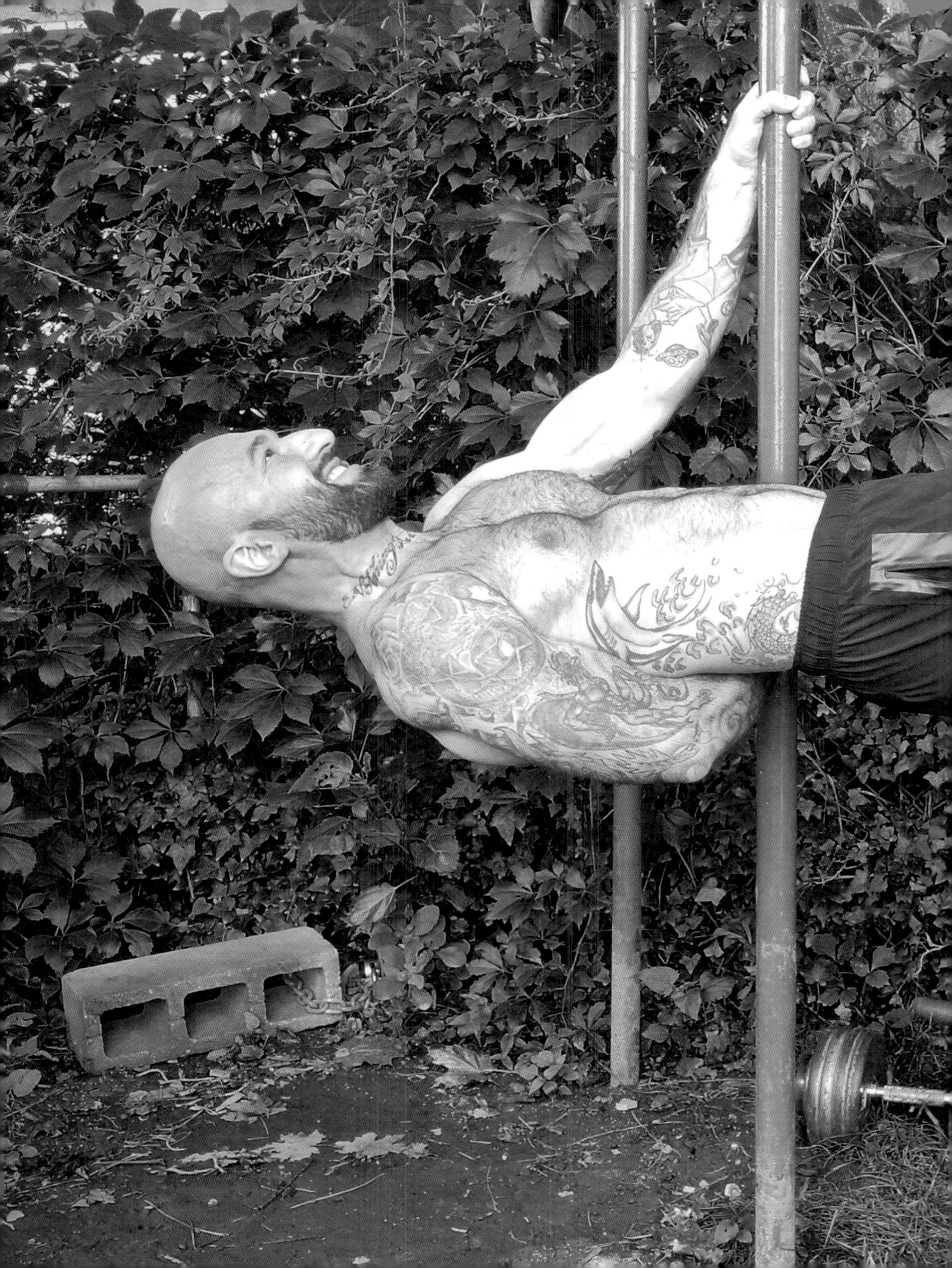

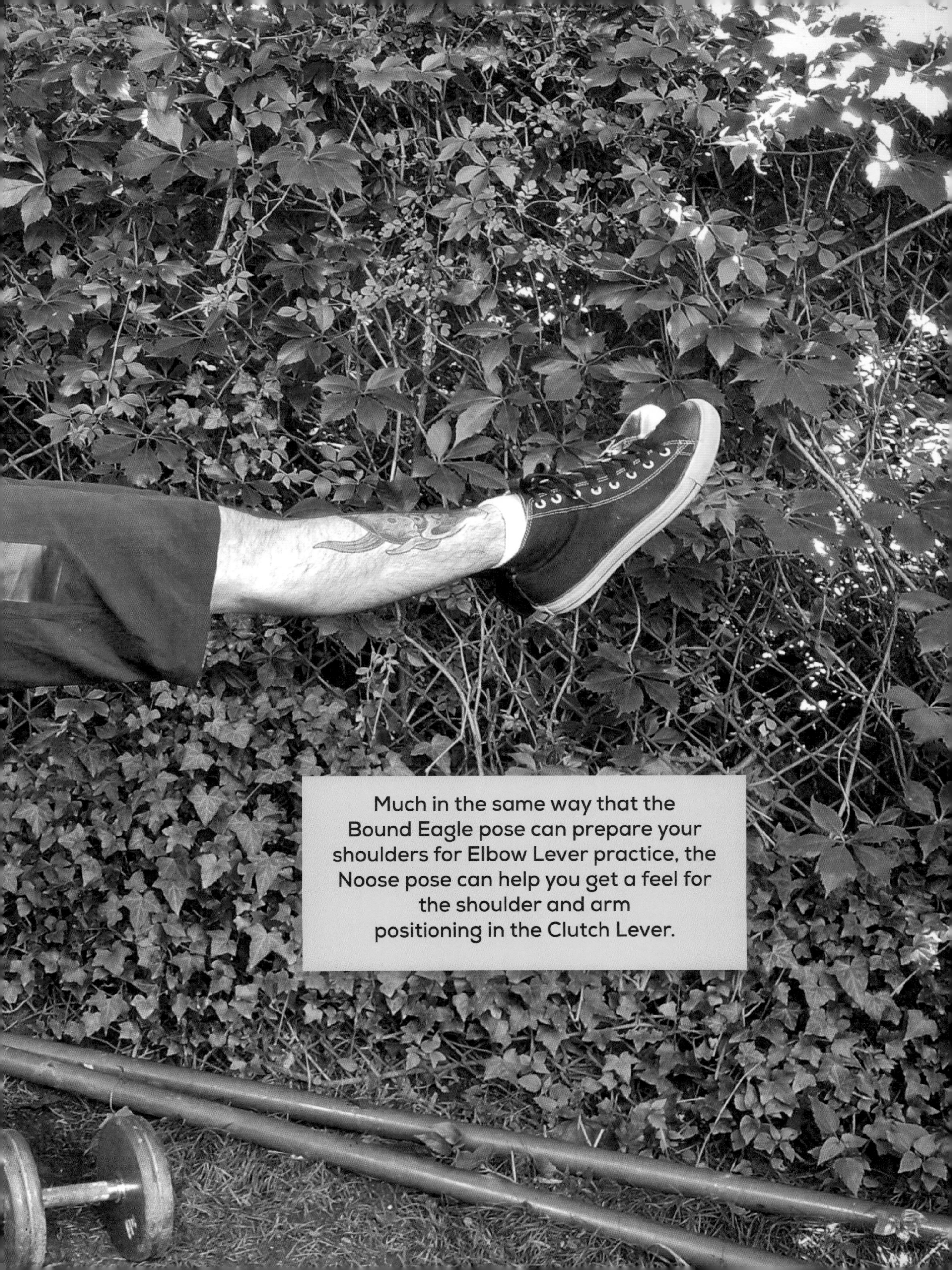

Much in the same way that the Bound Eagle pose can prepare your shoulders for Elbow Lever practice, the Noose pose can help you get a feel for the shoulder and arm positioning in the Clutch Lever.

# Downward Dog

Downward Dog is a great pose for building flexibility in the entire posterior chain. Begin on your hands and knees with your toes curled under your heels. Slowly lift your hips into the air while pressing your chest toward your thighs. Try to keep your back and arms as straight as possible while pressing your hands into the ground and reaching your hips into the air. Point your elbows toward your knees with your heels flat on the floor. Try to keep both your arms and legs straight. It's okay for beginners to allow the knees to bend and the heels to come off the floor. In time, work toward straightening the legs and pressing the feet flat. People with tight calves may find it helpful to bend one knee while straightening the other, alternating sides.

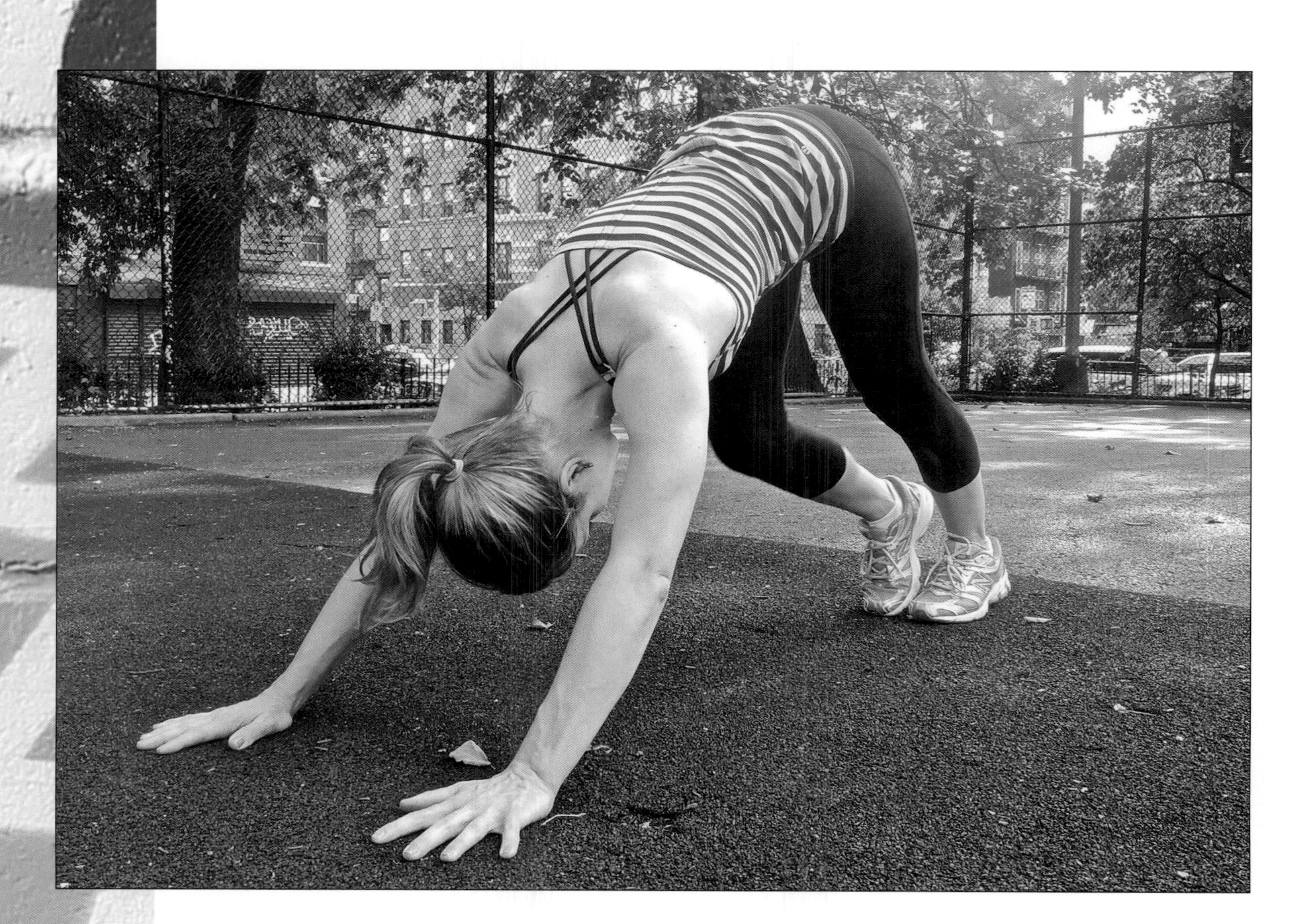

**Inhale:** Reach your hips into the air

**Exhale:** Press your chest toward your thighs

**Common Mistakes:** Overly rounded back, bent elbows

**Primary Muscle Groups:** Hamstrings, calves, shoulders, back

**Calisthenics Counterpart:** Pike Push-up

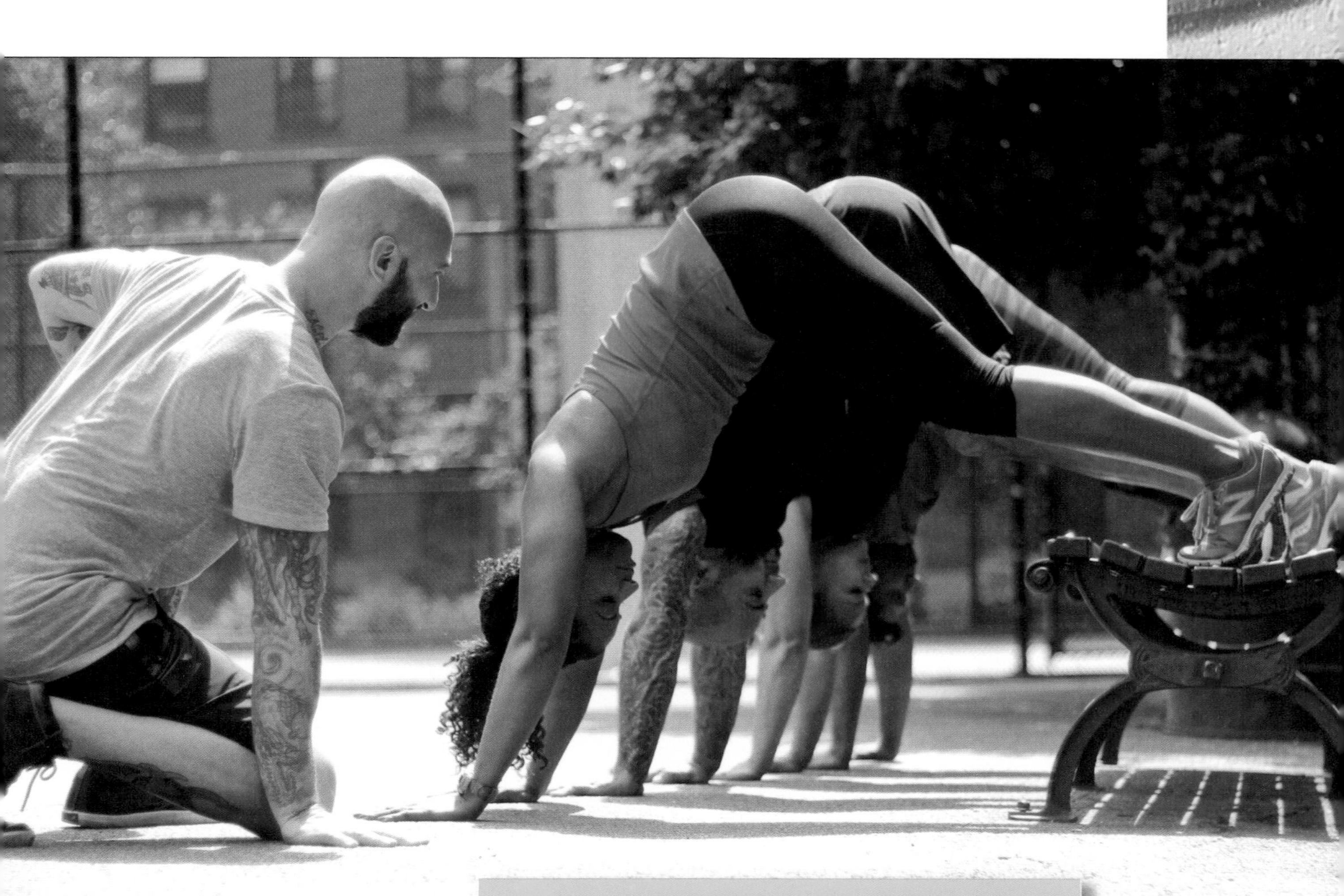

The similarities between the Downward Dog pose and bodyweight Pike Push-ups are easy to see.

# Wall Dog

The Wall Dog is a nice variation on Downward Dog that may be more appropriate for beginners or those who are particularly tight. Stand a few feet from a wall (or other sturdy vertical object) and bend over from your waist, placing your hands on the wall just above hip height, fingers pointed toward the ceiling. Press your chest toward the floor while pushing your hips away from the wall. Try to avoid bending your arms and/or legs while maintaining a flat back position.

**Inhale:** Lengthen your spine and extend your knees

**Exhale:** Press your chest toward the ground

**Common Mistakes:** Excessive rounding of the back, bent elbows

**Primary Muscle Groups:** Upper back, shoulders, hamstrings

**Calisthenics Counterpart:** Pike Push-up

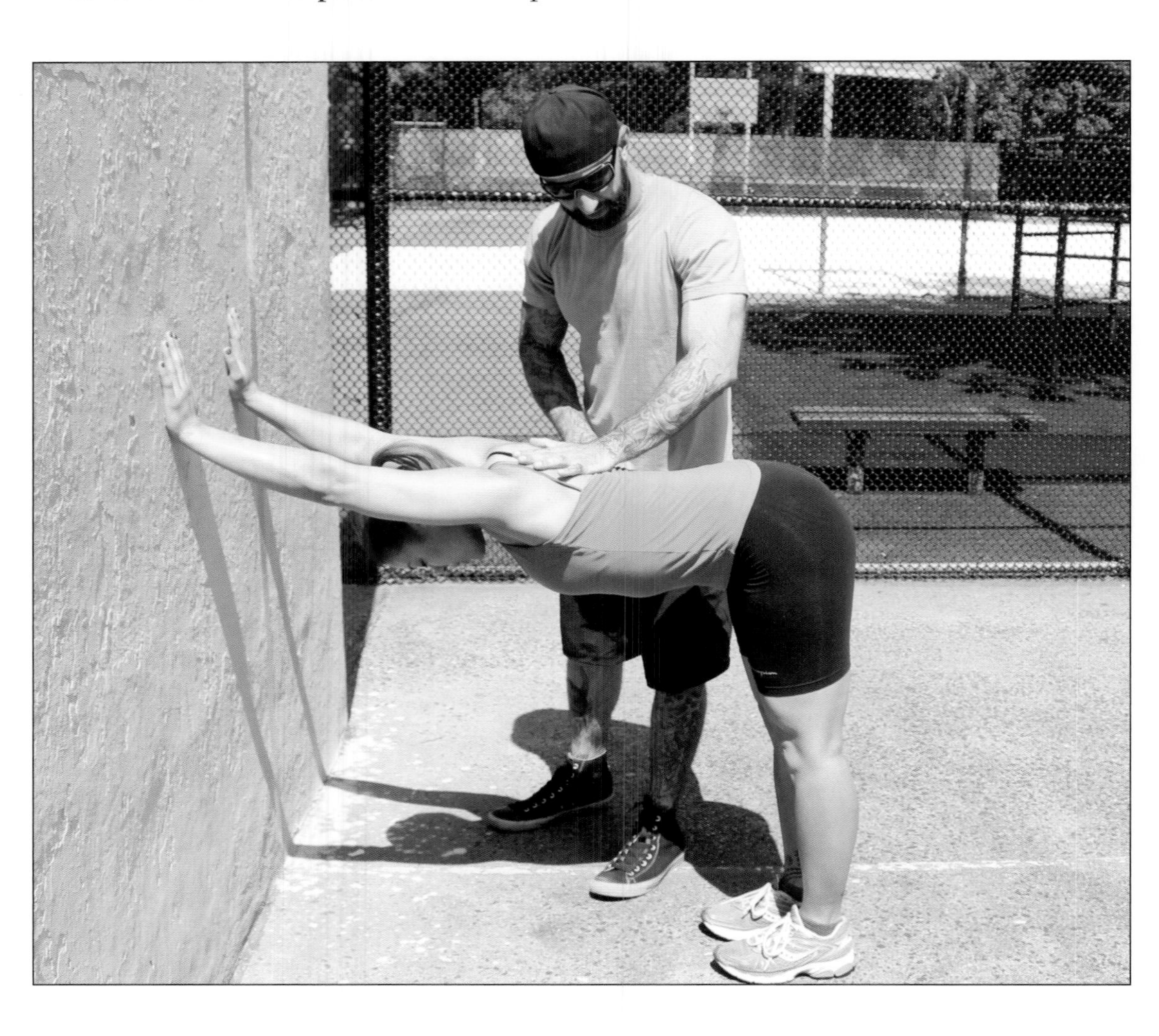

# Yoga Lunge

Though the Yoga Lunge emphasizes flexibility, it is very similar to the Walking Lunge typically seen in calisthenics. From the Statue position, take a big step forward with one leg (at least a leg's length.) Next bend your front knee while keeping your back leg as straight as possible. The heel of your back foot will come off the ground while your entire front foot remains flat. Your front knee should remain directly above your front ankle with the thigh parallel to the ground. Place your palms on the floor alongside your front foot or on top of your thigh. Hold for several breaths. When you are ready to switch sides, you can step your leg back while leaving your hands on the ground. You'll wind up in a Downward Dog during the transition. From here you can return to a Statue pose and repeat on the other side, or try to lunge the other leg forward from the Downward Dog position, placing the foot in between your hands. You may also add a sideways twist over your front knee for an added challenge.

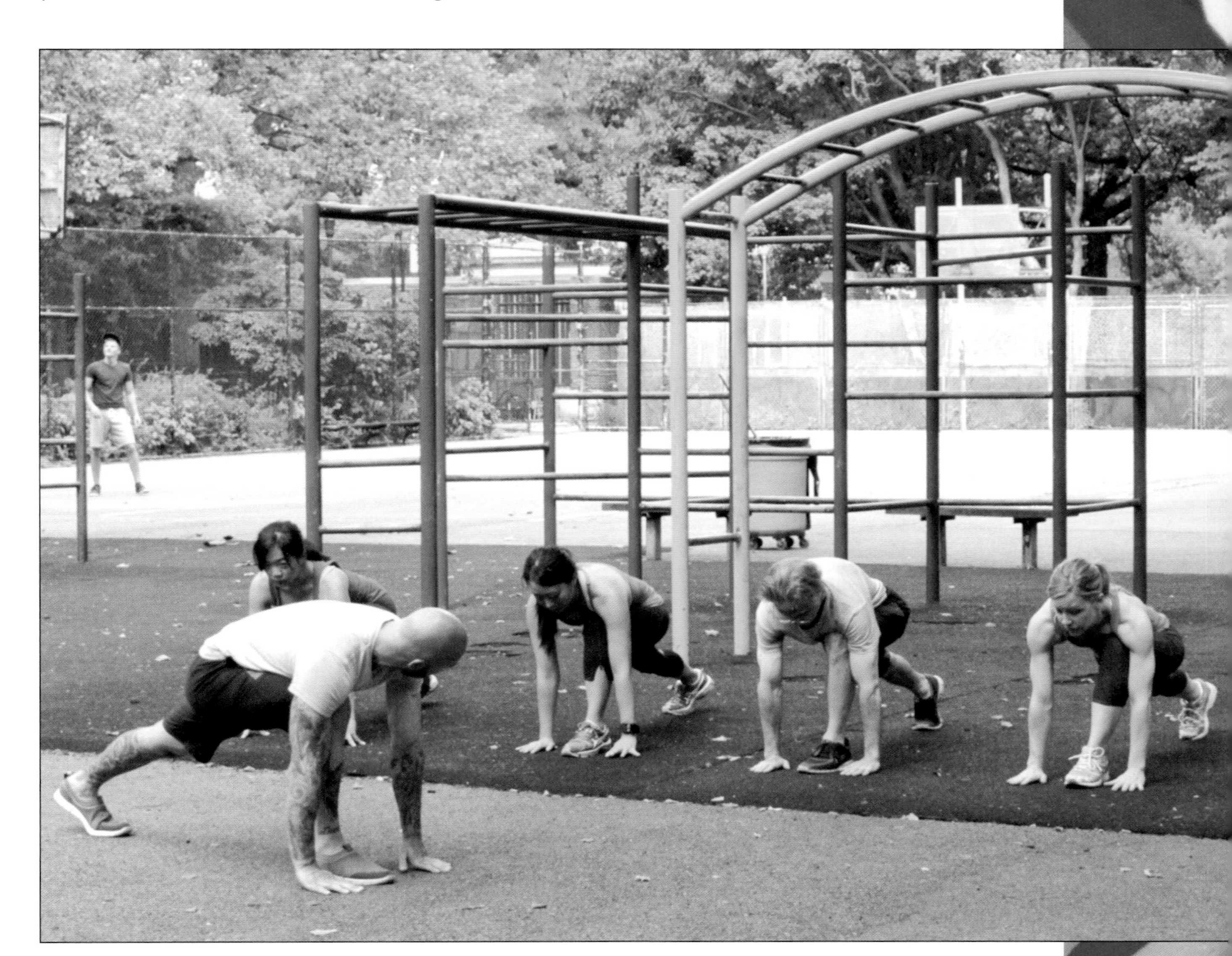

**Inhale:** Lengthen your spine

**Exhale:** Extend your back leg, pushing through the heel

**Common Mistakes:** Excessive bending of the back leg, torquing of the front knee

**Primary Muscle Groups:** Hips, hamstrings, calves

**Calisthenics Counterpart:** Walking Lunge

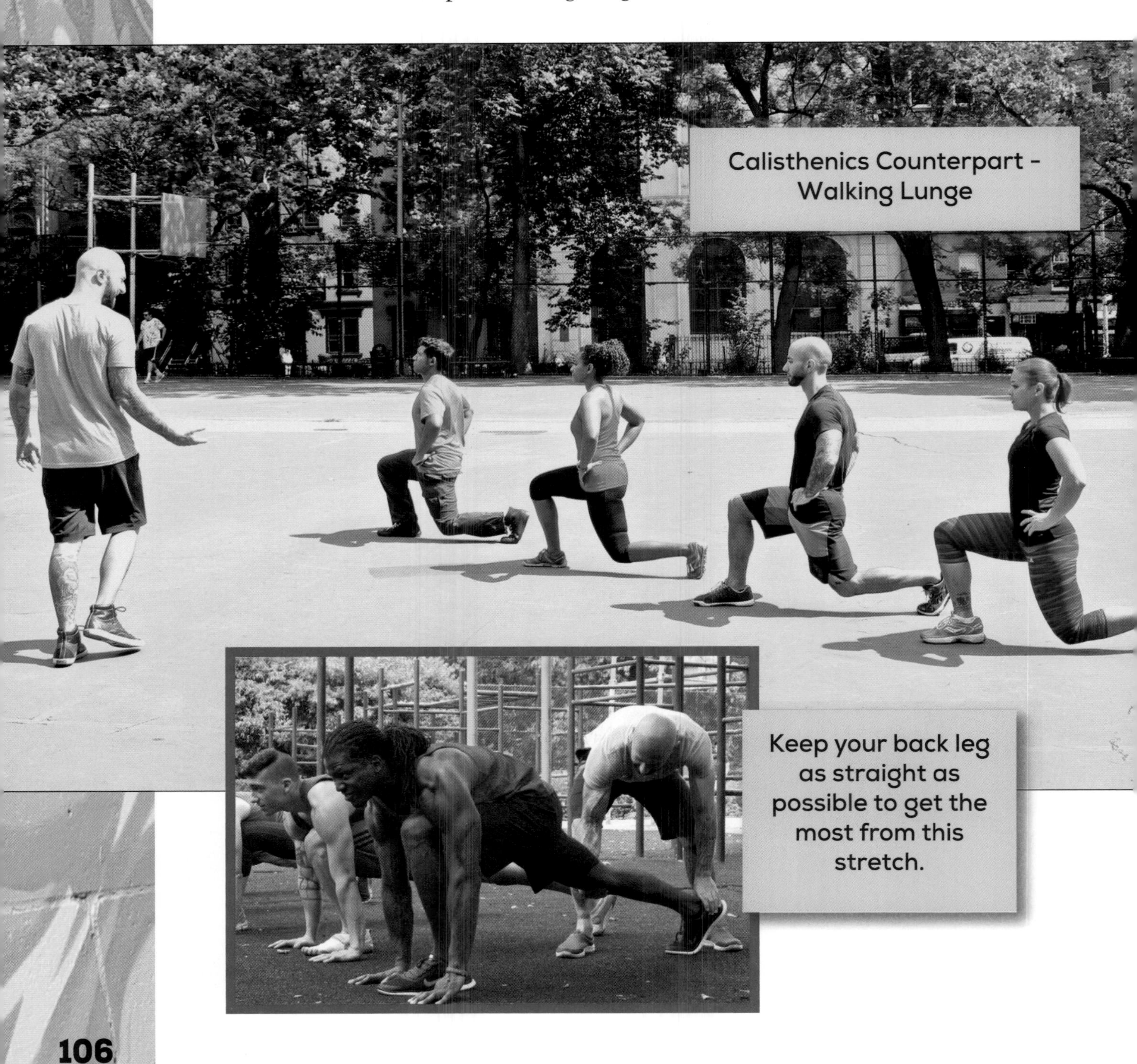

Calisthenics Counterpart -
Walking Lunge
Keep your back leg
as straight as
possible to get the
most from this
stretch.

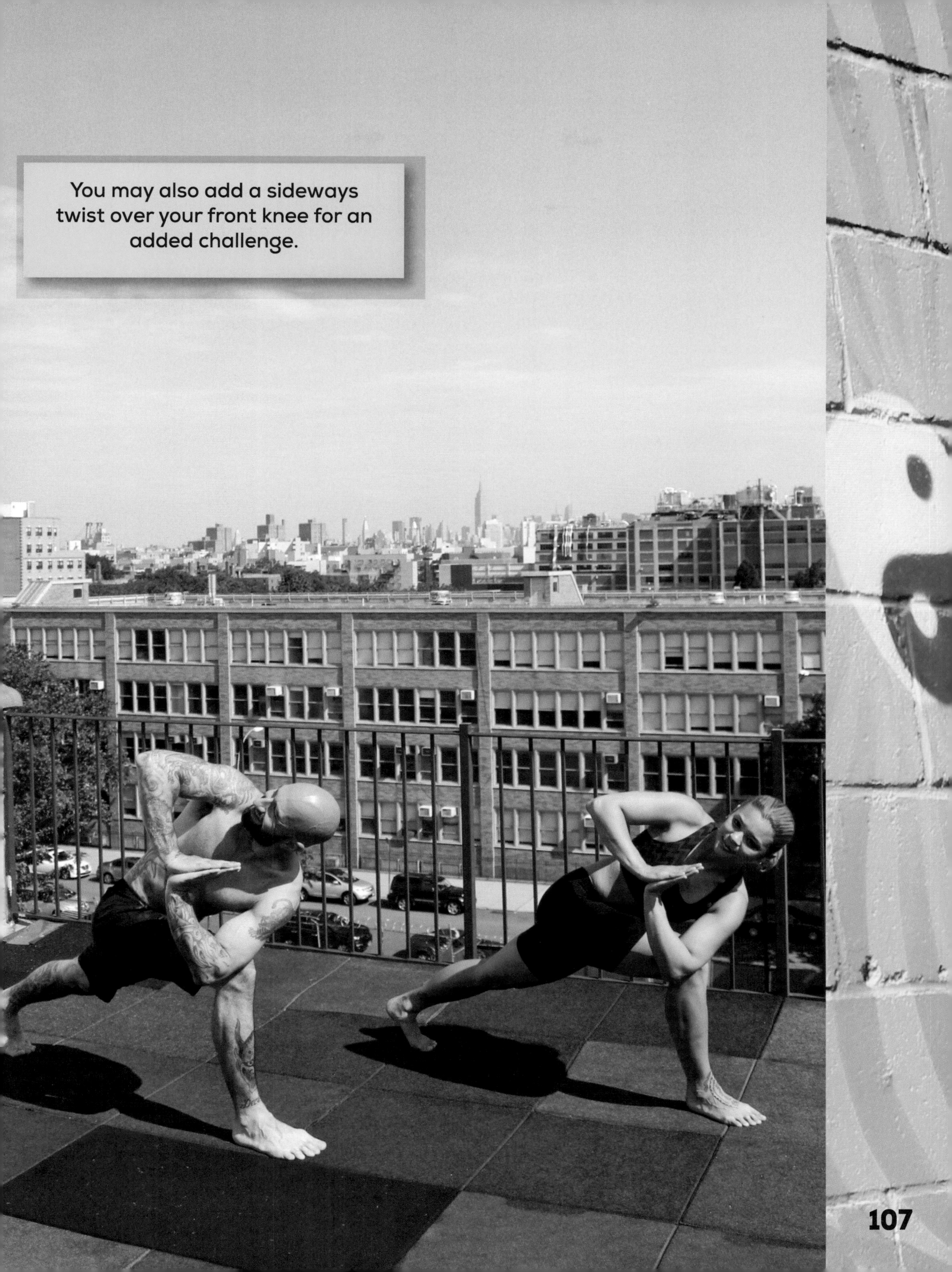

You may also add a sideways twist over your front knee for an added challenge.

## Cobra

Cobra is a gentle way for beginners to work on spinal mobility. Lie face down on the ground with your legs straight behind you and toes pointed. Your arms should be bent at the elbows so your palms are flat on the ground beneath your shoulders. Keep your elbows tucked in by your ribs as you lift your chest and look up while gently pressing down with your hands. Be careful not to press too hard or allow your shoulders to shrug. Engage your lower back and squeeze your glutes while pushing your hips into the ground, keeping your legs and feet together. You should feel a stretch through your abdominals and some light compression in your spine.

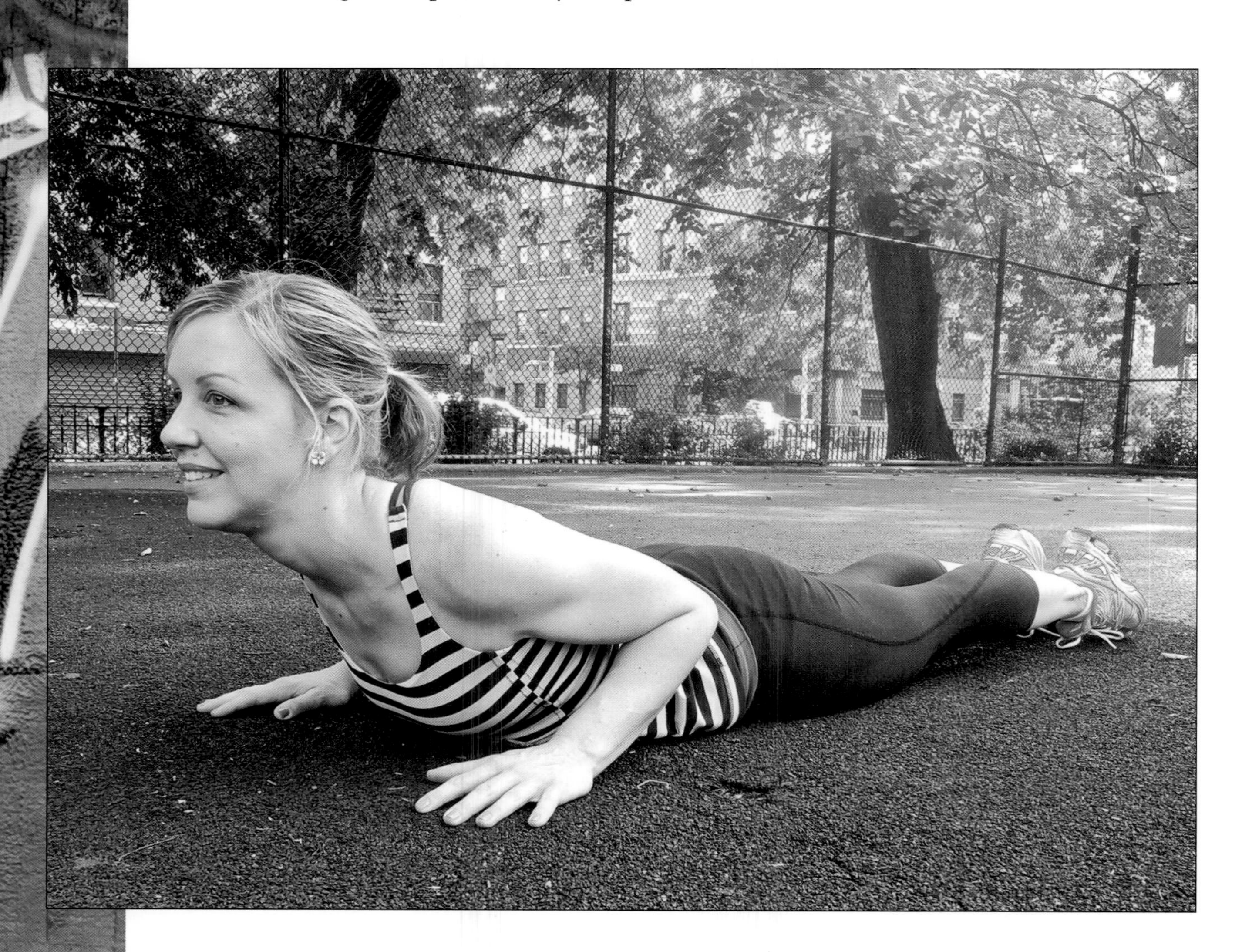

**Inhale:** Lengthen your spine and lift your chin

**Exhale:** Squeeze your shoulder blades down and back, lift your chest and tense your glutes

**Common Mistakes:** Shrugged shoulders, excessive triceps activation

**Primary Muscle Groups:** Abs, back, chest, neck

**Calisthenics Counterpart:** Neck Bridge

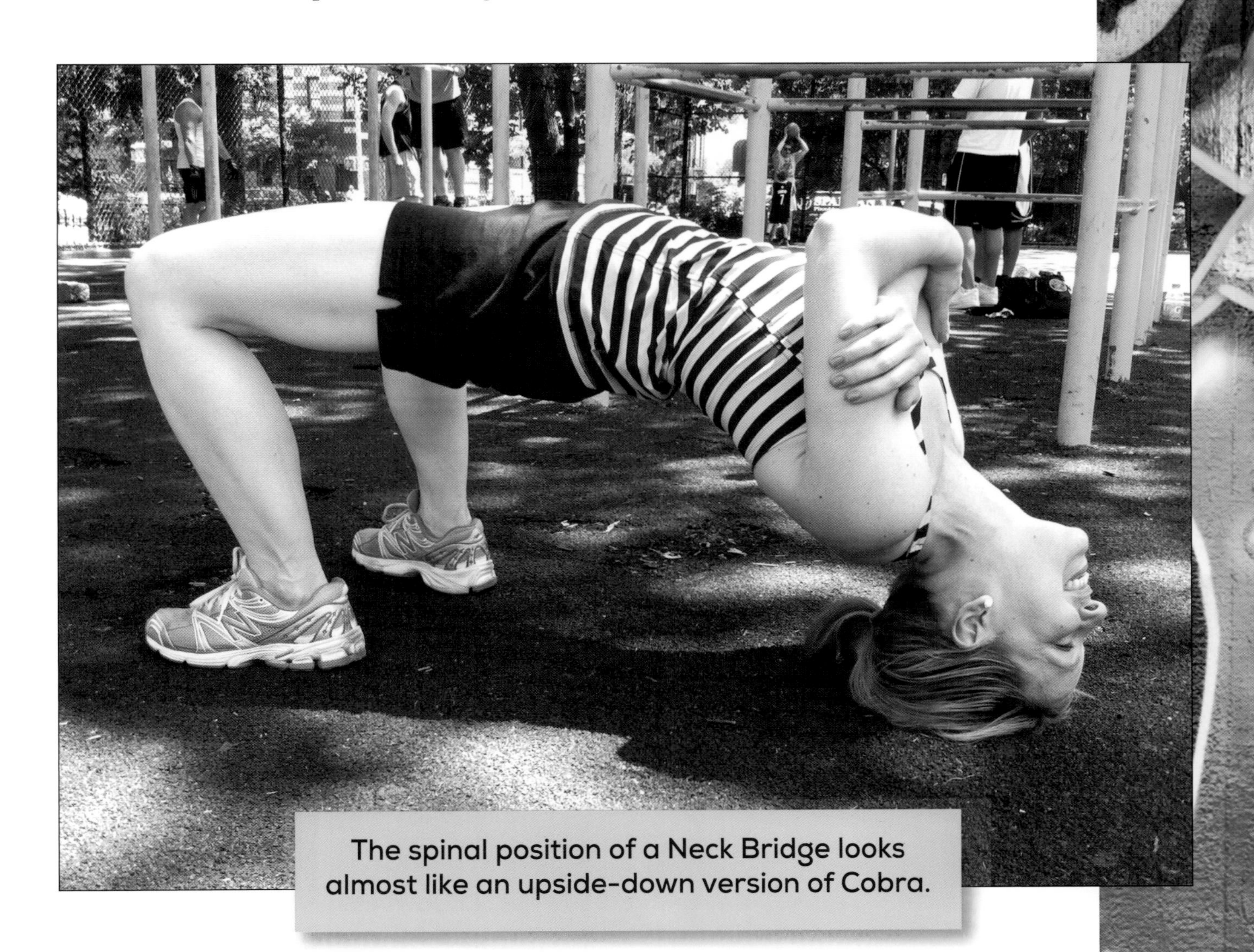

The spinal position of a Neck Bridge looks almost like an upside-down version of Cobra.

# Sphinx

Similar to Cobra, the Sphinx pose allows for a deeper stretch in the abdominals by moving the hands in front of the shoulders. Your elbows will wind up under your shoulders instead of by your ribs. This creates a deeper stretch through the upper back. Begin with your forearms on the ground and work toward straightening your arms without shrugging your shoulders. Keep your fingers pointed forward with your elbows close to your torso and pointed back.

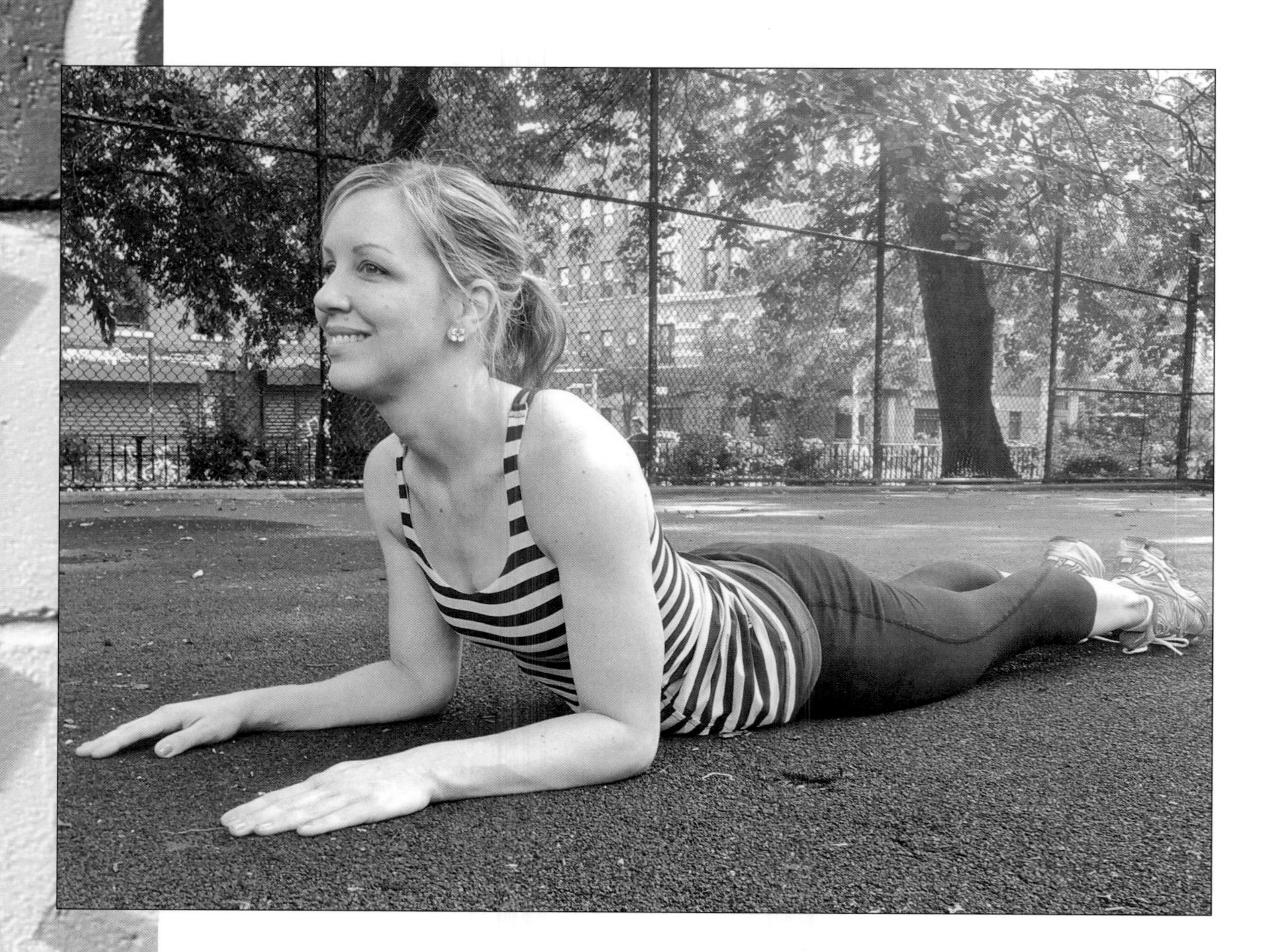

**Inhale:** Lengthen your spine and look upward

**Exhale:** Squeeze your shoulder blades down and back, lift your chest and tense your glutes

**Common Mistakes:** Shrugged shoulders, excessive triceps activation

**Primary Muscle Groups:** Abs, back, chest

**Calisthenics Counterpart:** Back Bridge

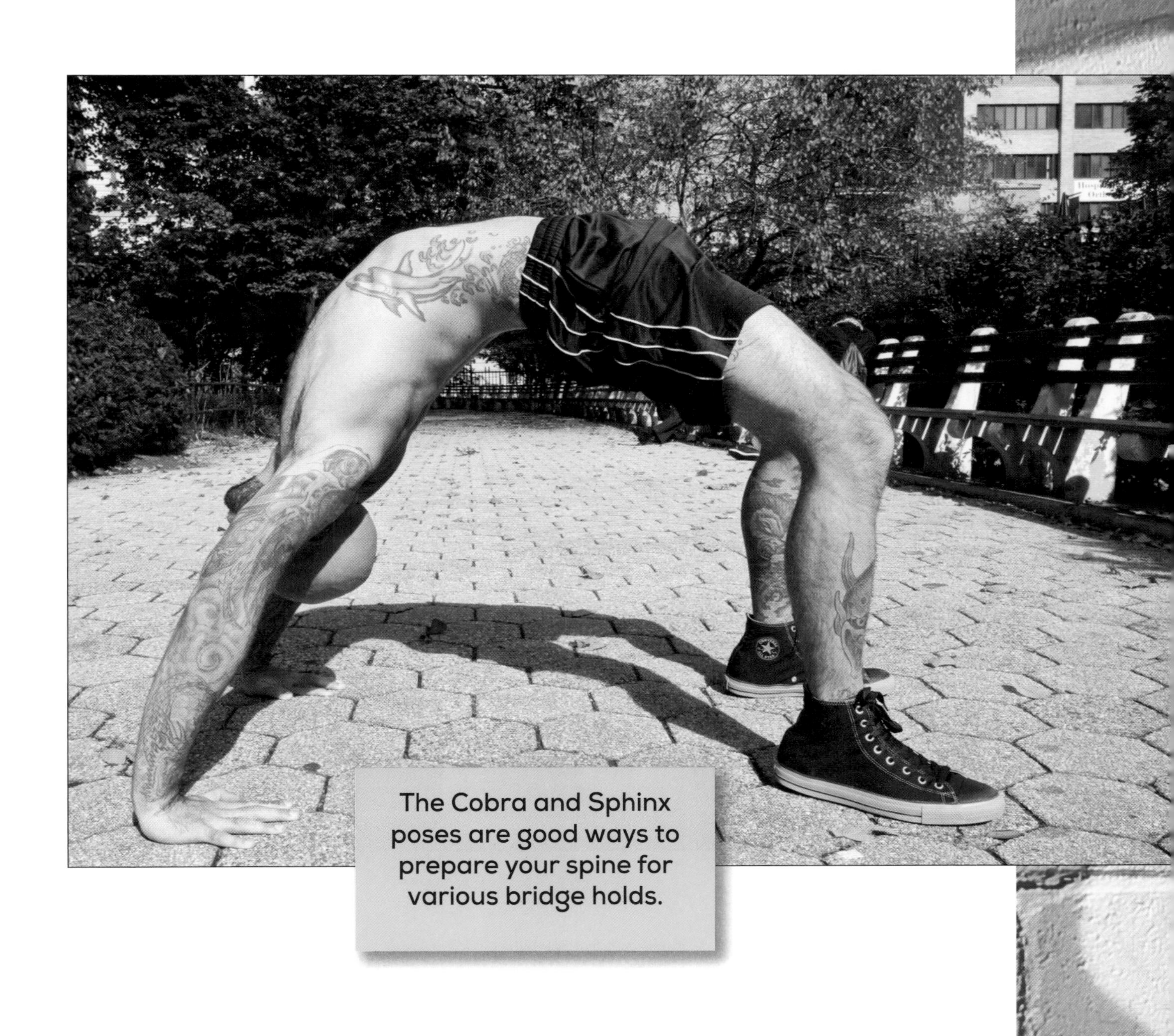

The Cobra and Sphinx poses are good ways to prepare your spine for various bridge holds.

# Updog

Similar to Cobra and Sphinx but with an even deeper stretch in the abdominals and further spinal compression, Updog is an advanced variation that will not be appropriate for most beginners. Just like Cobra, in Updog your hands are under your shoulders, only your elbows are fully extended with your hips remaining low to the ground. Remember to keep your shoulders retracted and depressed and lift your chest while pushing down through your hands.

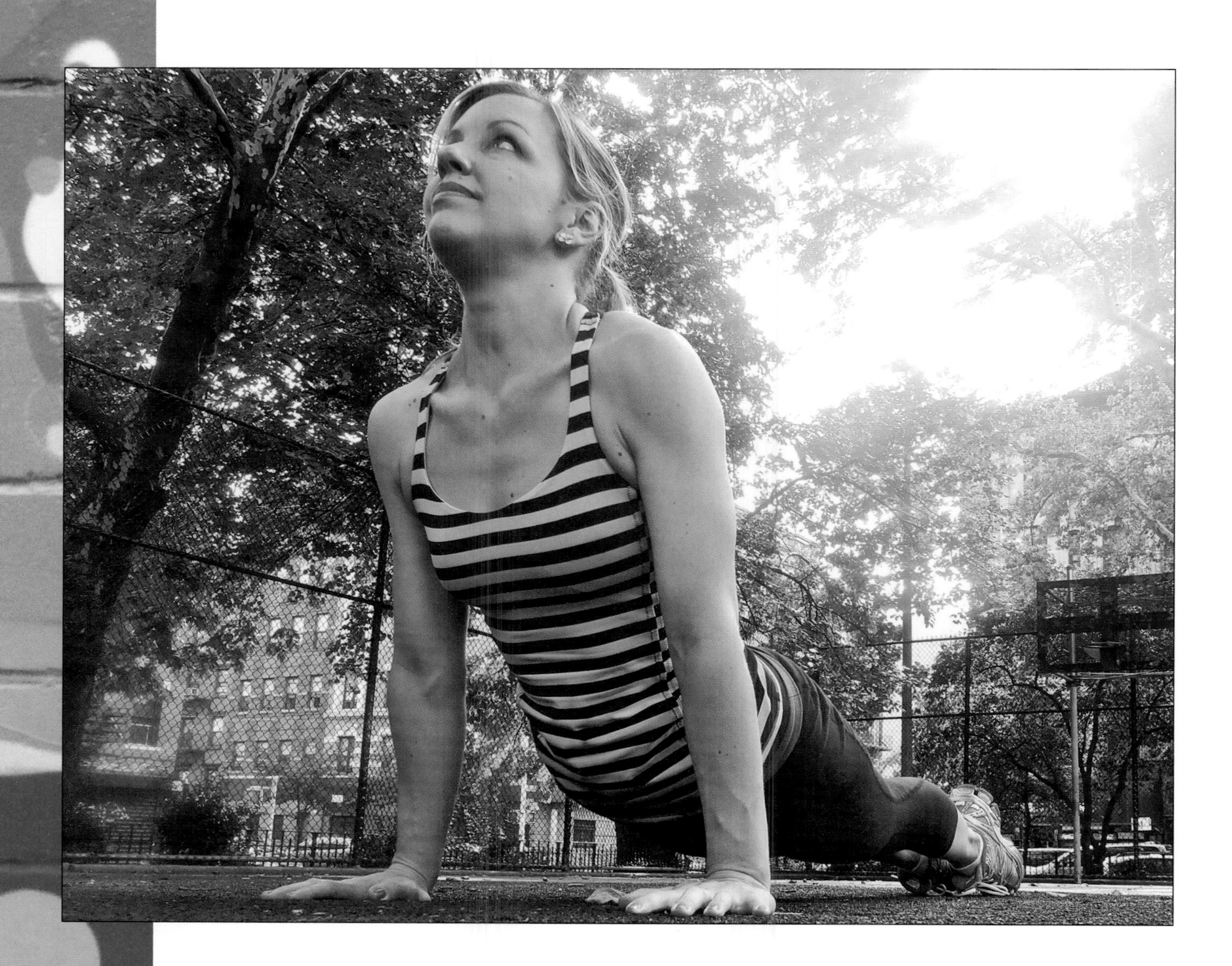

**Inhale:** Lengthen your spine and look up

**Exhale:** Squeeze your shoulder blades down and back, lift your chest and tense your glutes

**Common Mistakes:** Shrugged shoulders, excessive wrist flexion

**Primary Muscle Groups:** Abs, back, chest

**Calisthenics Counterpart:** Back Bridge

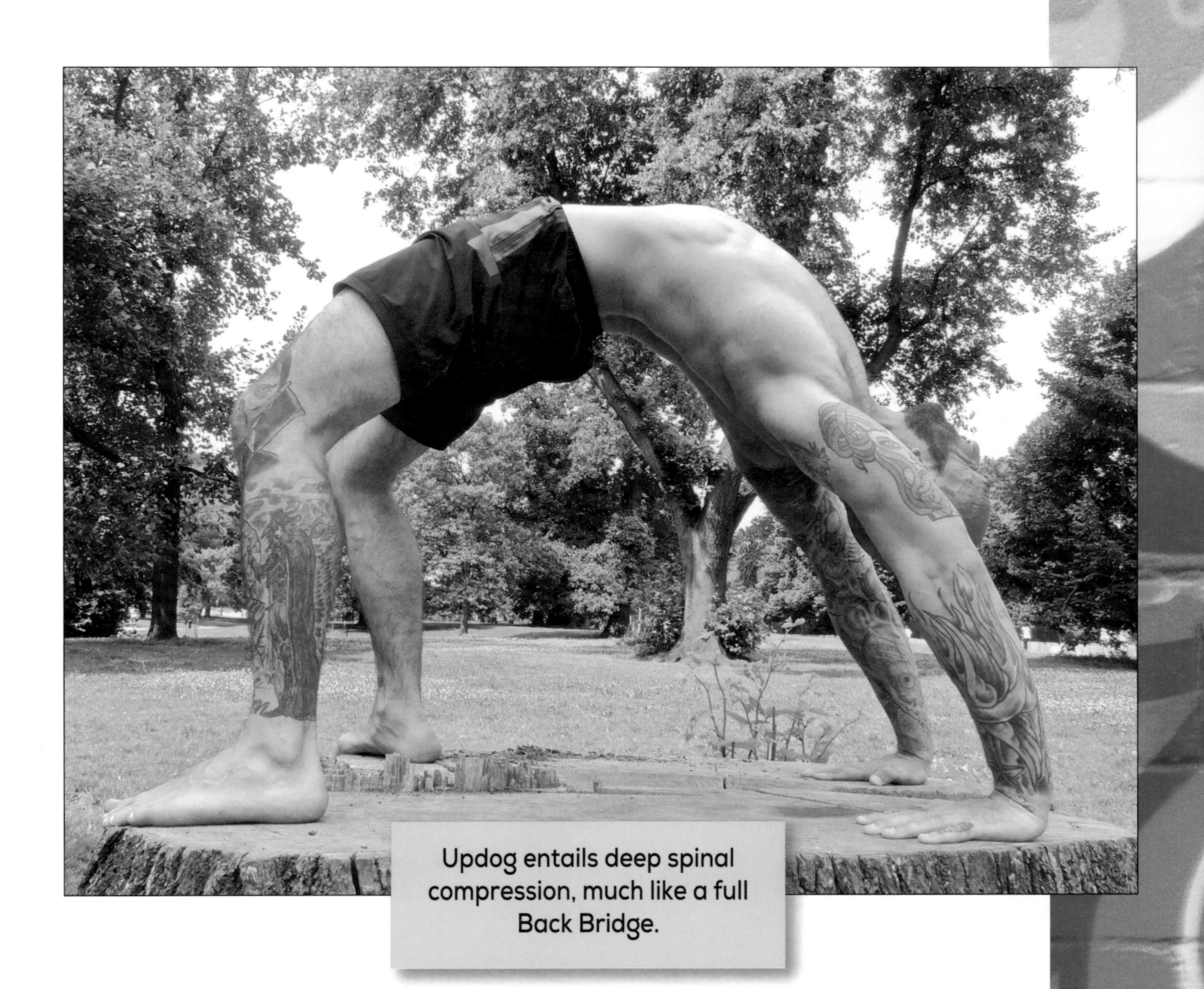

Updog entails deep spinal compression, much like a full Back Bridge.

# Child's Pose

Child's Pose is a great beginner stretch for the hips and hamstrings as well as the upper back and shoulders. Begin by kneeling on the ground, then slowly sit back until your buttocks rest on your heels. Open your knees while keeping your ankles close to each other, then lean forward from your hips. Walk your hands all the way out away from your body so that your chest winds up in between your thighs with your arms resting on the ground straight in front of you. Slide your hips back toward your heels to deepen the stretch.

**Inhale:** Lengthen your spine and reach your arms away from your body

**Exhale:** Press your hips back and your chest down

**Common Mistakes:** Excessive elbow bending, knees too close together

**Primary Muscle Groups:** Hips, hamstrings, upper-back, shoulders

**Calisthenics Counterpart:** Tuck Lever

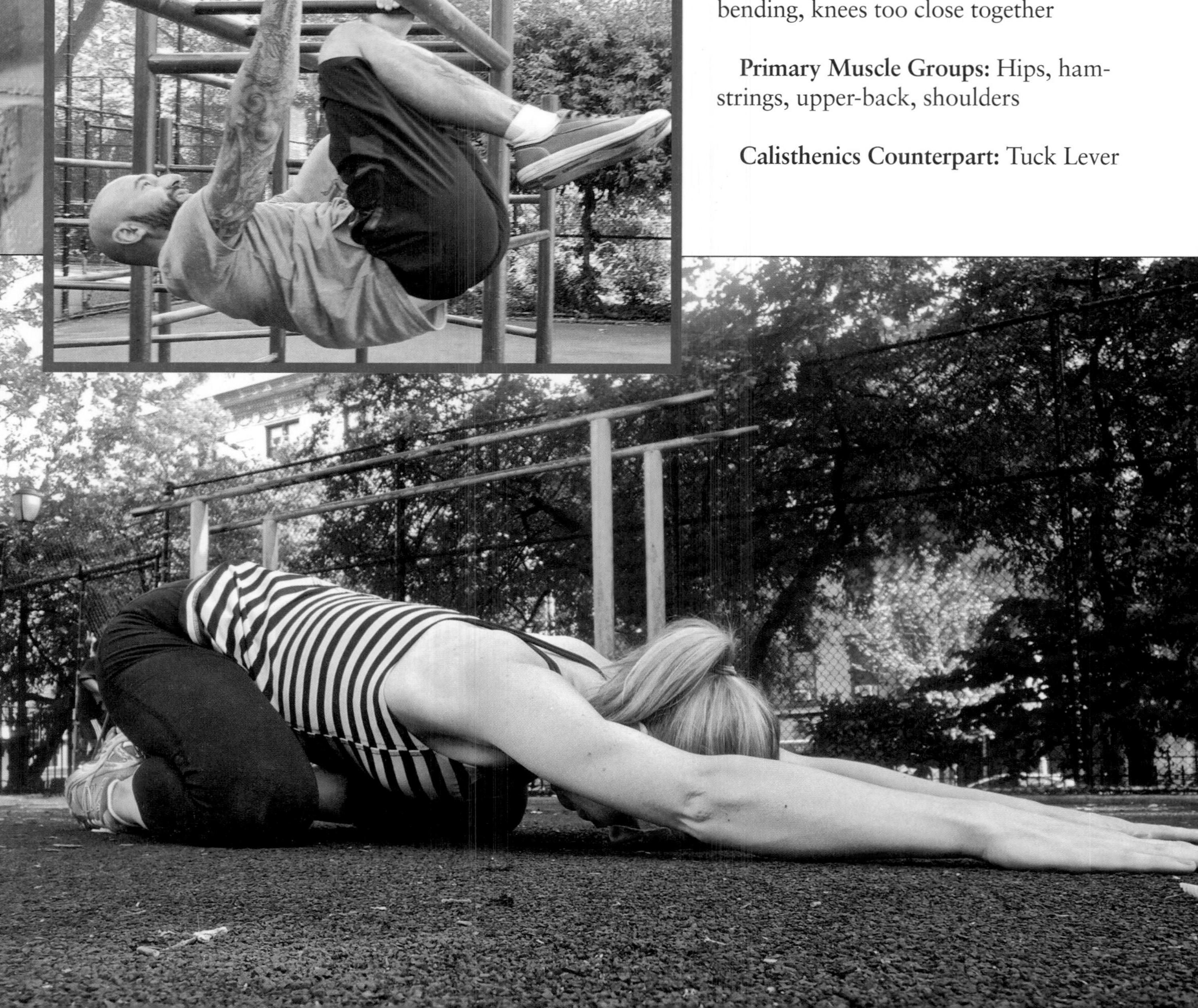

# Inchworm

Similar to Child's Pose, the Inchworm puts a deeper emphasis on the thoracic region of the spine. Instead of sliding your hips down to your heels like you would in Child's Pose, raise them in the air directly above your knees. This will give you greater leverage to press your chest down toward the ground, further opening your upper back and shoulders.

**Inhale:** Lift your hips and reach your arms away from your body

**Exhale:** Press your chest all the way to the ground

**Common Mistakes:** Hips too low, excessive elbow bending

**Primary Muscle Groups:** Upper back, shoulders

**Calisthenics Counterpart:** Back Bridge

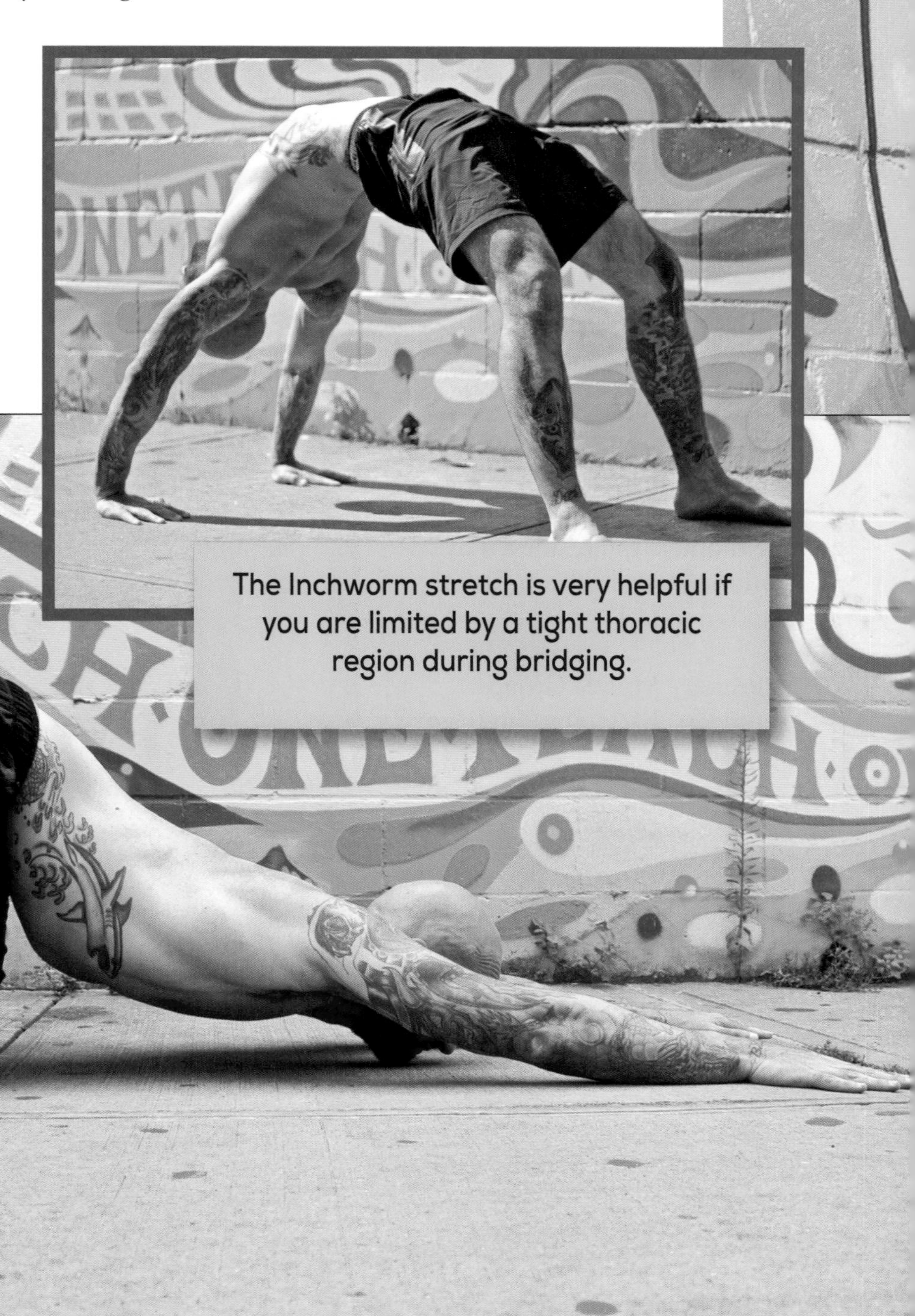

The Inchworm stretch is very helpful if you are limited by a tight thoracic region during bridging.

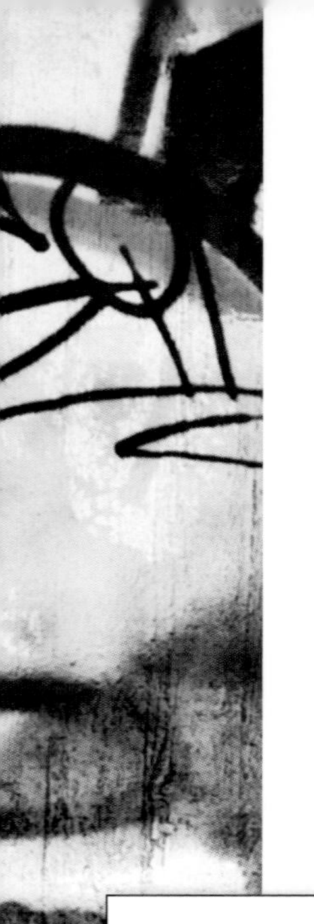

# Wheel

This is one move that isn't much different whether you're practicing traditional yoga or participating in the modern day phenomenon known as "Street Workout." The Wheel or Back Bridge is such an essential bodyweight exercise, that like the Squat and Push-up, its ubiquity transcends modalities.

As we've seen already, the Wheel pose involves holding yourself face-up on your hands and feet with your body in a deep arch. The Wheel pose requires harmony between all the muscles of the posterior chain as well as adequate flexibility, particularly in the upper back and shoulders, where many of us are prone to tightness. Be careful with this move, especially if you have particularly tight shoulders or issues with your lower back.

**Inhale:** Lift your hips, lengthen your spine and push your body away from the ground

**Exhale:** Press your chest up and out while squeezing your glutes and hamstrings

**Common Mistakes:** Insufficient extension through the thoracic spine, uneven distribution of weight through the hands and feet

**Primary Muscle Groups:** Shoulders, back, abs, hip flexors

**Calisthenics Counterpart:** Back Bridge

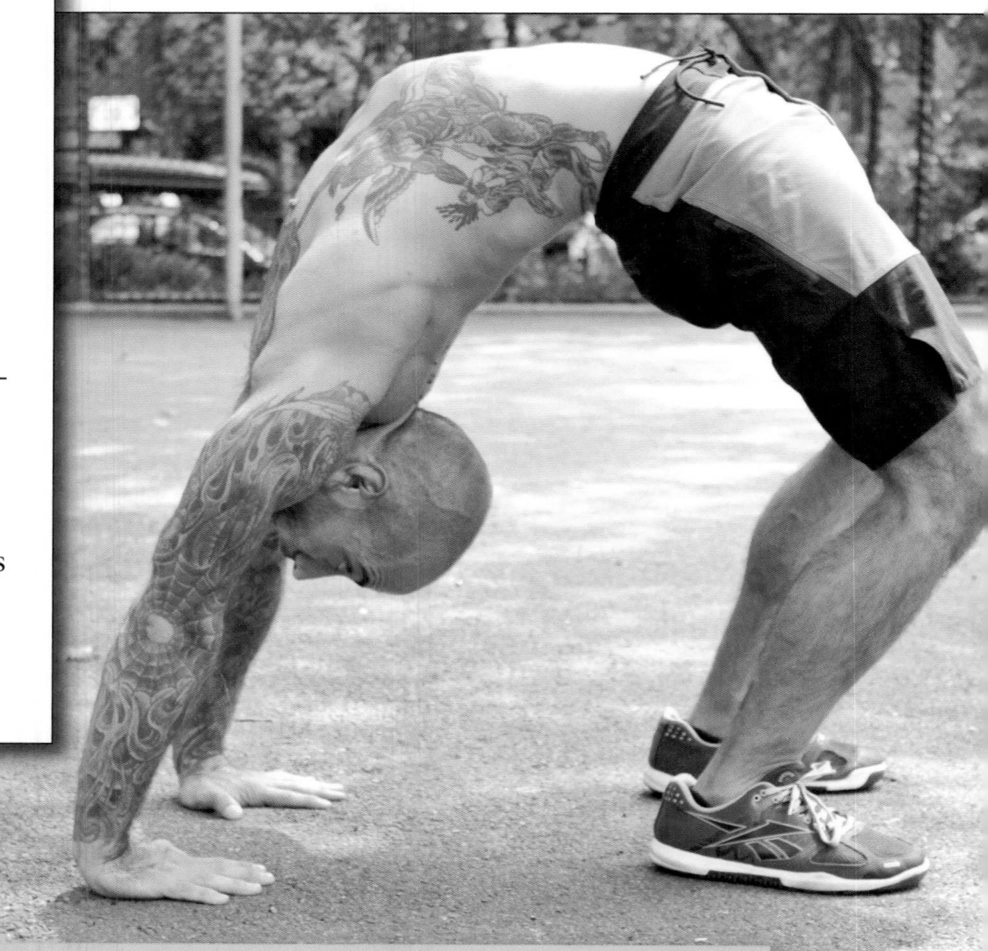

This is one move that isn't much different whether you're practicing traditional yoga or participating in the modern day phenomenon known as "Street Workout."

# Upward Bow

The Upward Bow is another fantastic bridge variant. Lie face down on the ground with your arms stretched out to the sides, then engage your lower back and glutes to lift your chest off the floor. Now bend your knees toward your backside and reach your arms behind you. Try to grab the inside of your ankles with your hands, while keeping your shoulder blades pinched together and thumbs pointed up. Squeeze your knees together, kick your feet into your hands and press your chest forward.

**Inhale:** Lengthen your spine and lift yourself away from the ground

**Exhale:** Kick your feet into your hands while squeezing your glutes and legs

**Common Mistakes:** Insufficient extension through the thoracic spine

**Primary Muscle Groups:** Shoulders, back, abs, hip flexors

**Calisthenics Counterpart:** Back Bridge

The Upward Bow is another fantastic bridge variant.

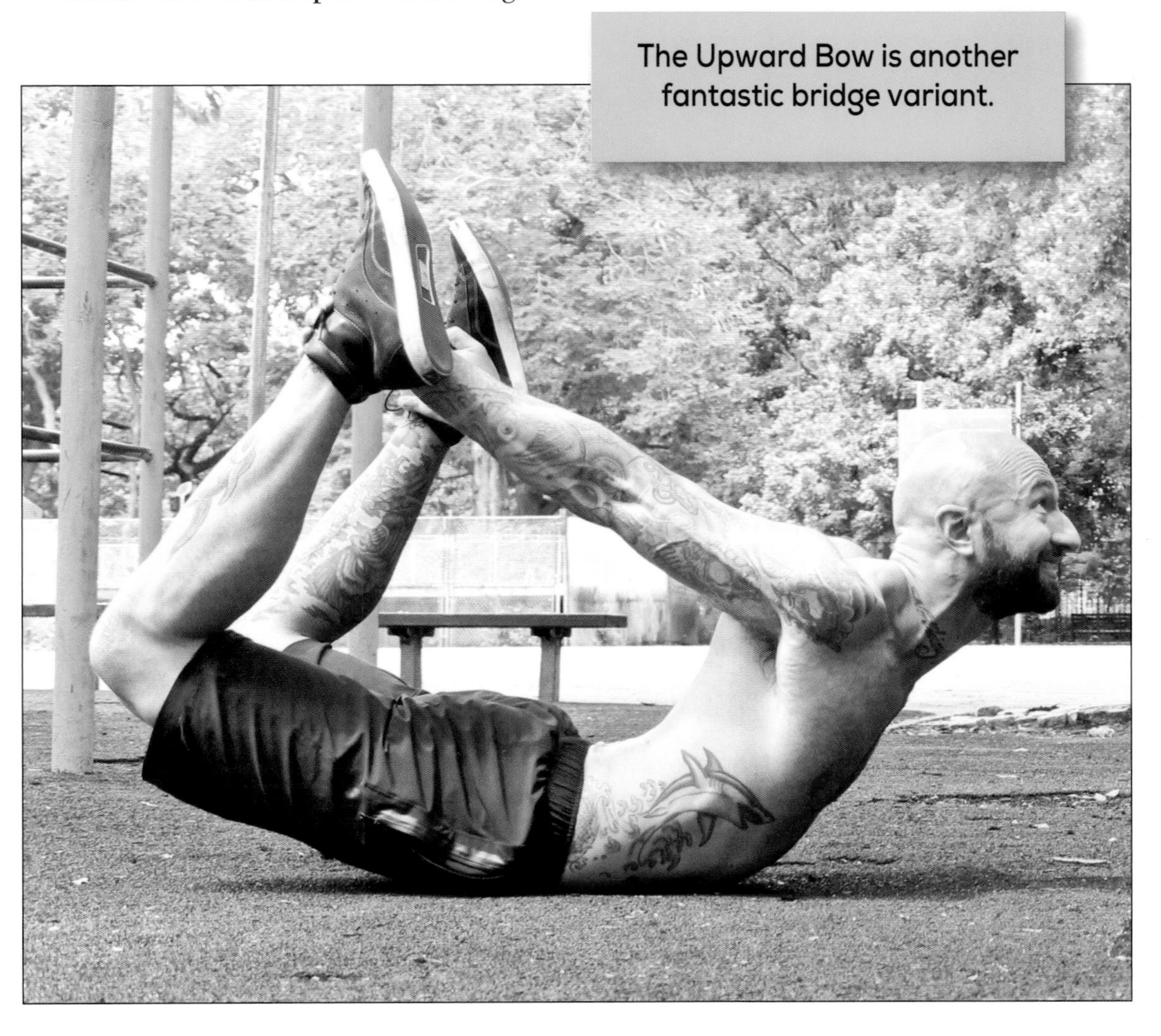

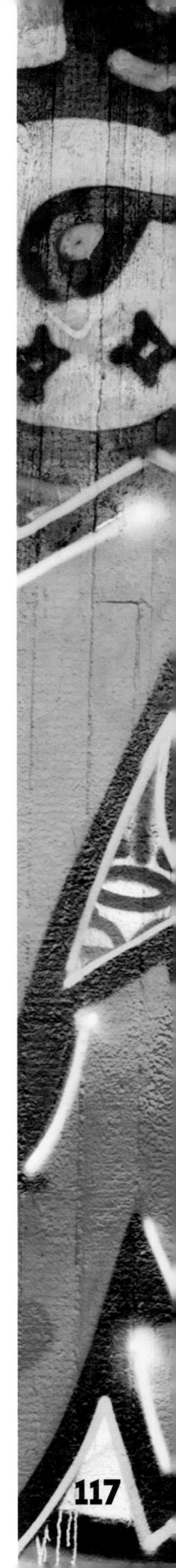

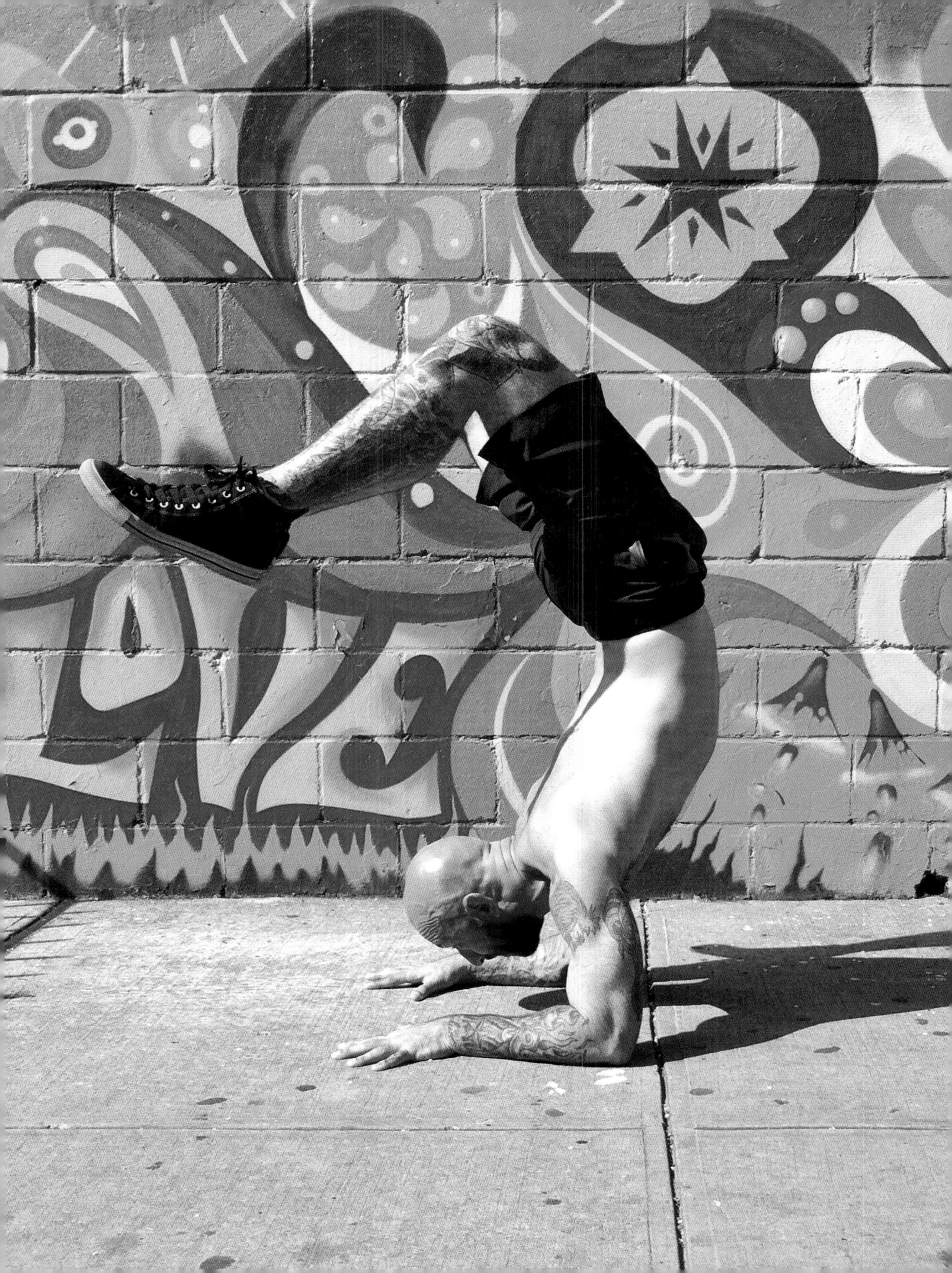

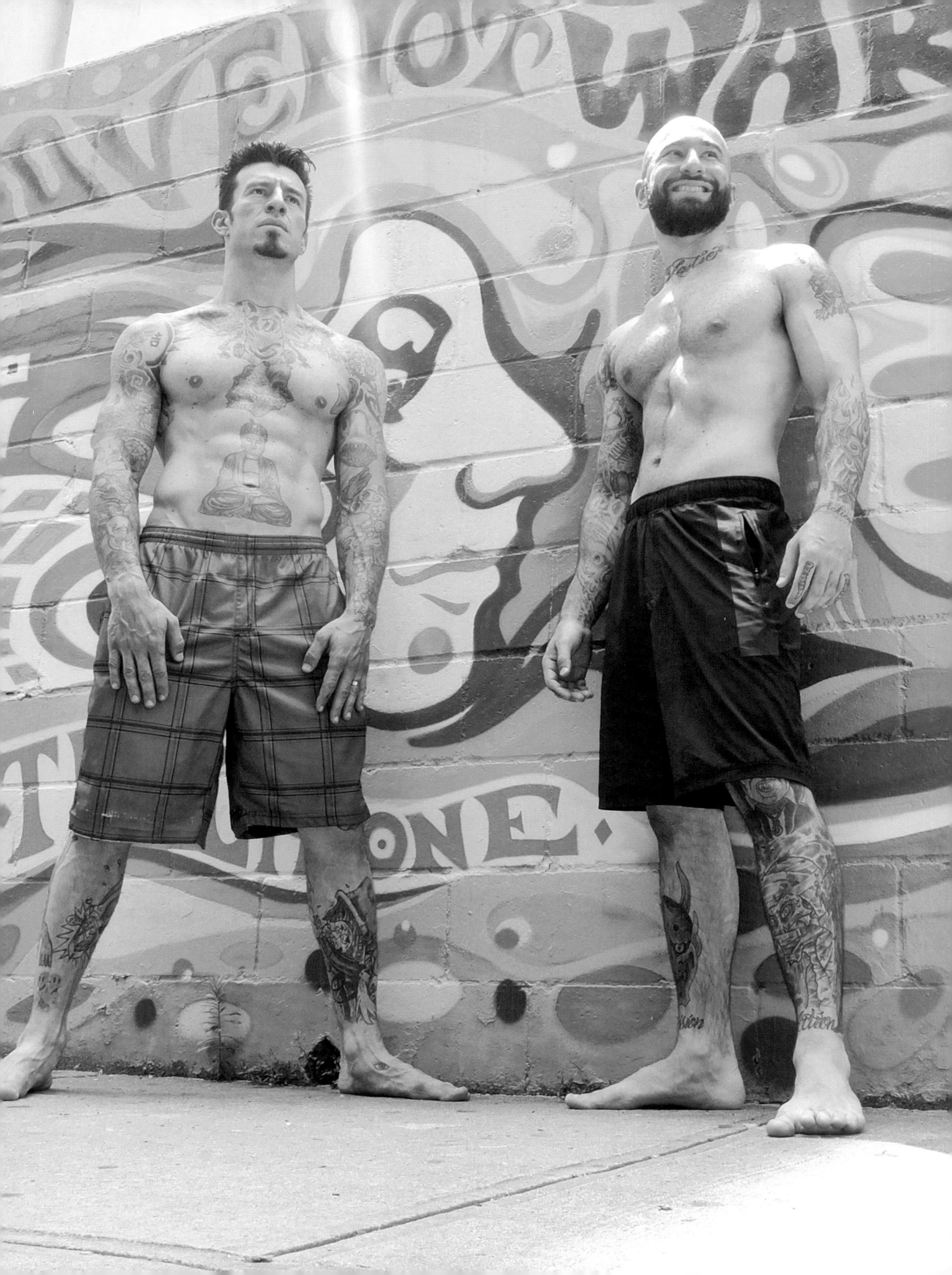

## Camel

Similar to the Upward Bow, Camel pose is another useful stretch for the trunk and spine. Kneel on the ground with your feet pointed straight behind you (or toes curled under if you prefer). Your legs should be hip distance apart with your knees bent to 90 degrees. Slowly begin arching your spine while looking behind your back. Lift your sternum and reach your arms behind your body, pinching your shoulder blades together. Rotate your arms so your elbows are facing inward and palms are facing outward. Grab the heel of your foot with an open palm grip, drop your head all the way back and push your chest out.

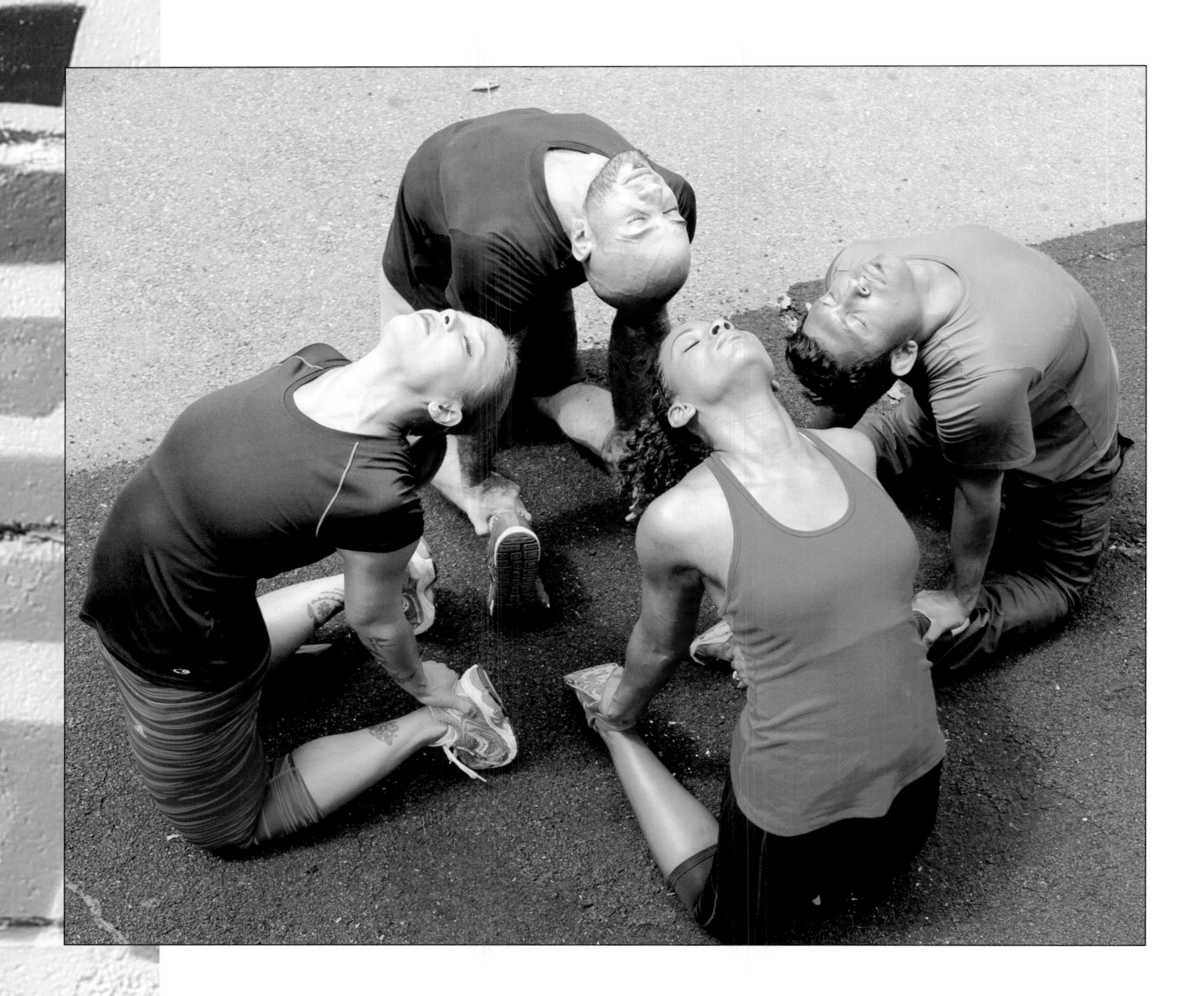

**Inhale:** Lengthen your spine and push your chest out

**Exhale:** Drop your head while squeezing your shoulder blades down and back

**Common Mistakes:** Shrugged shoulders, holding the breath

**Primary Muscle Groups:** Chest, shoulders, abs, hip flexors

**Calisthenics Counterpart:** Back Bridge

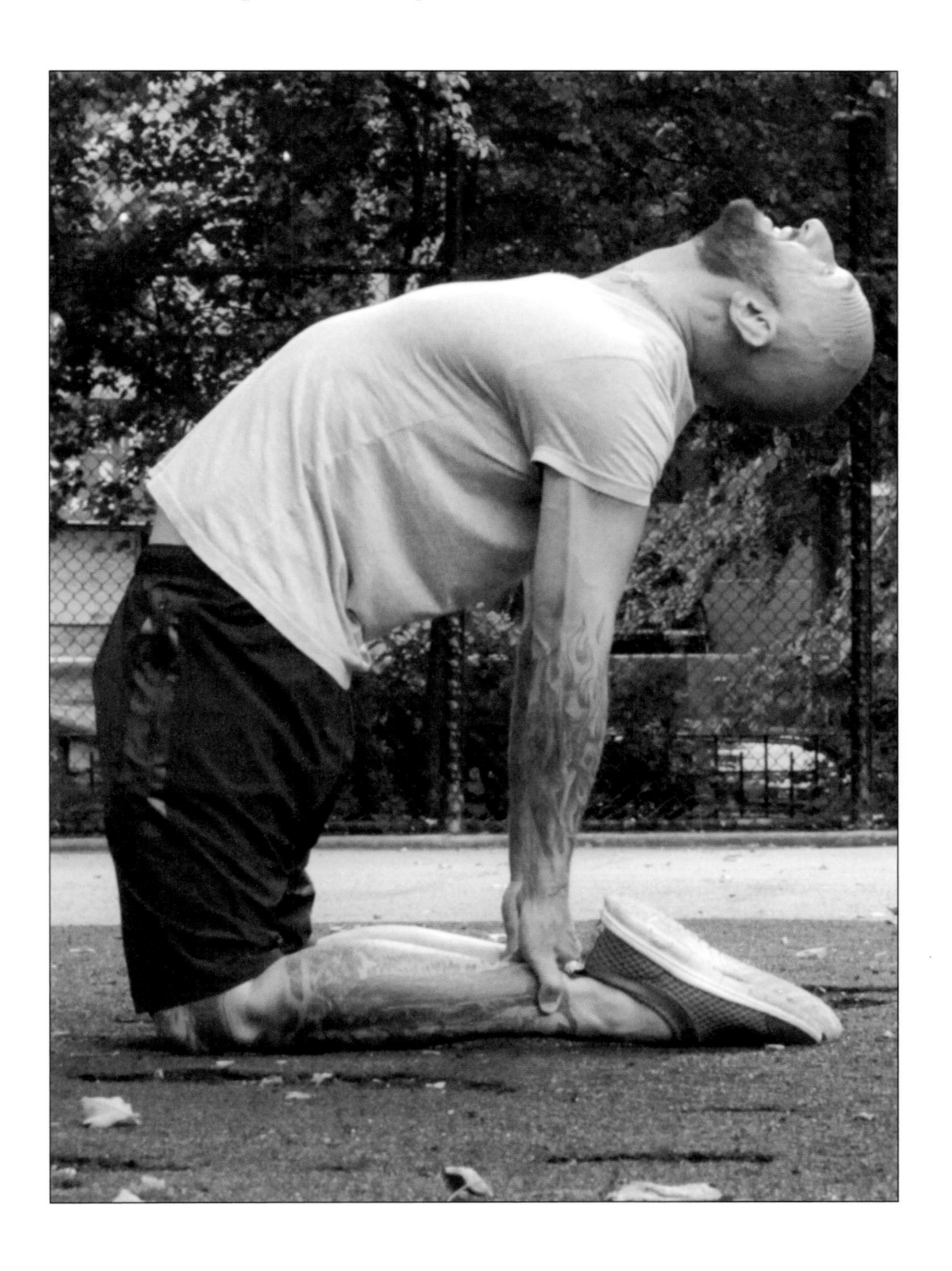

## Seated Forward Bend

The Seated Forward Bend or gym-class "toe touch" is a great stretch for the lower body. Sit on the floor with both legs extended straight in front of you, knees facing upward. Lift your chest and reach your arms overhead. Slowly hinge forward from the waist, reaching your hands toward your feet. If you cannot reach your feet, rest your hands on your thighs or grab your shins and gently pull yourself forward. If you can easily reach past your toes, aim toward getting your face to rest on your shins.

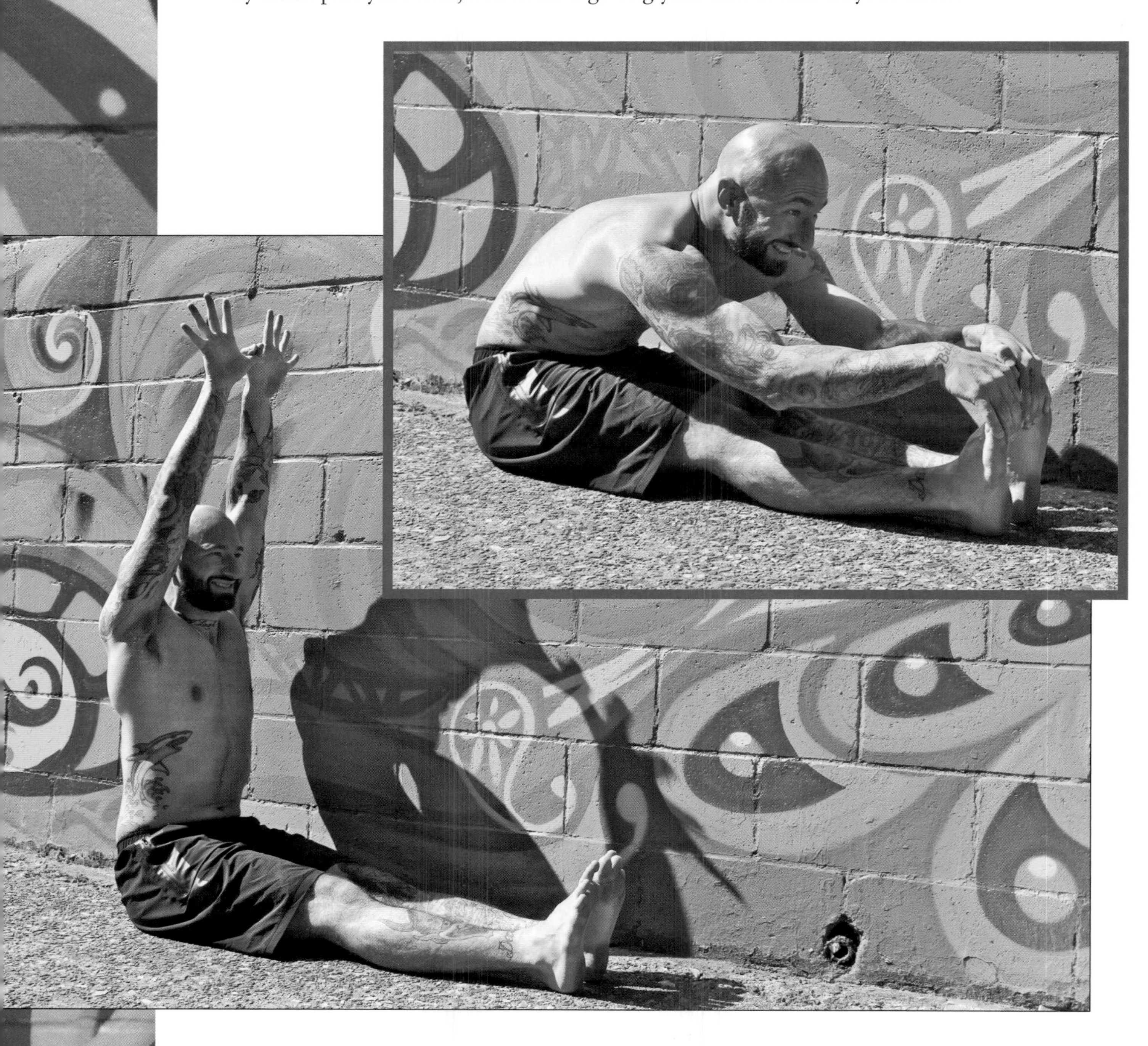

**Inhale:** Lengthen your spine and lift your chest

**Exhale:** Fold forward from the hips while reaching past your toes, taking as much of the stretch as possible in your hamstrings

**Common Mistakes:** Excessive rounding of the spine, external rotation of the legs (toes flaring out to the sides)

**Primary Muscle Groups:** Hamstrings, calves, lower back, hips

**Calisthenics Counterpart:** L-sit

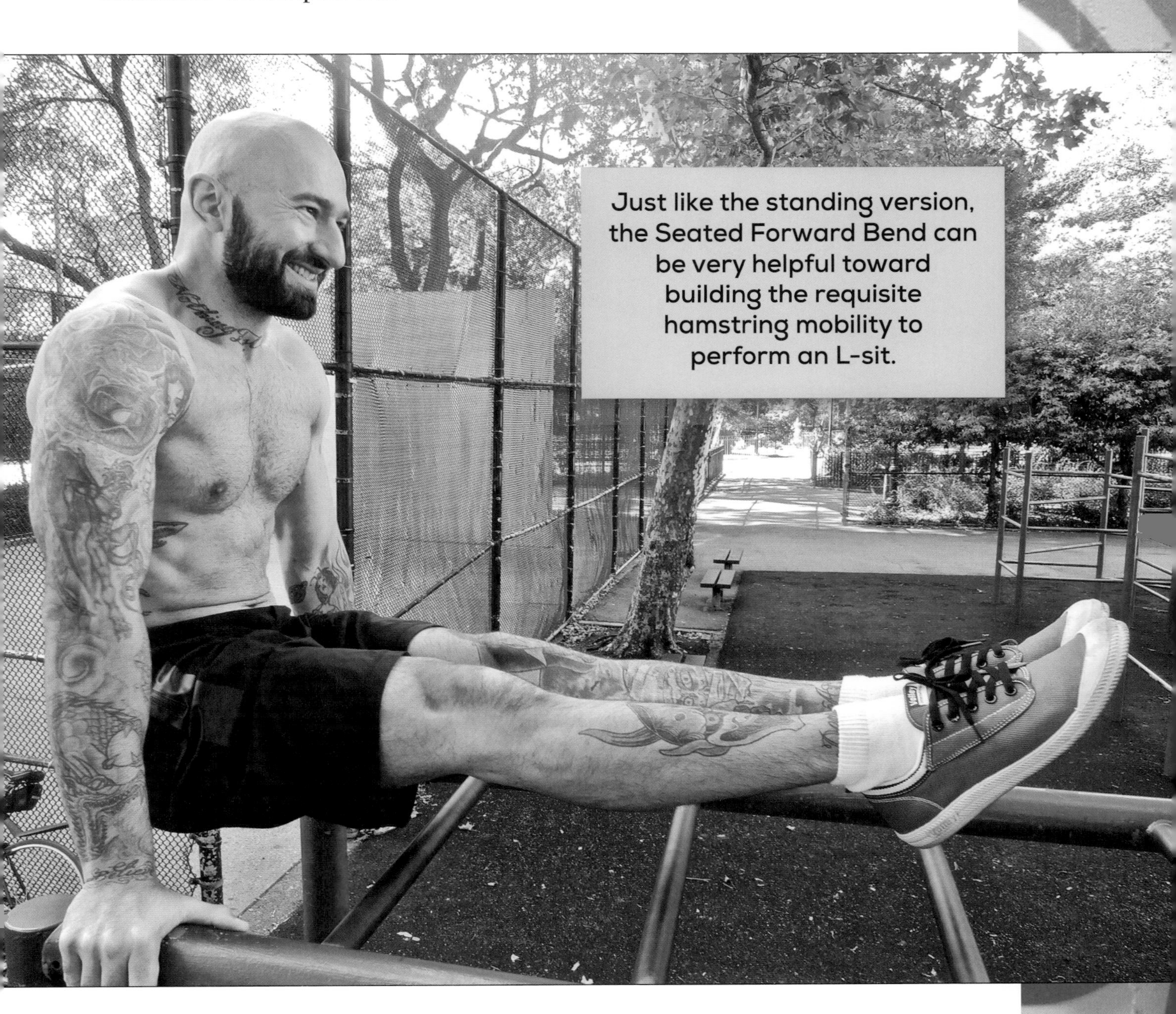

Just like the standing version, the Seated Forward Bend can be very helpful toward building the requisite hamstring mobility to perform an L-sit.

# Half Straddle

The Half Straddle is another great pose for beginners. Sit on the floor with your right leg extended straight out to the side. Now bend your left leg so your left foot winds up near your right inner thigh with your left leg remaining near the ground. Point the toes of your right foot straight into the air. Slowly lean forward from the waist while twisting through your trunk to reach your hands toward your right foot. Switch legs and repeat on the opposite side.

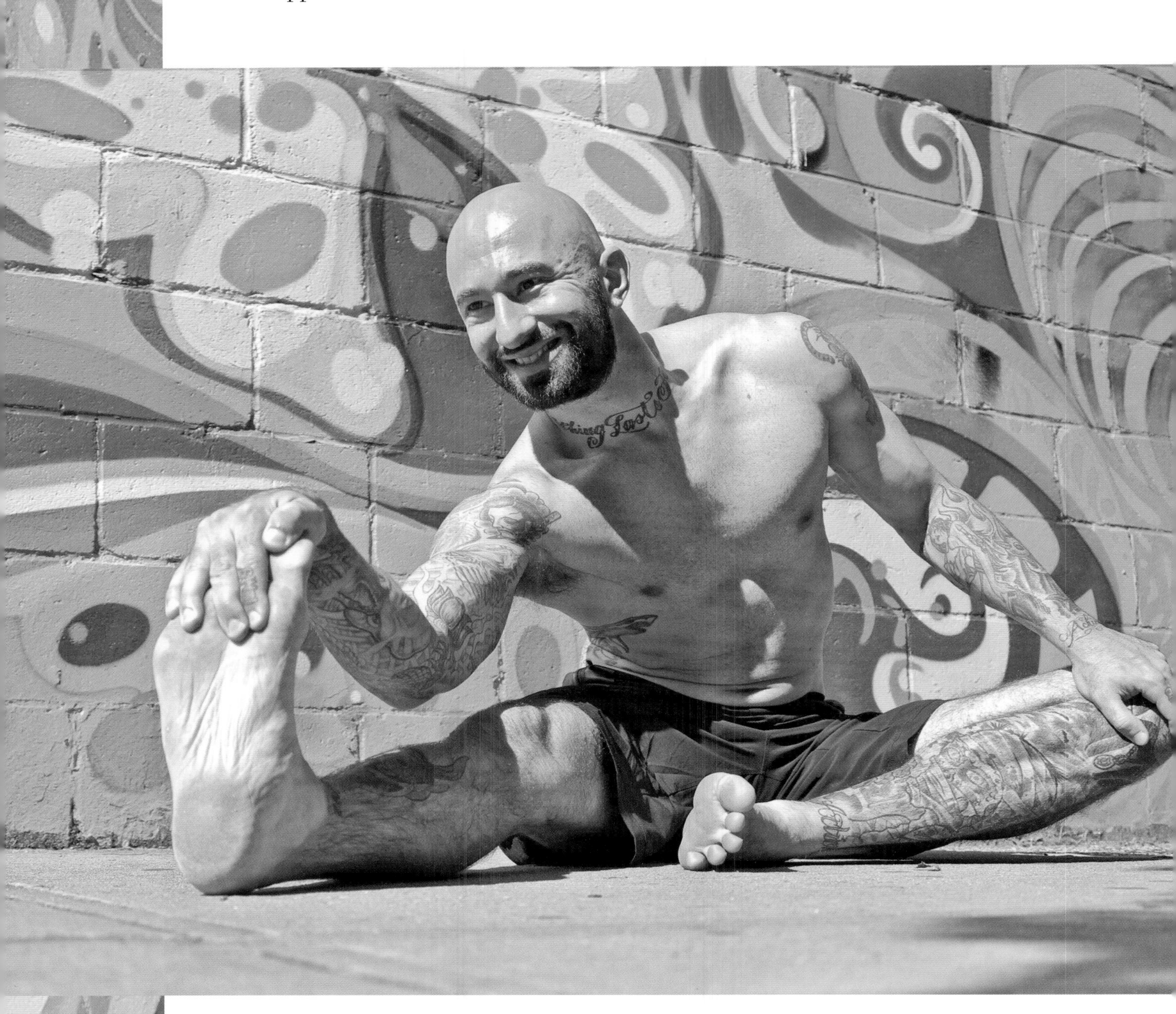

**Inhale:** Lift your chest and straighten your back while filling your belly with air

**Exhale:** Reach past your toes while thinking about bringing your elbow toward the knee of your extended leg

**Common Mistakes:** Excessive arching of the spine, external rotation of the extended leg (toes flaring out to the side)

**Primary Muscle Groups:** Hamstrings, calves, lower back, hips

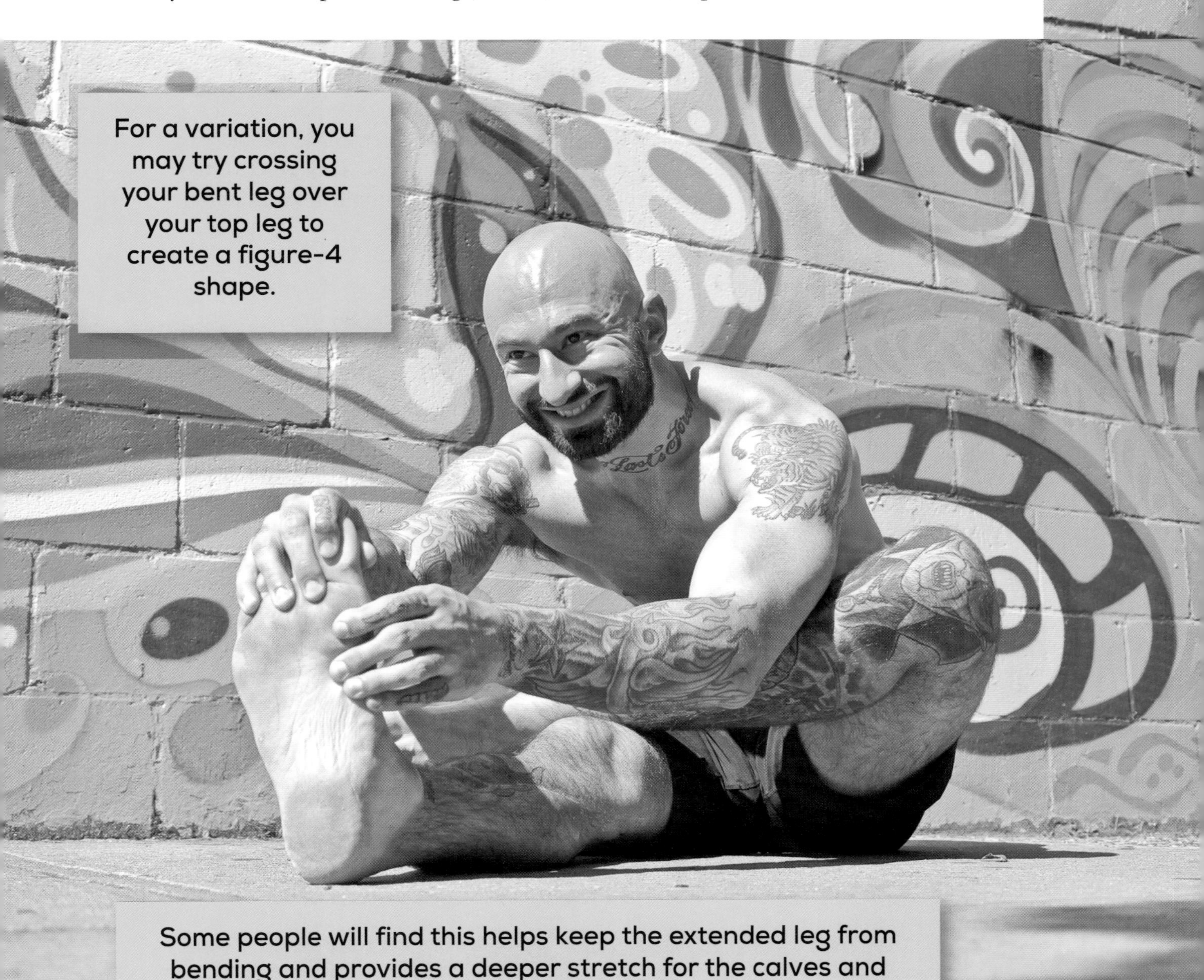

For a variation, you may try crossing your bent leg over your top leg to create a figure-4 shape.

Some people will find this helps keep the extended leg from bending and provides a deeper stretch for the calves and hamstrings. It also might give you a deeper stretch in the hip on the side of the bent leg.

# Full Straddle

Also known as a Side Split, achieving a Full Straddle requires patience and persistence. From the Half Straddle position, extend your bent leg so both legs are straight and spread as far apart as possible. Sit up with your chest tall and point your toes, keeping your legs straight. Think about rotating your hips outward - you want the backs of your thighs in contact with the ground rather than your inner thighs. Begin to lean forward as far as possible, hinging from your hips while reaching your arms out in front. Gradually work toward leaning farther forward and opening your legs wider.

For many, simply getting your legs to form a 90 degree angle to each other is going to be an adequate range of motion. If you decide to work toward a full side split remember to be patient. For some it will come fairly naturally, while others will need to put forth a lot of dedicated effort. With consistent practice, however, most people can gradually progress toward increasing the angle to a full 180 degrees. This process may take anywhere from a few weeks to several years depending on a number of variables.

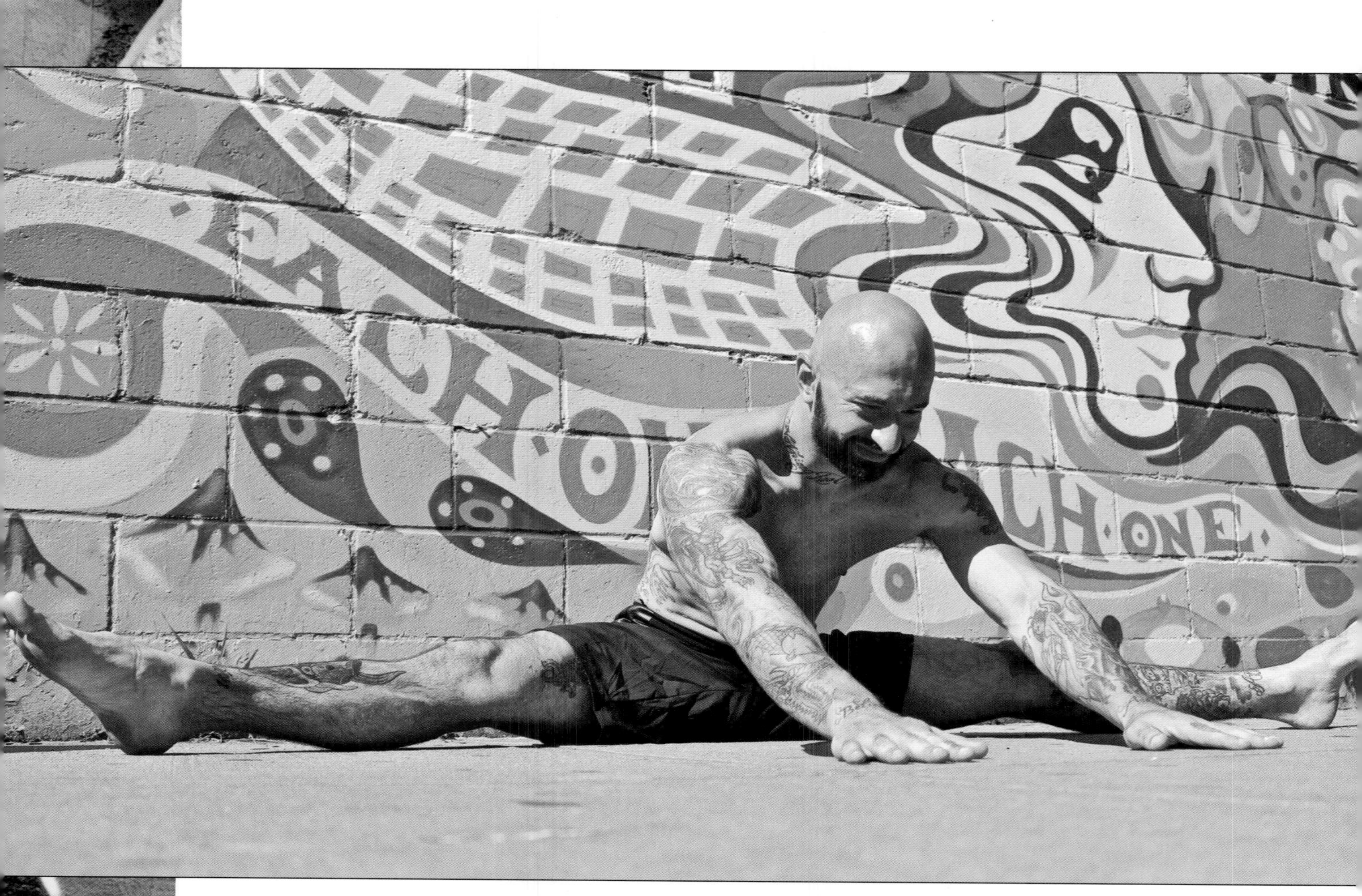

**Inhale:** Lift your chest and think about elongating your spine and legs

**Exhale:** Bend forward from the hips

**Common Mistakes:** Excessive rounding of the lower back, hips too far in front of torso (try to keep your buttocks away from the ground as much as possible)

**Primary Muscle Groups:** Groin, inner thighs, hamstrings, hips

**Calisthenics Counterpart:** Straddle Lever

The ability to perform a straddle is helpful for several lever variations.

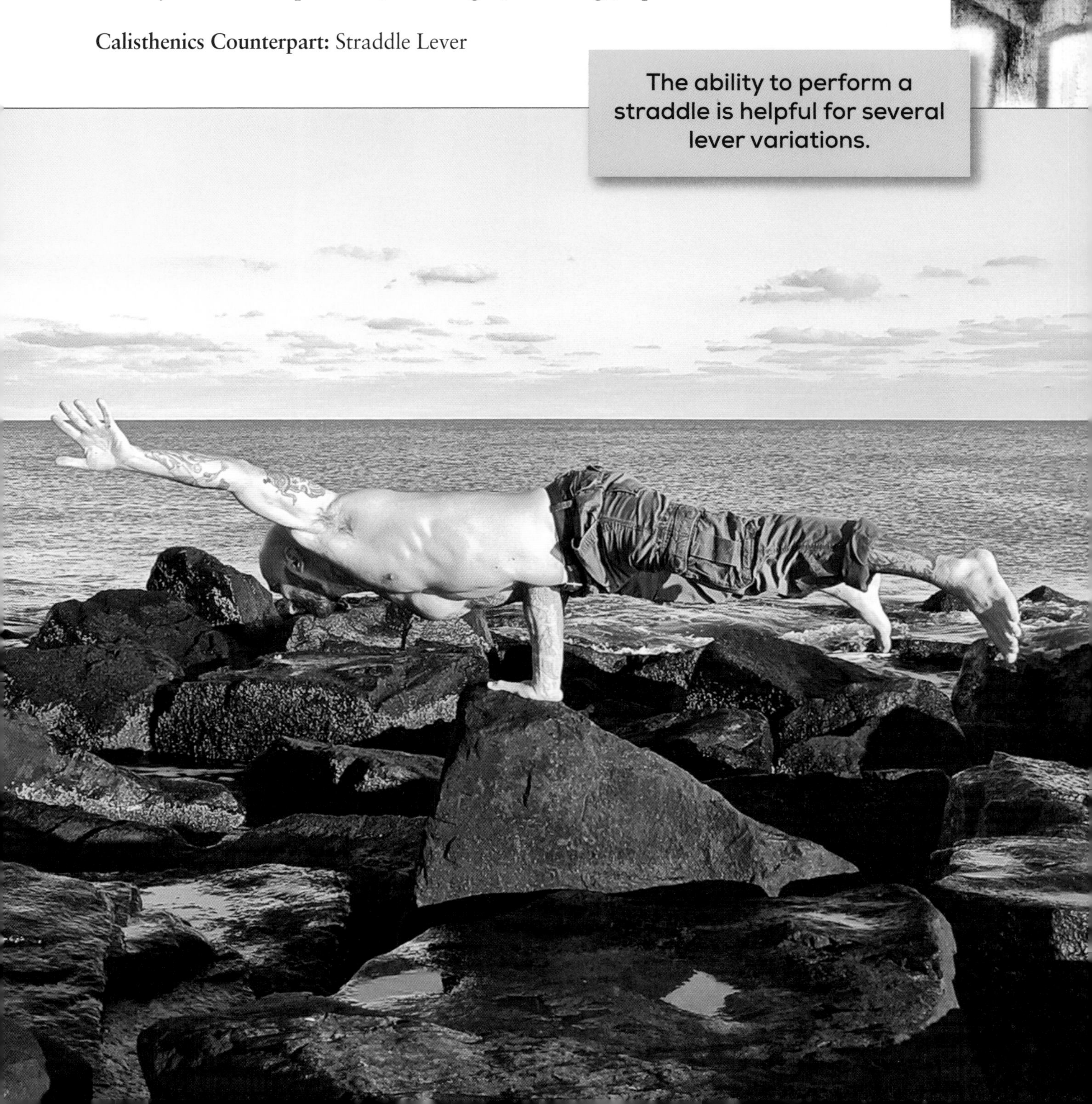

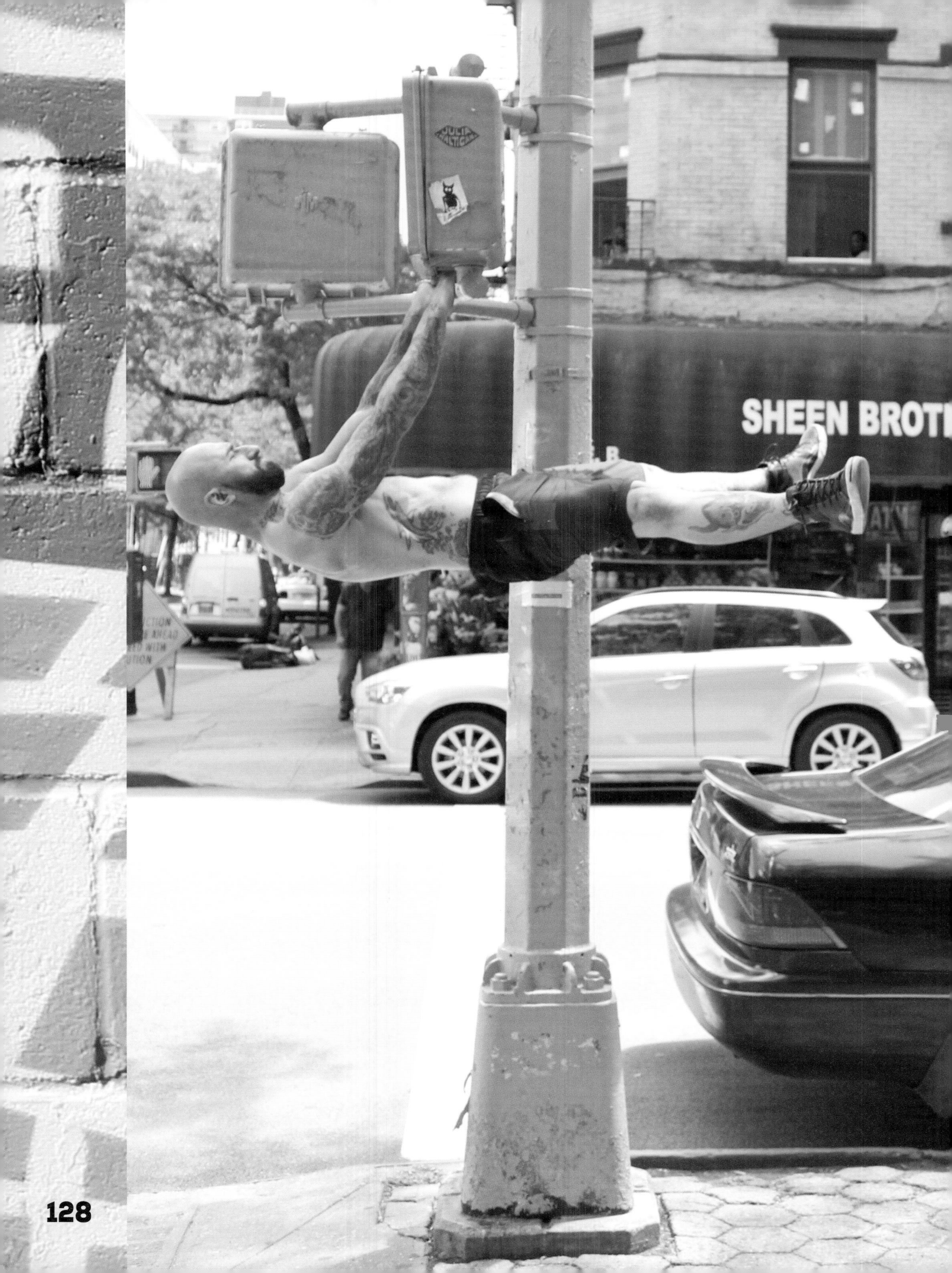
SHEEN BROT

# Wall Straddle

The Wall Straddle is a very useful stretch for anyone working toward the Full Straddle. Position your body so you're lying on your back with your legs inverted against a wall and your chest facing the ceiling. Slowly open your legs, keeping your hips as close to the wall as possible. Wiggle your feet lower toward the ground, using the wall for leverage. Point your toes, squeeze your quads and assist with your arms as needed. This can be a very useful technique to help increase your range of motion toward achieving a Full Straddle.

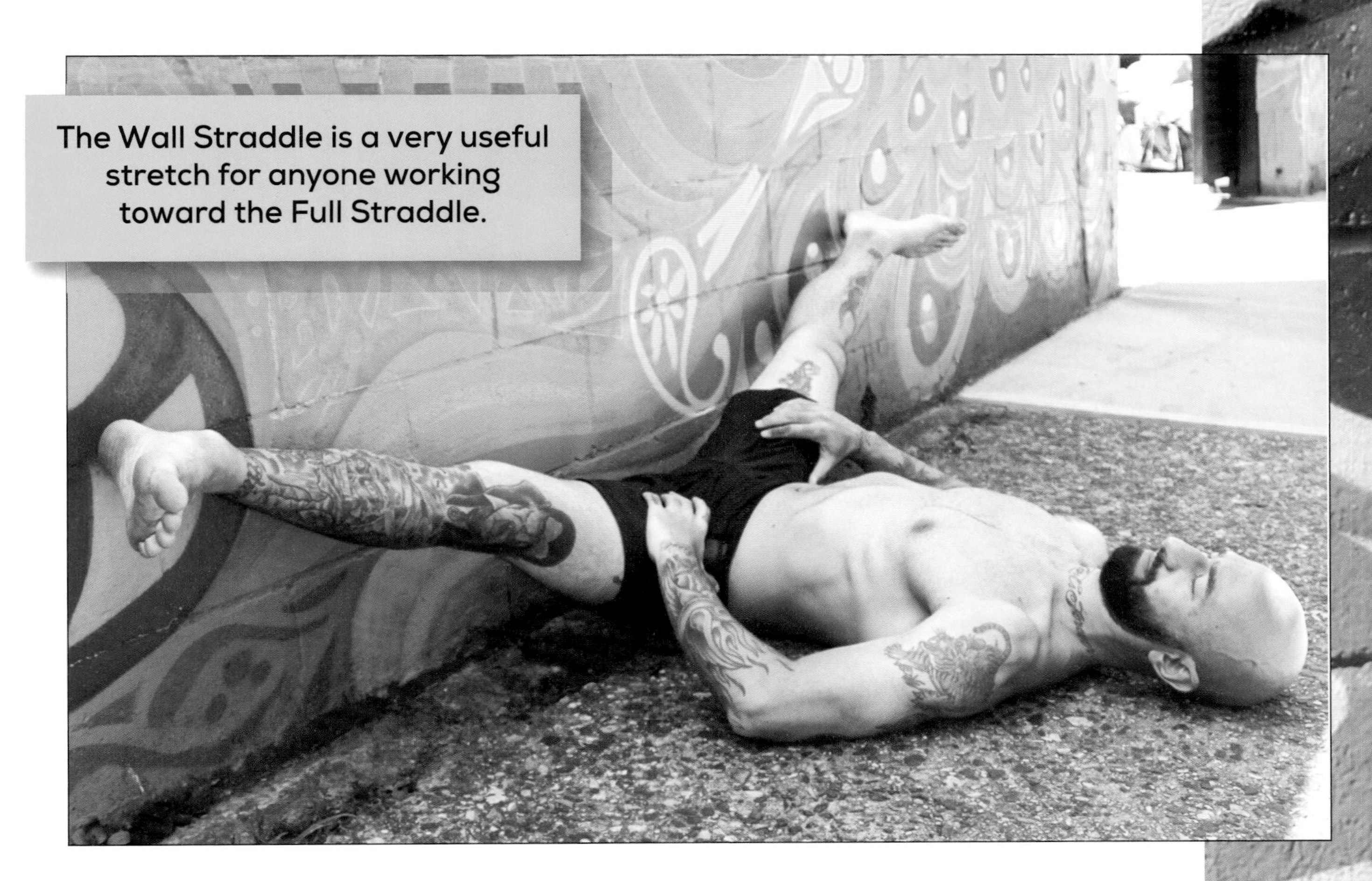


**Inhale:** Lengthen your spine and legs

**Exhale:** Gently open your legs wider

**Common Mistakes:** Hips too far away from the wall

**Primary Muscle Groups:** Groin, inner thighs, hamstrings, hips

**Calisthenics Counterpart:** Straddle Lever

# Butterfly

The Butterfly is a great hip and groin stretch for beginners. Sit upright and bend your knees to bring the soles of your feet together. Let your legs fall outward with the sides of your feet resting on the floor. Gently press your heels together and try to open your legs as wide as possible. Though many people will find their knees ride up close to their shoulders when starting out, aim toward getting them closer to the floor over time.

**Inhale:** Sit up straight and lengthen your spine

**Exhale:** Press your feet together and pitch your chest forward

**Common Mistakes:** Excessive rounding of the spine

**Primary Muscle Groups:** Groin, hips, inner thighs

**Calisthenics Counterpart:** Straddle Lever

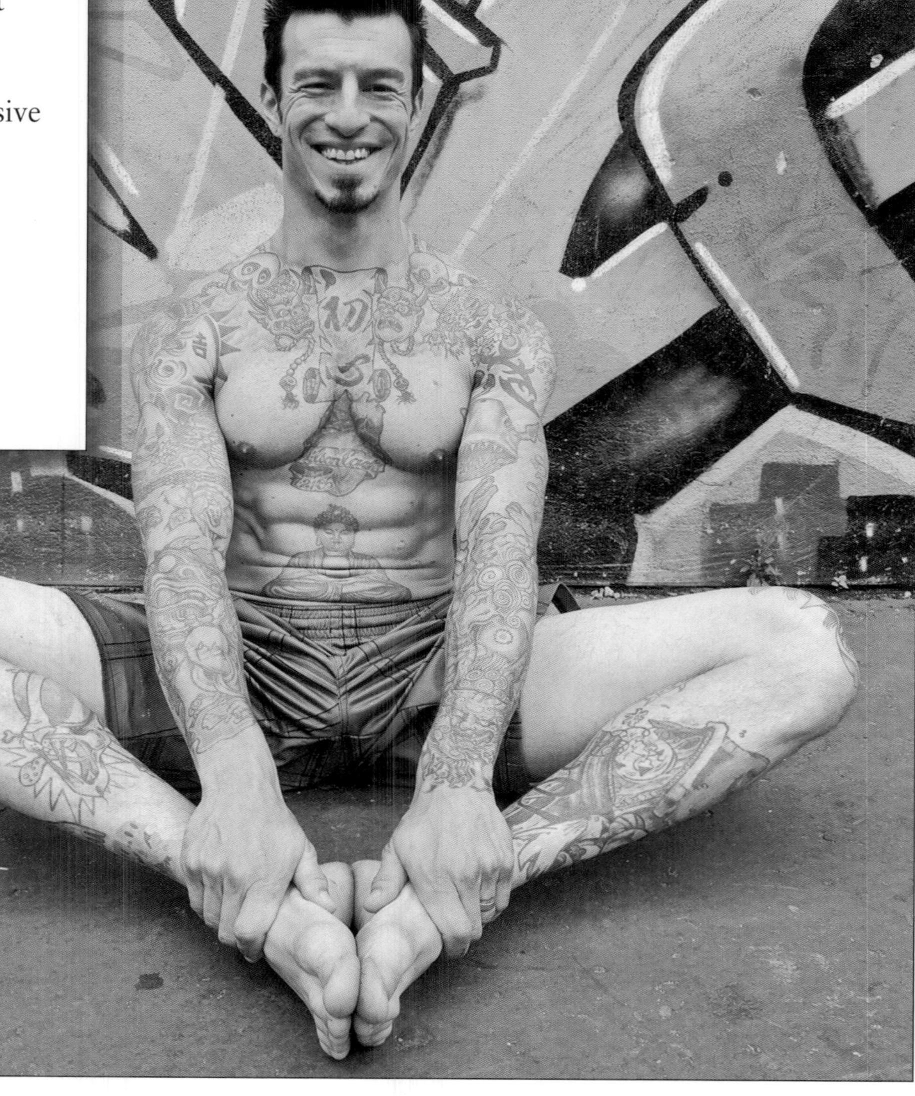

# Frog

The Frog pose is almost like an inverted version of the Butterfly. Begin in an "all-fours" position on your hands and knees with your back flat. Now drop down to your forearms and slowly slide your knees and legs out to the sides. Try to get your torso and inner thighs as close as possible to being flat on the ground. You may find it helpful to slowly flex and extend your hips and knees to get deeper into the stretch.

**Inhale:** Lengthen your spine and fill your belly with air

**Exhale:** Slowly try to open your knees wider

**Common Mistakes:** Excessive compression of the lower back

**Primary Muscle Groups:** Groin, hips, inner thighs

**Calisthenics Counterpart:** Straddle Lever

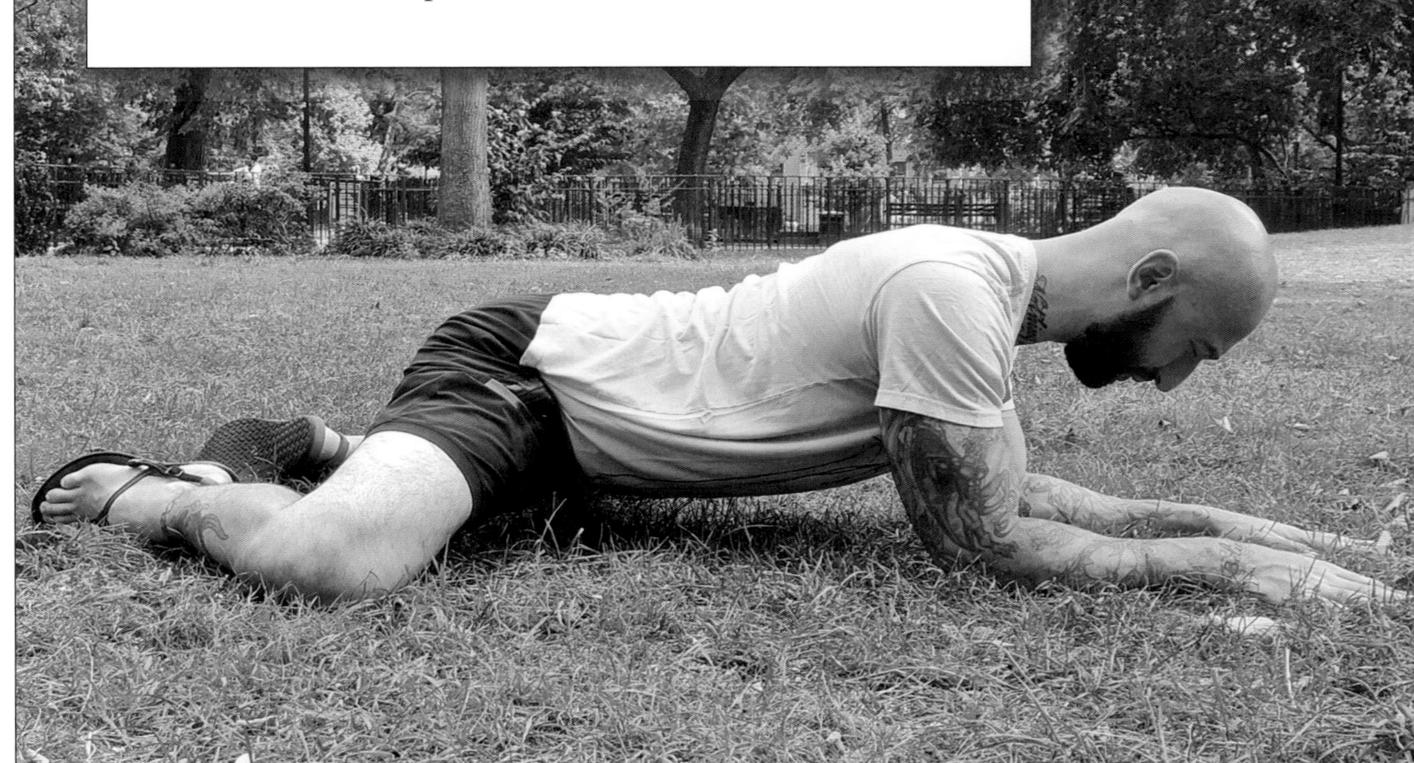

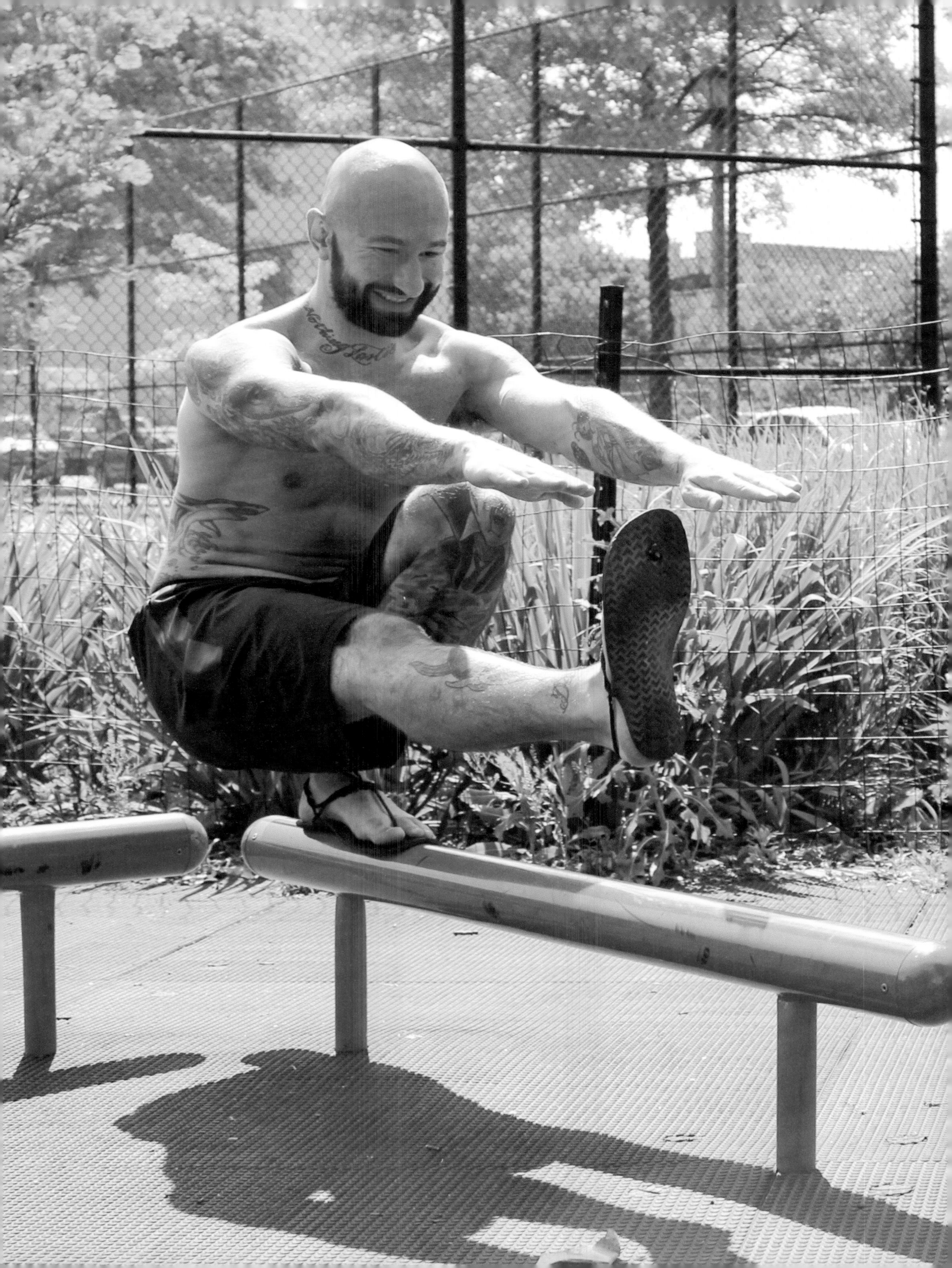

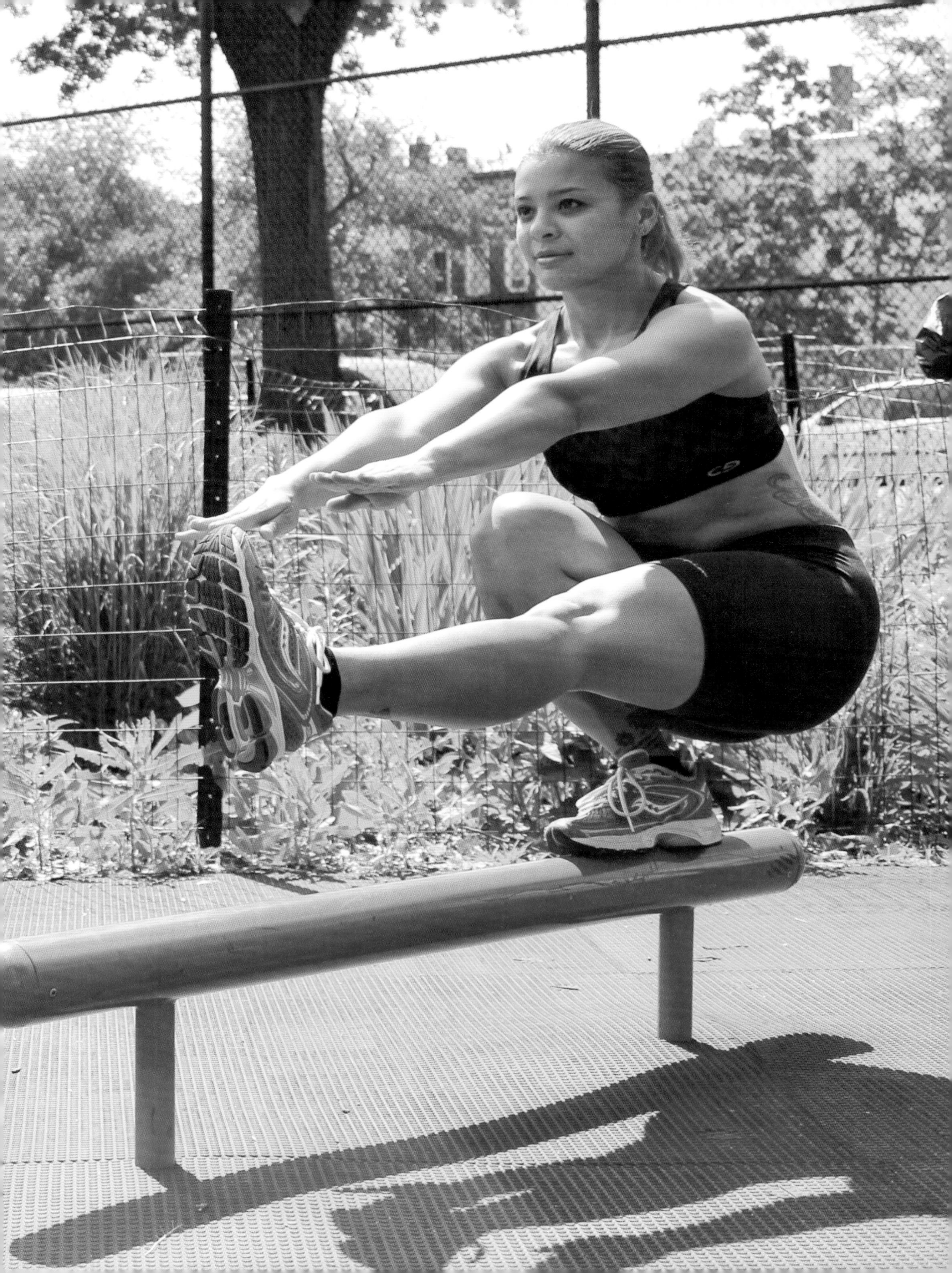

# Ankle to Knee Pose

The Ankle to Knee Pose is a great way to ease into deep hip stretching. Sit on the floor and bring your left leg in front of you with a deep bend in the knee. Gently press your outer thigh and knee to the ground with your hands. Now rotate your right leg to bring the outside of your right ankle to rest on top of your left knee. At first, you may have a lot of space between your shins. Use your arms for assistance to gently work toward bringing your shins to rest parallel on top of one another with each ankle touching the opposite knee. Hold for several breaths then switch sides.

**Inhale:** Sit up straight and relax your hips

**Exhale:** Gently press your knee down toward your opposite ankle

**Common Mistakes:** Excessive knee torque instead of hip rotation, hunched back and shoulders

**Primary Muscle Groups:** Hips

**Calisthenics Counterpart:** Cross-legged Pistol Squat

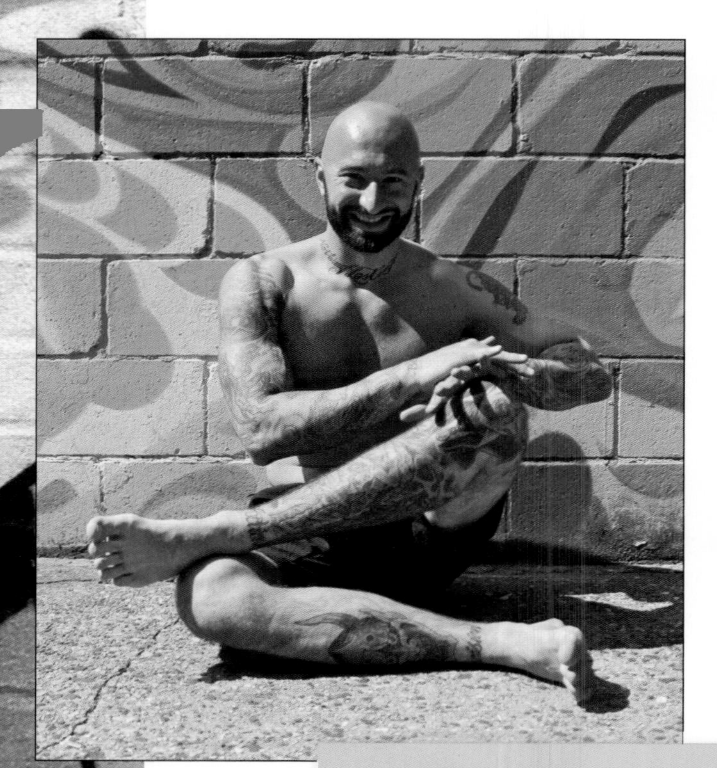

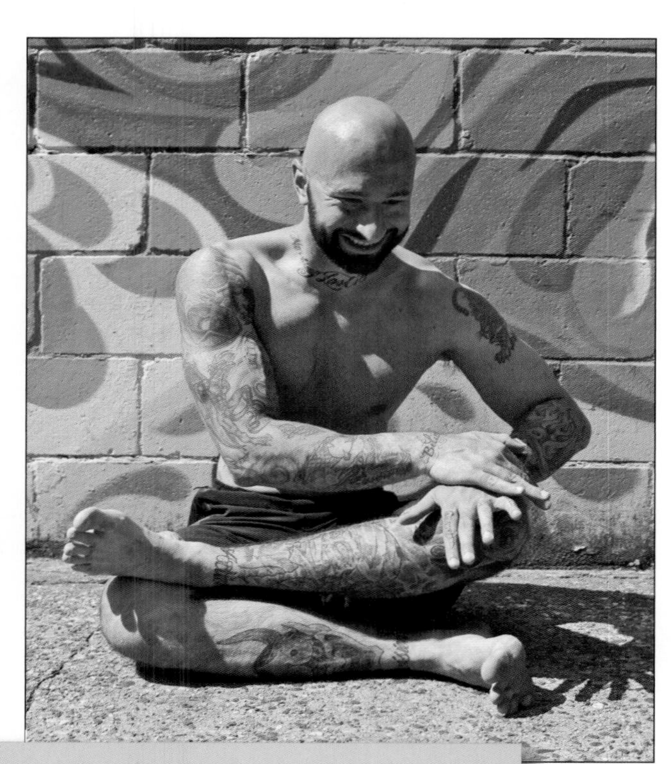

Use your arms for assistance to gently work toward bringing your shins to rest parallel on top of one another with each ankle touching the opposite knee.

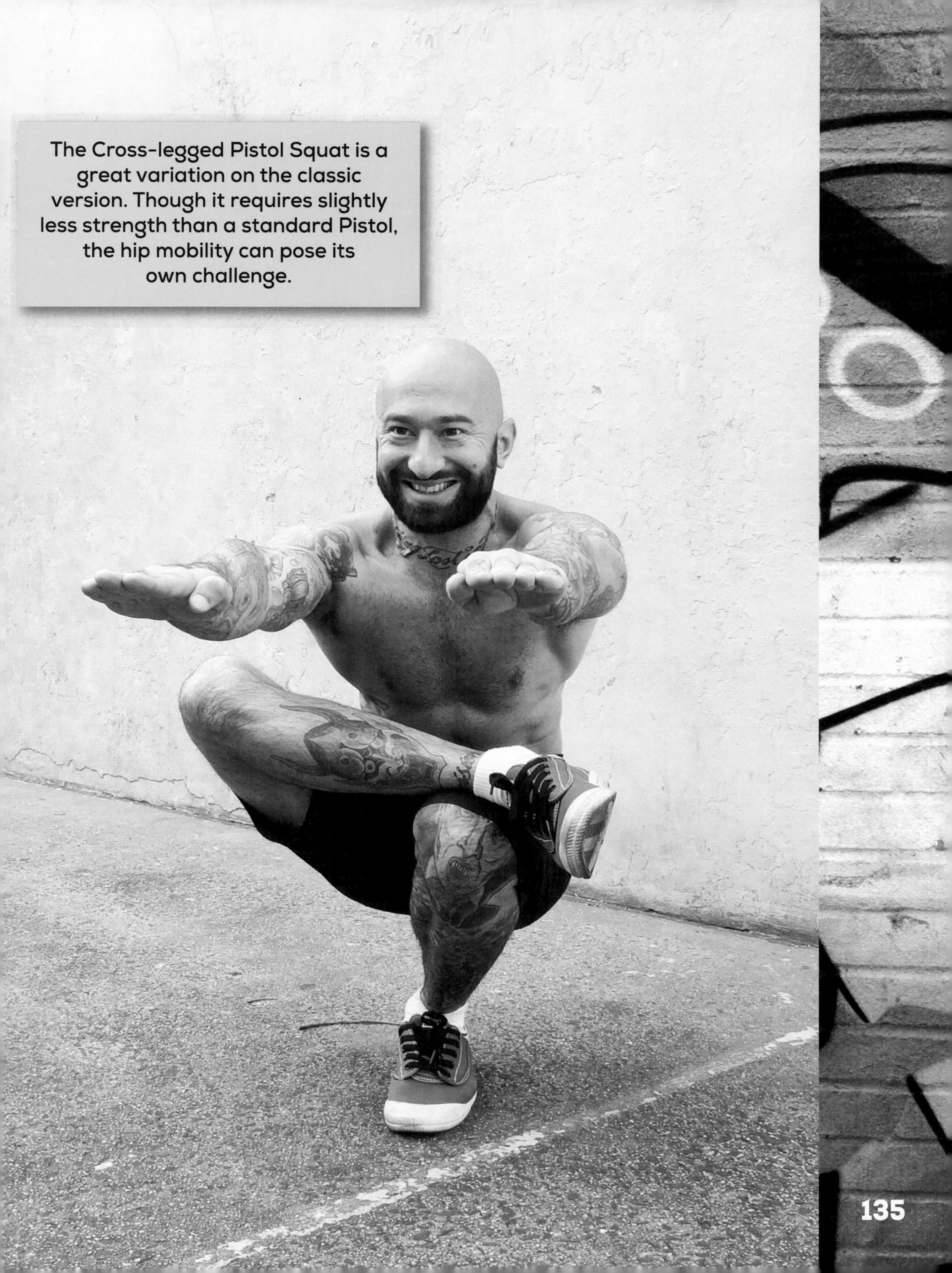

The Cross-legged Pistol Squat is a great variation on the classic version. Though it requires slightly less strength than a standard Pistol, the hip mobility can pose its own challenge.

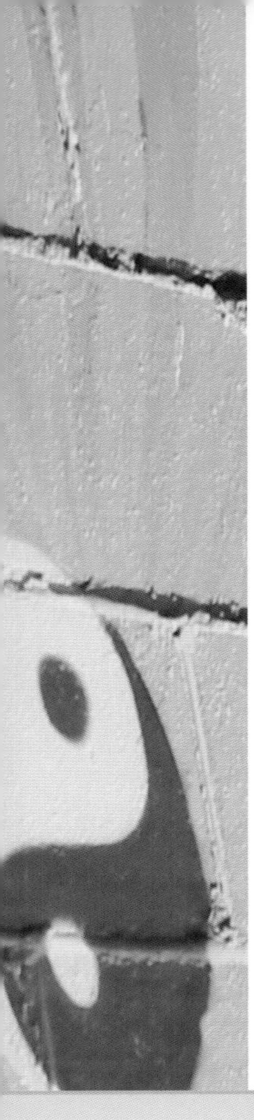

# Half Lotus

The Half Lotus is a hip-opener similar to the Ankle to Knee Pose, except with a deeper knee bend. Instead of placing your ankle on top of your opposite knee, slide it all the way up into your hip crease. Though you may not get the full range of motion for some time, wiggle your foot as far up as you can toward your hip (without causing any knee discomfort). The bottom leg should be in a deep bend as well. Hold for several breaths then switch sides.

**Inhale:** Lift the crown of your head and lengthen your spine

**Exhale:** Relax your hips and reach your knees away from your body

**Common Mistakes:** Excessive knee torque instead of hip rotation, hunched back and shoulders

**Primary Muscle Groups:** Hips, quads

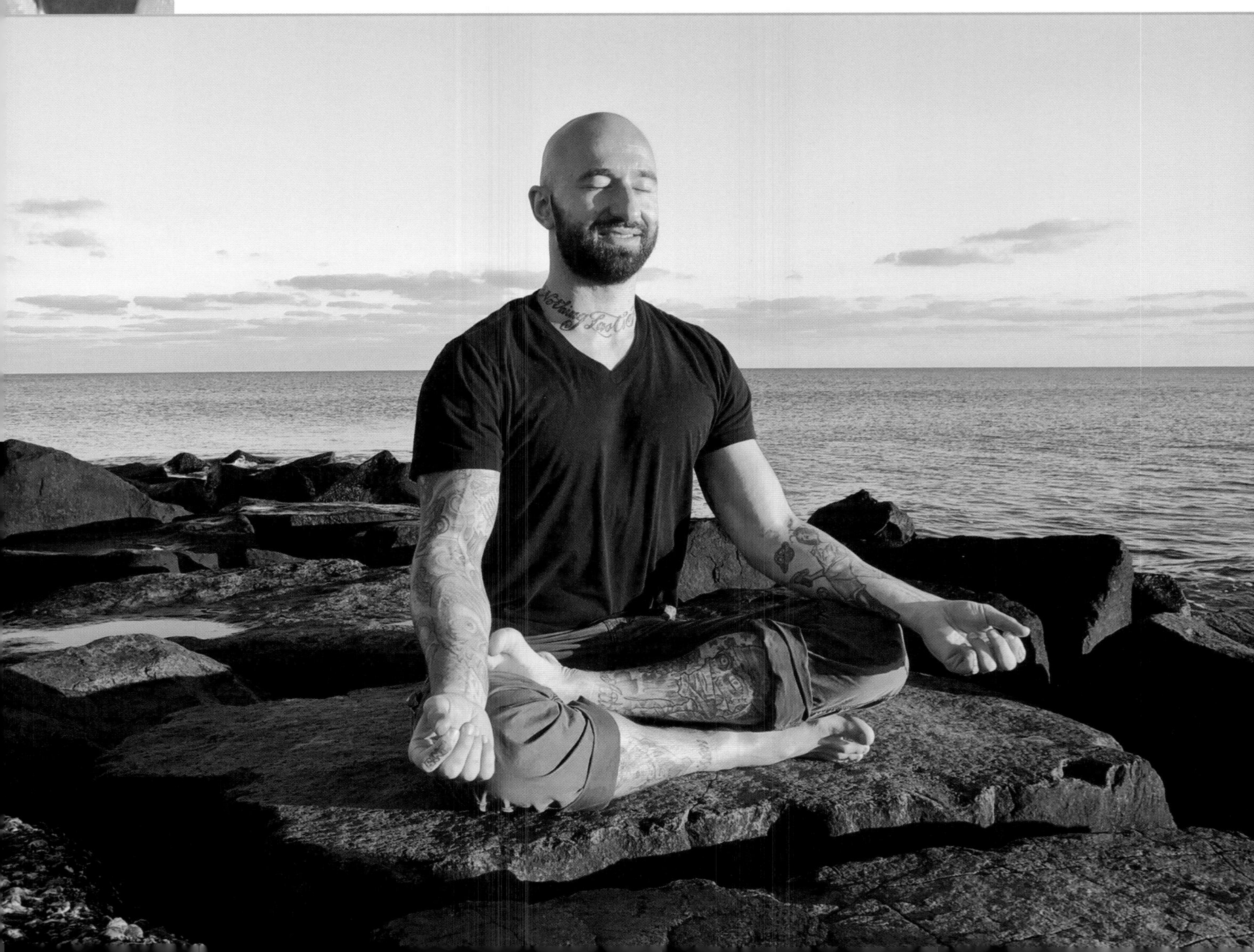

# Full Lotus

The Full Lotus is one of the most famous poses in yoga. From the Half Lotus position, lift your lower leg up and over your top leg, so the instep of each foot comes to rest in the opposite side's hip crease. Be mindful to take the stretch in your hips to avoid putting pressure on your knee joints.

**Inhale:** Lengthen your spine and fill your belly with air

**Exhale:** Rotate your hips and knees away from your body to relax deeper into the stretch

**Common Mistakes:** Torquing the knees due to tight hips, hunched back and shoulders

**Primary Muscle Groups:** Hips, glutes, quads

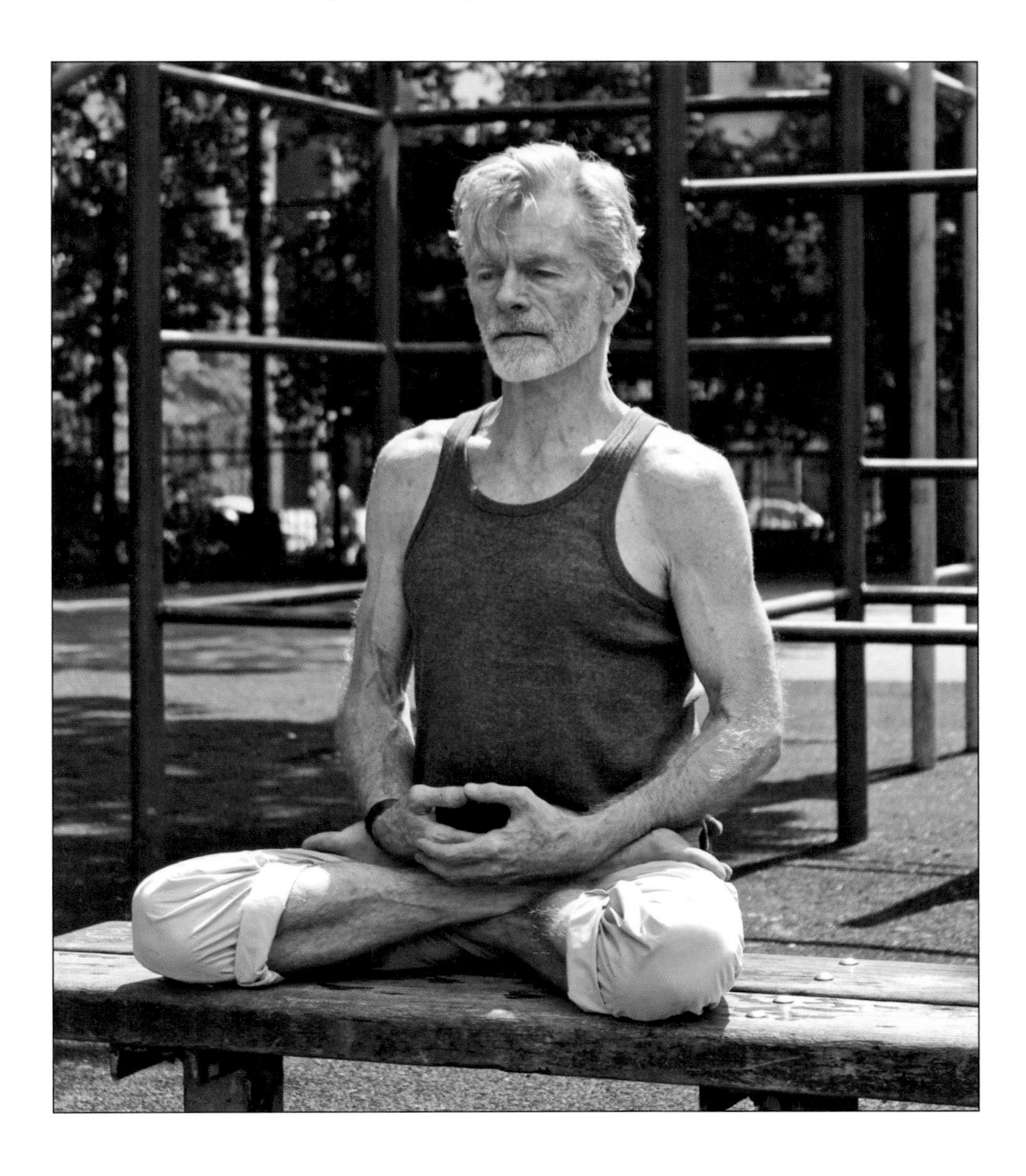

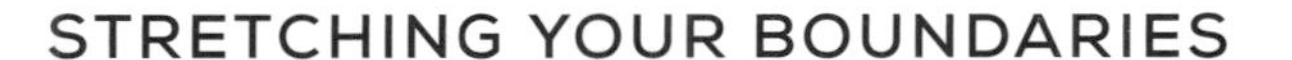

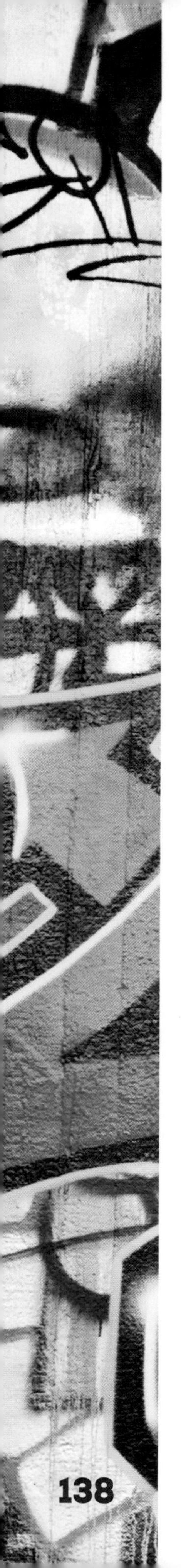

# Cow Face

This advanced hip opener is similar to the Ankle to Knee Pose, but provides an even deeper stretch. Instead of stacking your ankle on top of your knee, the aim is to stack your knees on top of each other, with each foot winding up next to the opposite hip. Cow Face pose is a very deep hip opener that's not appropriate for beginners.

**Inhale:** Lengthen your spine

**Exhale:** Gently ease your legs farther across one another

**Common Mistakes:** Hunched back and shoulders, excessive knee torque instead of hip rotation

**Primary Muscle Groups:** Hips, glutes

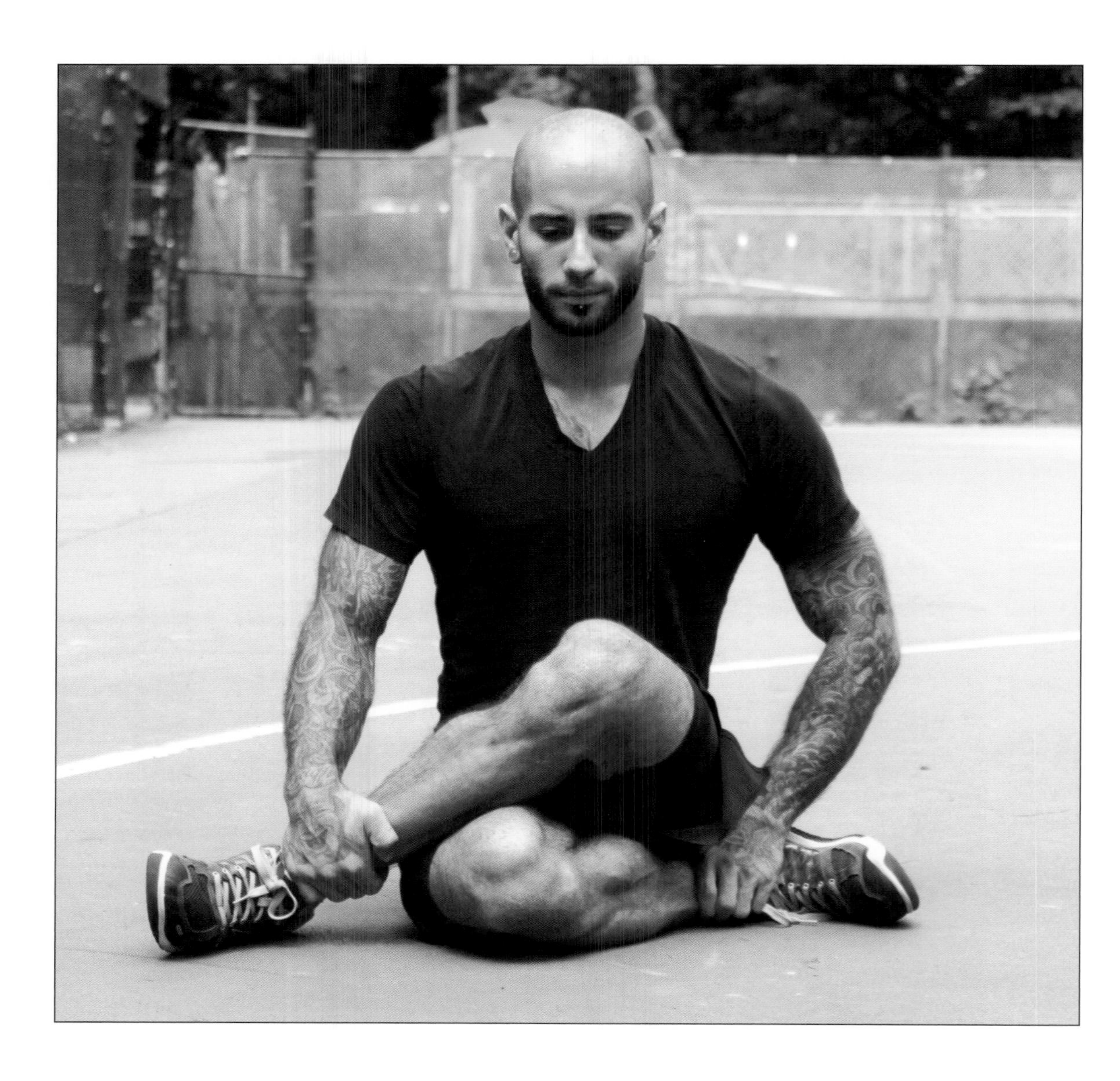

# Lying Knee to Chest

The Lying Knee to Chest stretch is like a grounded version of the Standing Single Leg Foot Hold. Lie on your back and bring your left knee toward your torso, grabbing your lower leg with both hands. Try to get your fingers interlaced around your shin. You can curl your upper back off the floor if you need to in order to get your grip. Once you have a solid grasp around your leg, lie back and attempt to get your back totally flat on the ground. Think about pulling your knee around your rib cage toward your left armpit, rather than bringing it straight up against your chest. Hug your elbows to your sides and keep your opposite leg straight. Repeat on the right side.

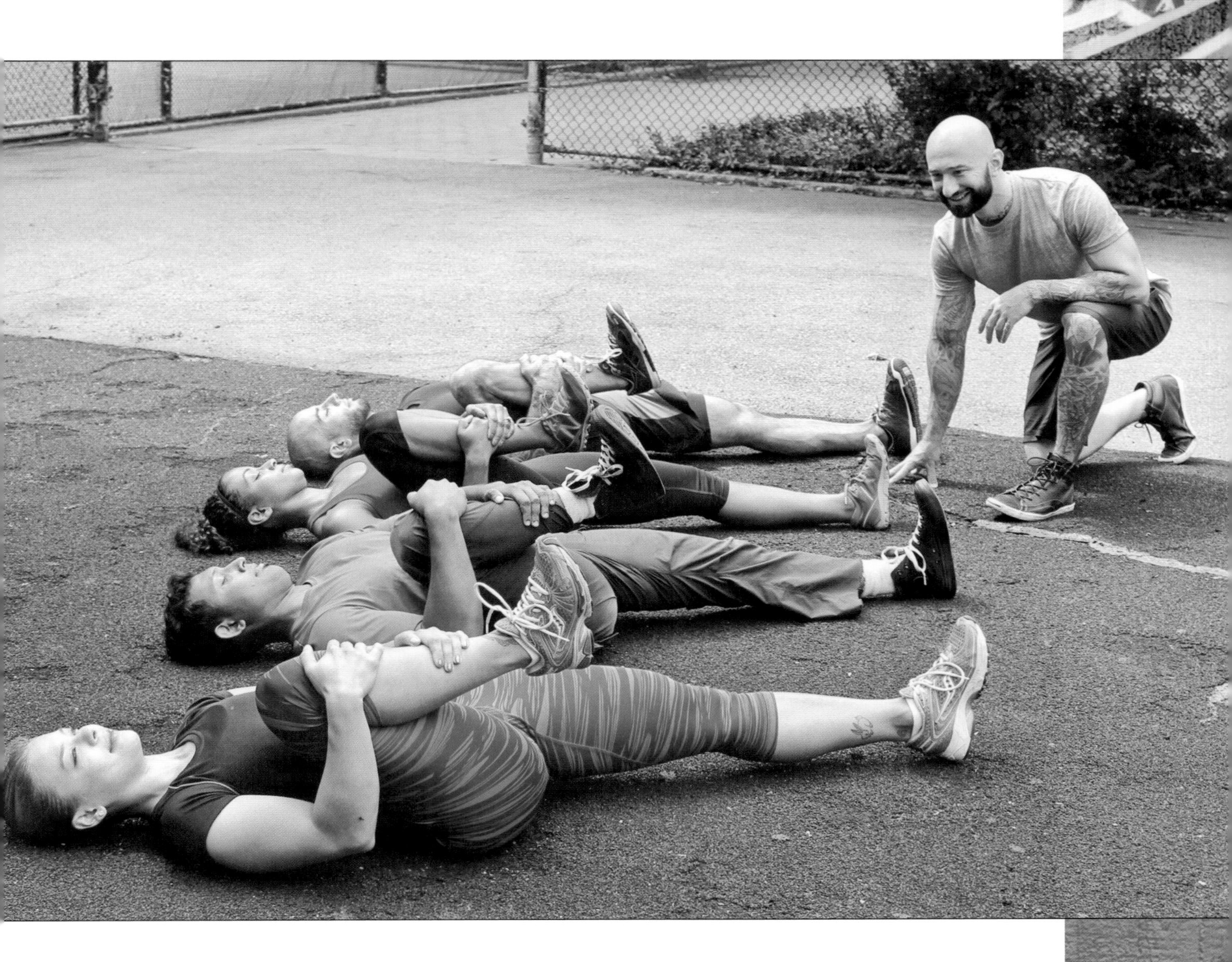

**Inhale:** Lengthen your spine

**Exhale:** Pull your knee deeper toward your armpit

**Common Mistakes:** Pulling the knee straight to the chest

**Primary Muscle Groups:** Hips, hamstrings

**Calisthenics Counterpart:** Half Tuck Lever

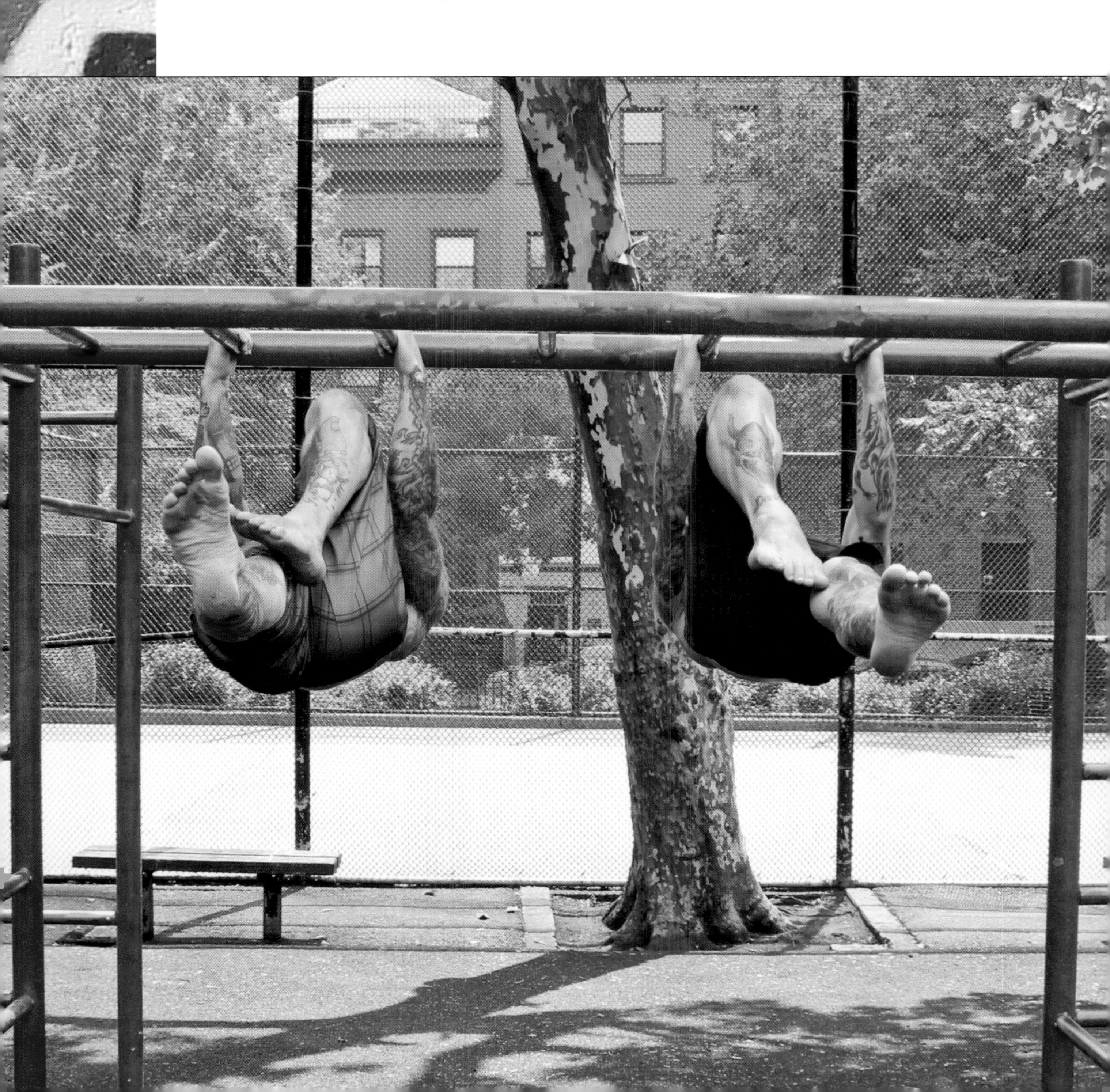

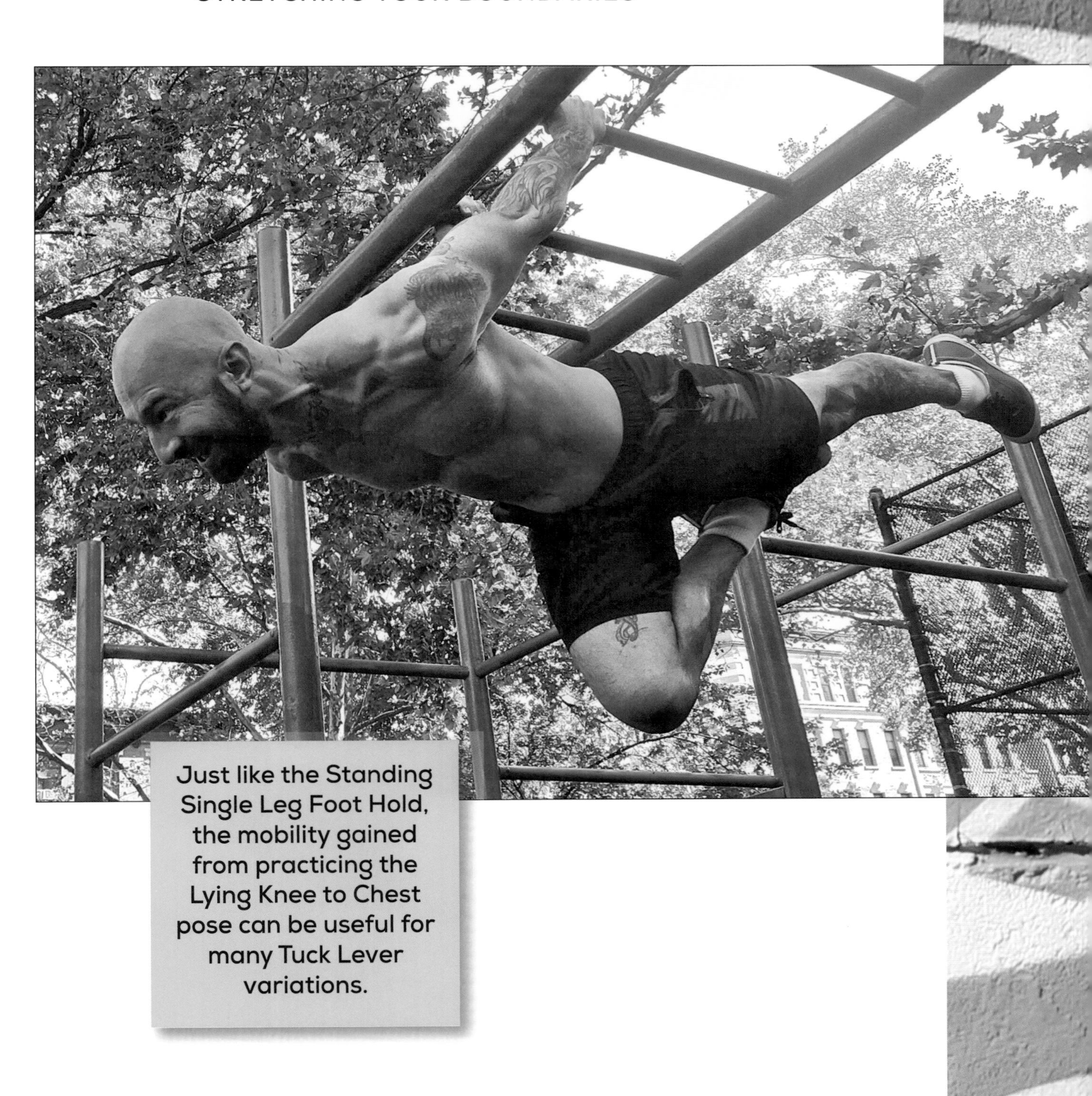

Just like the Standing Single Leg Foot Hold, the mobility gained from practicing the Lying Knee to Chest pose can be useful for many Tuck Lever variations.

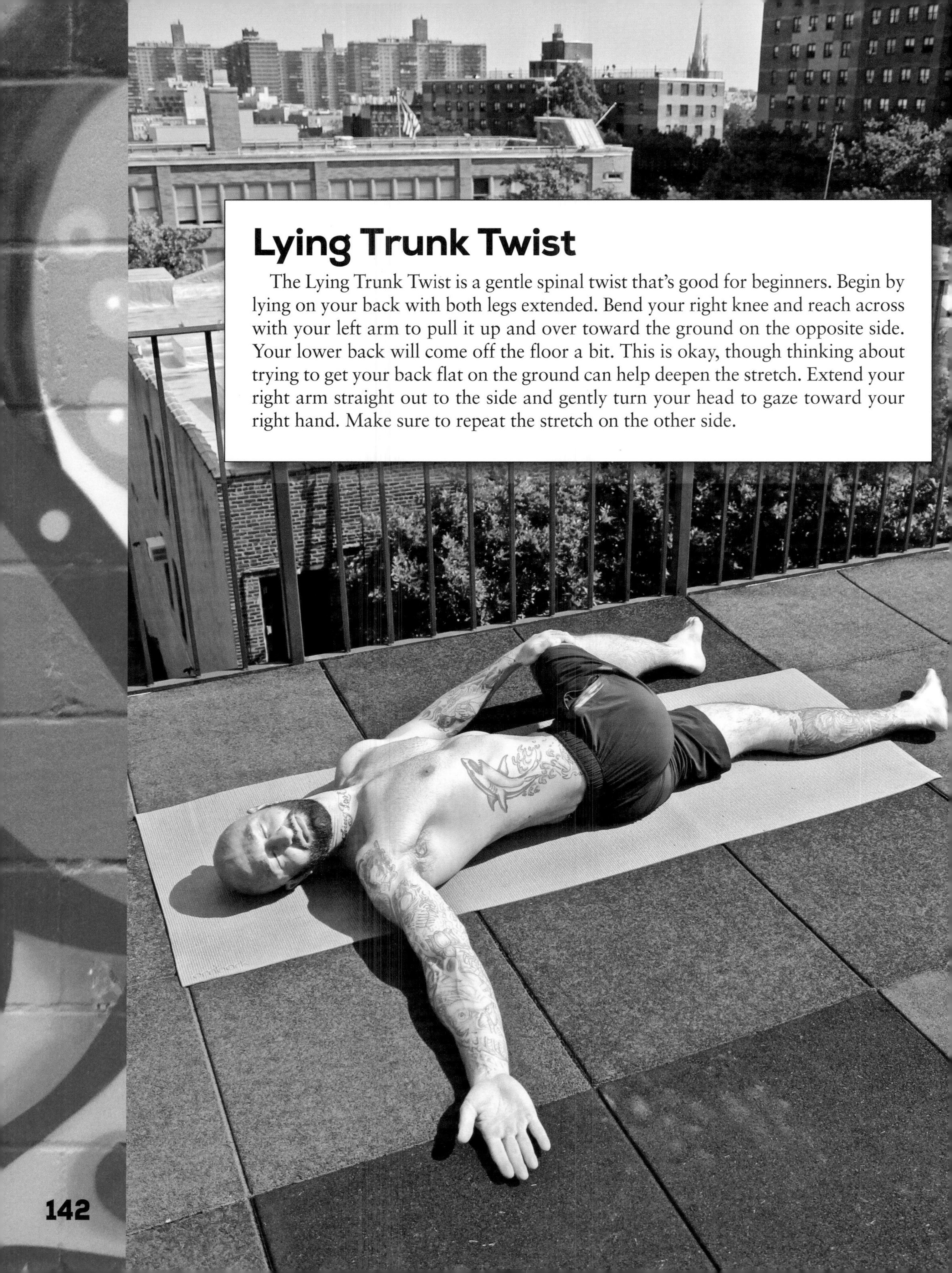

# Lying Trunk Twist

The Lying Trunk Twist is a gentle spinal twist that's good for beginners. Begin by lying on your back with both legs extended. Bend your right knee and reach across with your left arm to pull it up and over toward the ground on the opposite side. Your lower back will come off the floor a bit. This is okay, though thinking about trying to get your back flat on the ground can help deepen the stretch. Extend your right arm straight out to the side and gently turn your head to gaze toward your right hand. Make sure to repeat the stretch on the other side.

**Inhale:** Reach your free arm out to the side and lengthen your spine

**Exhale:** Gently pull your knee further across your body

**Common Mistakes:** Back strain due to placing excessive pressure on the bent knee

**Primary Muscle Groups:** Trunk, hips, glutes

**Calisthenics Counterpart:** Twisting Hanging Knee Raise

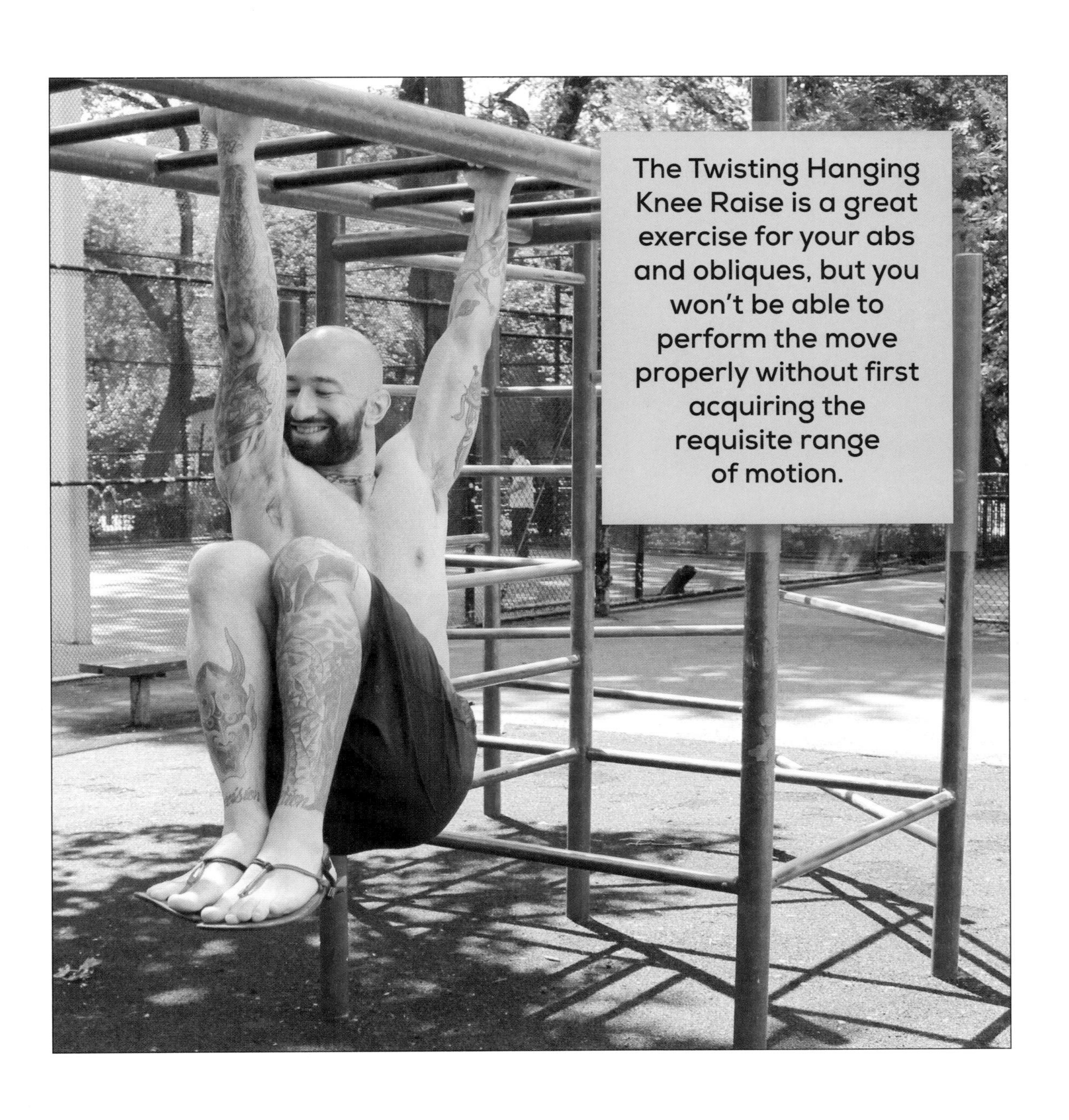

The Twisting Hanging Knee Raise is a great exercise for your abs and obliques, but you won't be able to perform the move properly without first acquiring the requisite range of motion.

# Seated Trunk Twist

The Seated Trunk Twist is a slightly more difficult spinal twist than the lying version. Sit on the ground with both legs extended straight in front of you. Now bend your right leg and cross it over the left, placing your right foot flat on the floor. From here, twist your trunk and reach your left arm out in front of your right knee. Your right hand should be placed palm down on the floor a few inches behind your back as you twist and look over your right shoulder. From here you can bend your left leg as well, tucking the foot beneath your opposite hip. For an added stretch, reach your right hand behind your back while threading your left hand through the opening beneath your right knee, bringing your hands into a bind (or gripping a cloth between the hands if a bind is not yet attainable). Make sure to repeat the stretch on both sides.

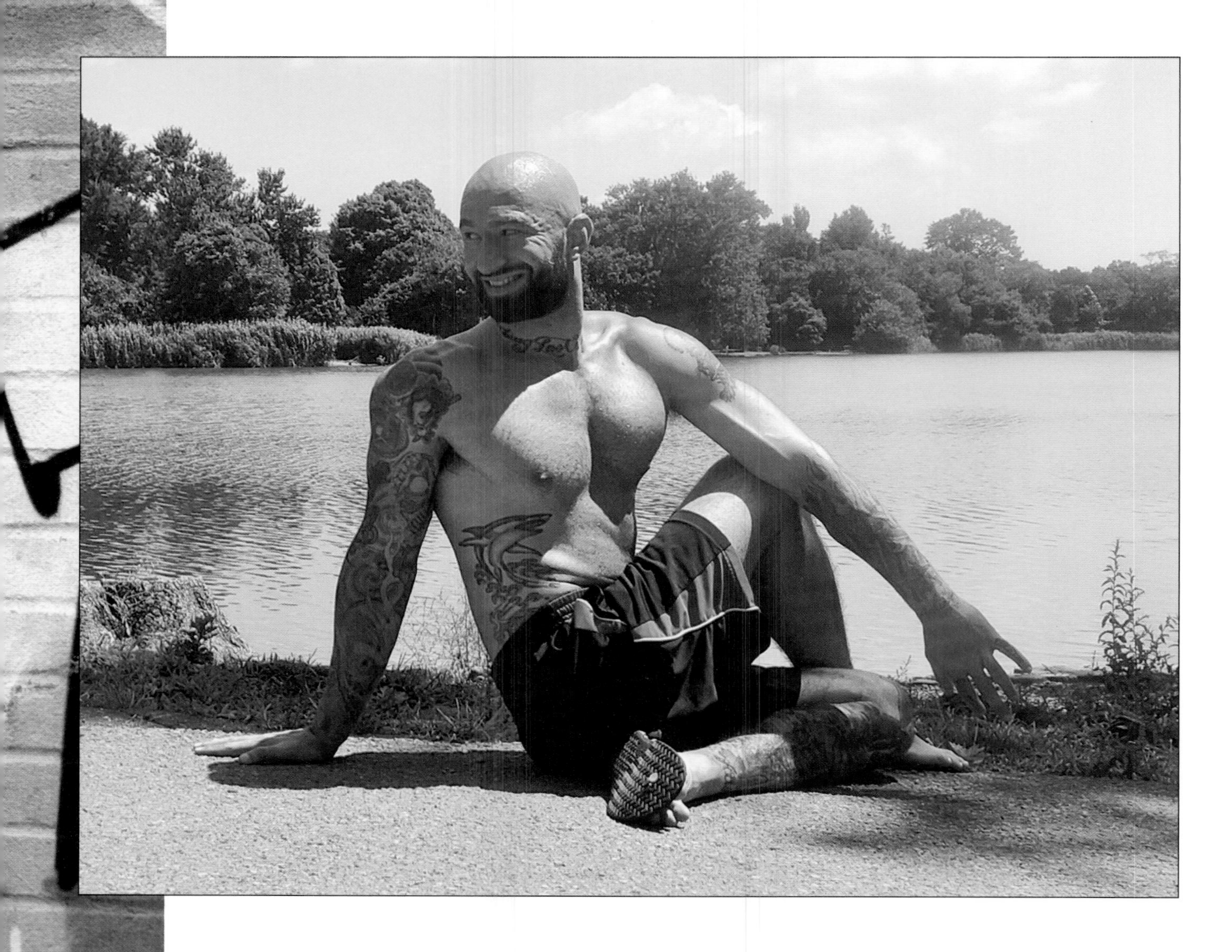

**Inhale:** Lengthen your spine

**Exhale:** Twist from your trunk and look over your shoulder

**Common Mistakes:** Hunched back, shrugged shoulders

**Primary Muscle Groups:** Hips, glutes, trunk, shoulders and spine

**Calisthenics Counterpart:** Twisting Hanging Knee Raise

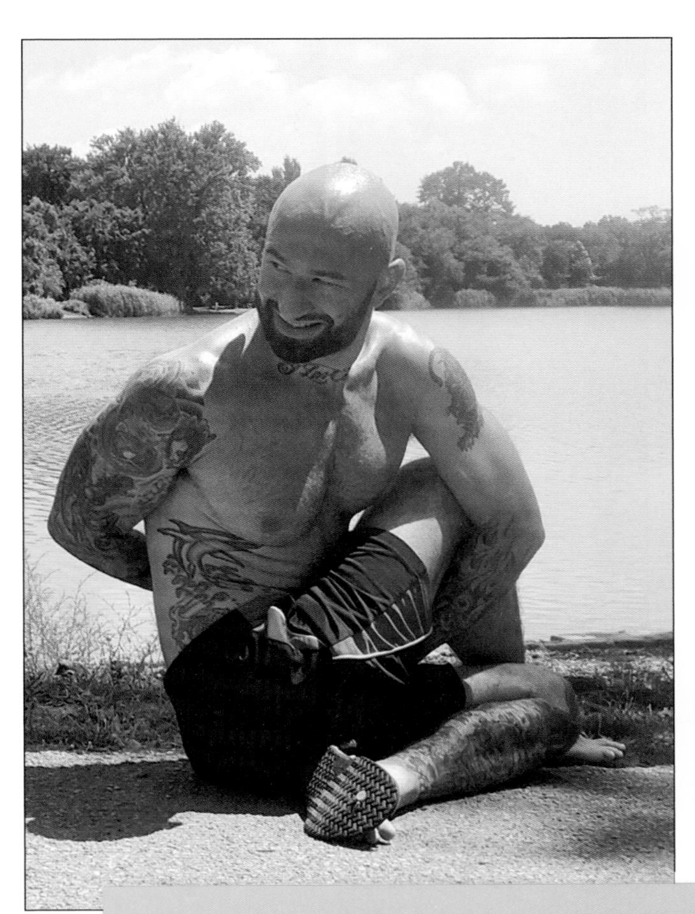

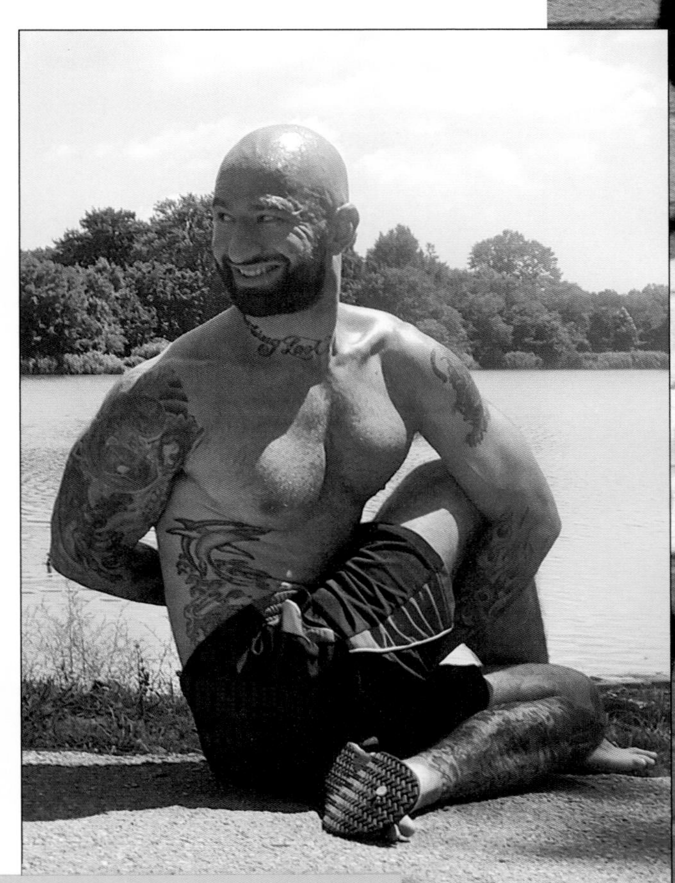

For an added stretch, reach your right hand behind your back while threading your left hand through the opening beneath your right knee, bringing your hands into a bind.

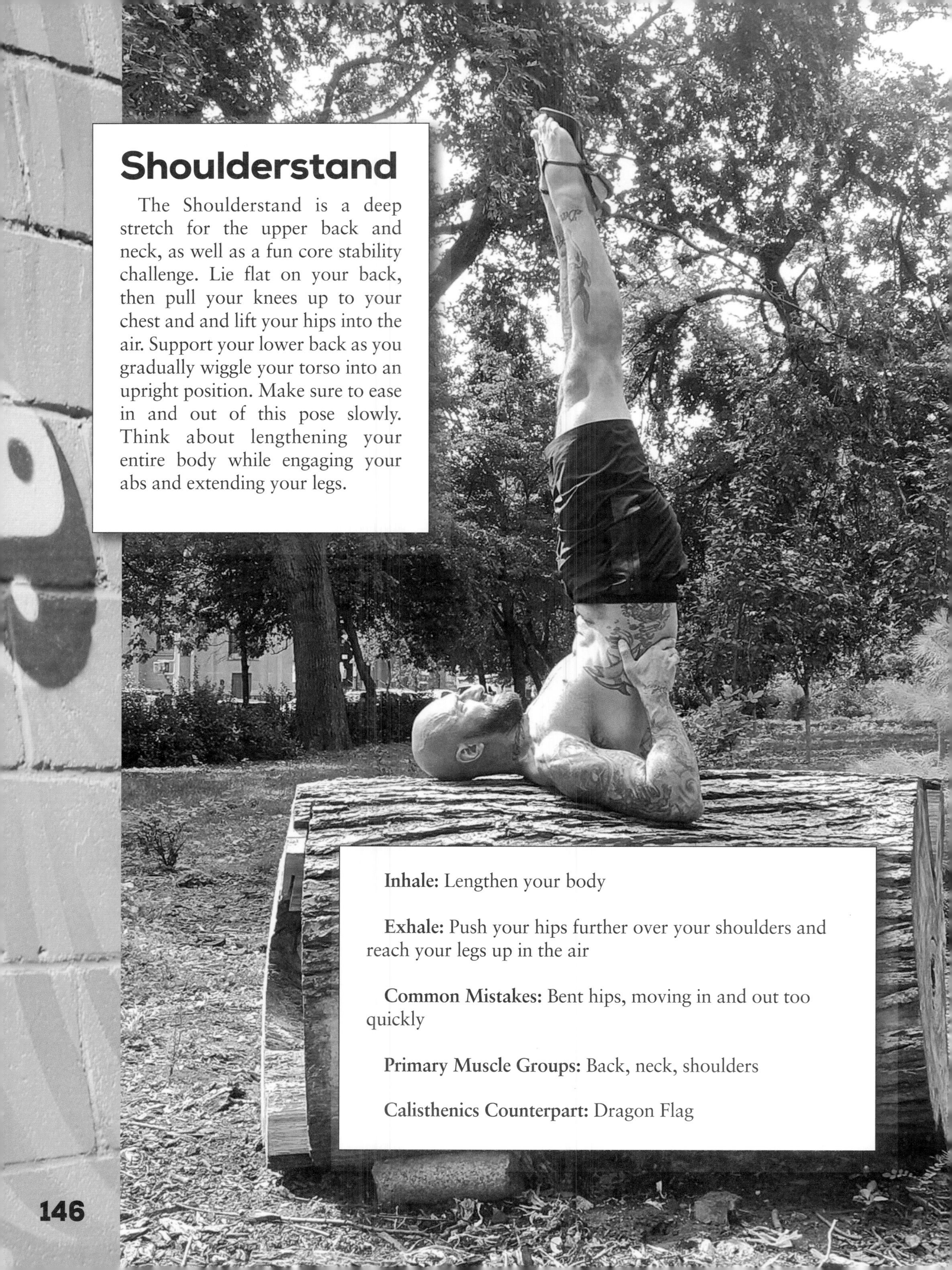

# Shoulderstand

The Shoulderstand is a deep stretch for the upper back and neck, as well as a fun core stability challenge. Lie flat on your back, then pull your knees up to your chest and and lift your hips into the air. Support your lower back as you gradually wiggle your torso into an upright position. Make sure to ease in and out of this pose slowly. Think about lengthening your entire body while engaging your abs and extending your legs.

**Inhale:** Lengthen your body

**Exhale:** Push your hips further over your shoulders and reach your legs up in the air

**Common Mistakes:** Bent hips, moving in and out too quickly

**Primary Muscle Groups:** Back, neck, shoulders

**Calisthenics Counterpart:** Dragon Flag

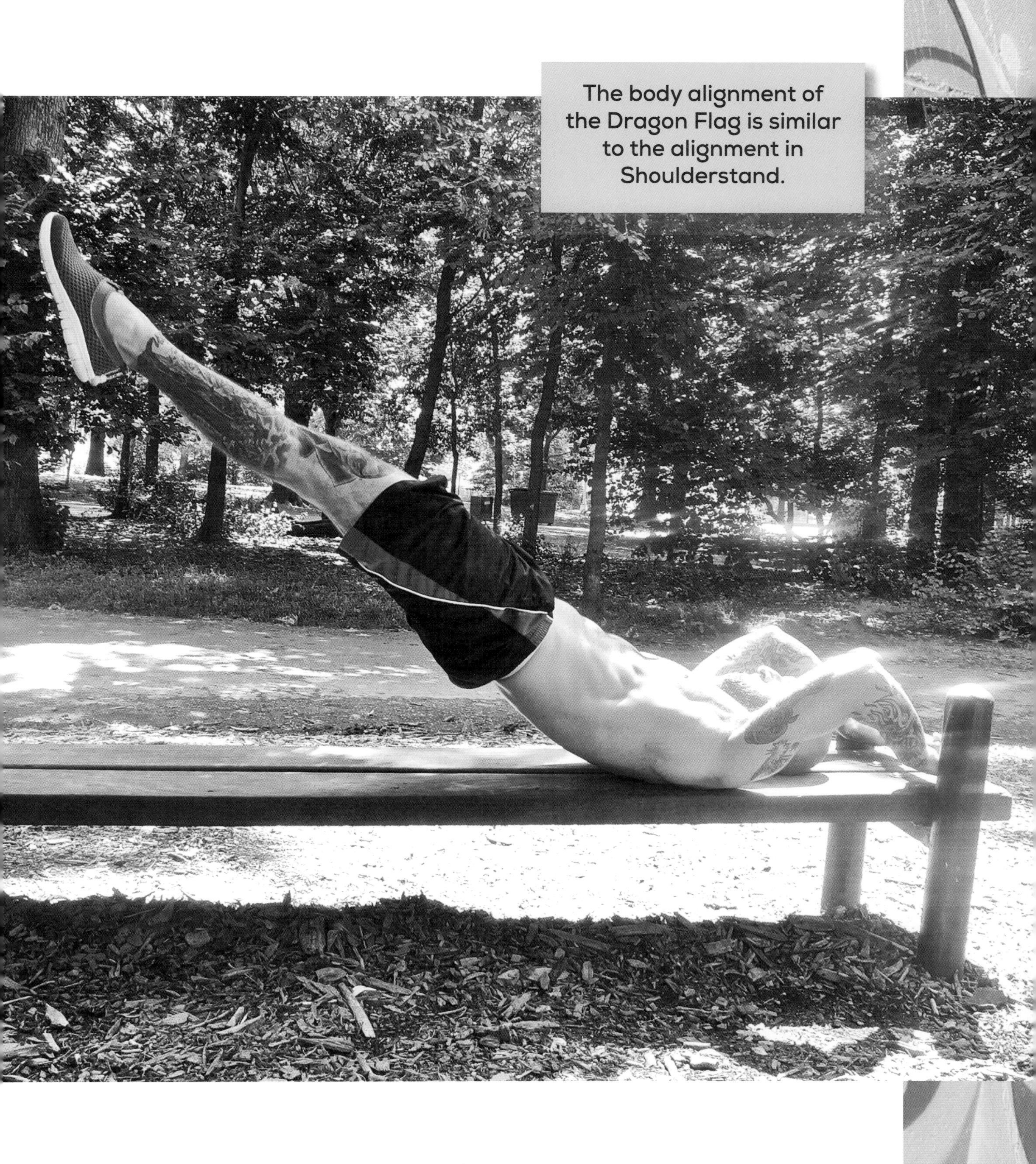

The body alignment of the Dragon Flag is similar to the alignment in Shoulderstand.

# Plow

The Plow pose is an intense stretch for the entire posterior chain. From the Shoulderstand position, slowly lower your legs behind your head. Take your arms away from your hips and lay them flat on the floor with your palms down. You may need to bend your knees at first. Over time, work toward getting your legs straighter. You may also find it helpful to practice lowering your legs from the Shoulderstand position one at a time.

**Inhale:** Lift your hips as high as you can

**Exhale:** Reach your legs farther behind your body and relax deeper into the stretch

**Common Mistakes:** Moving in and out too quickly

**Primary Muscle Groups:** Back, neck, shoulders, hamstrings

**Calisthenics Counterpart:** Skin the Cat

Just like its standing version, the shoulder mobility gained from the Plow pose is helpful for the Skin the Cat exercise.

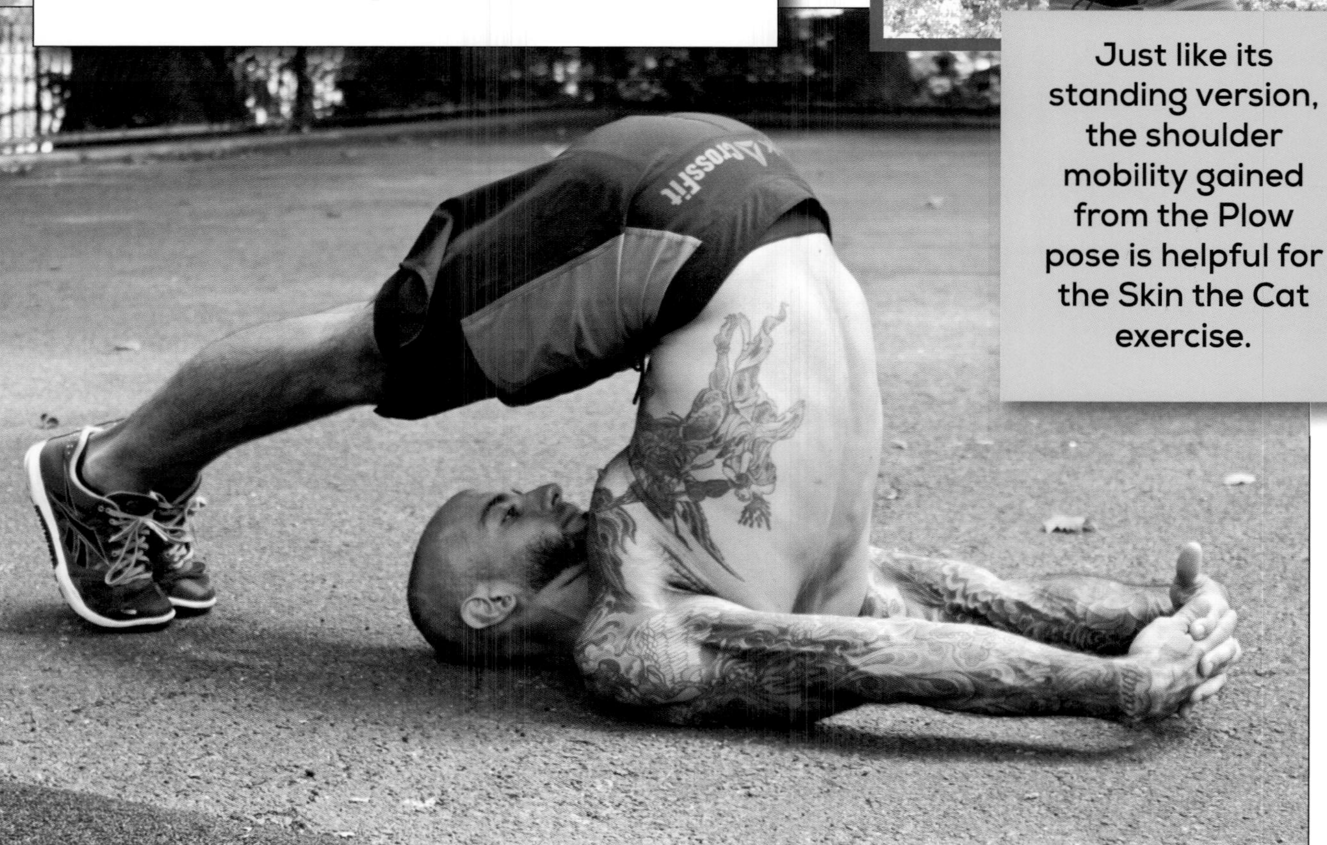

# Dead Man's Pose

It is traditional to end any type of formal yoga practice with what is often called the "Corpse Pose" or as I like to call it, Dead Man's Pose. Simply lie flat on your back with your arms at your sides in the anatomical position. The idea is to take a moment to let your practice sink in both physically and mentally. This is a time for quiet reflection and an opportunity to bring awareness to all parts of your body. Take your time to relax into this position for as long as you like. When you return to "normal activity" do so slowly and gradually. Ideally, you'll feel refreshed and invigorated.

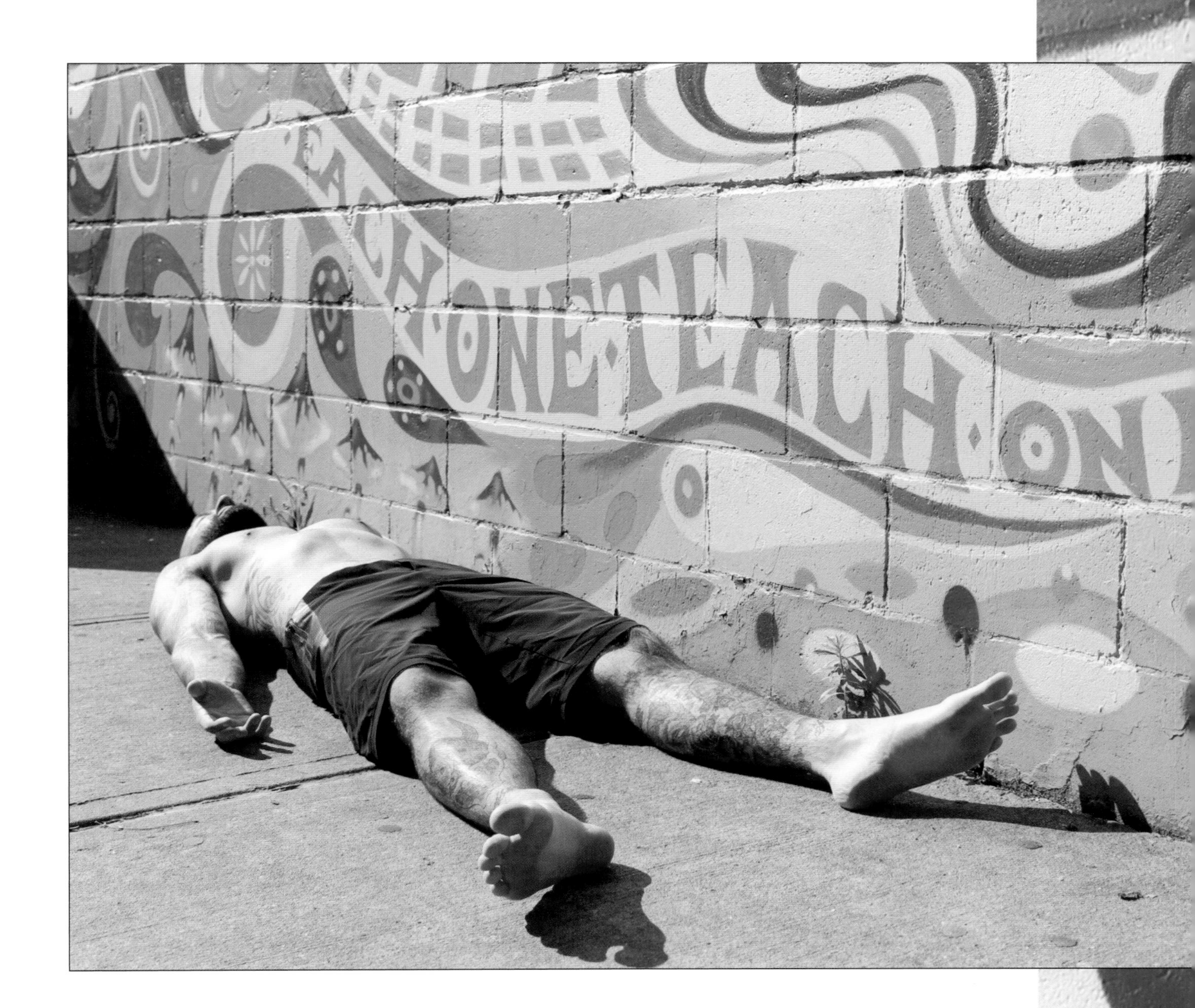

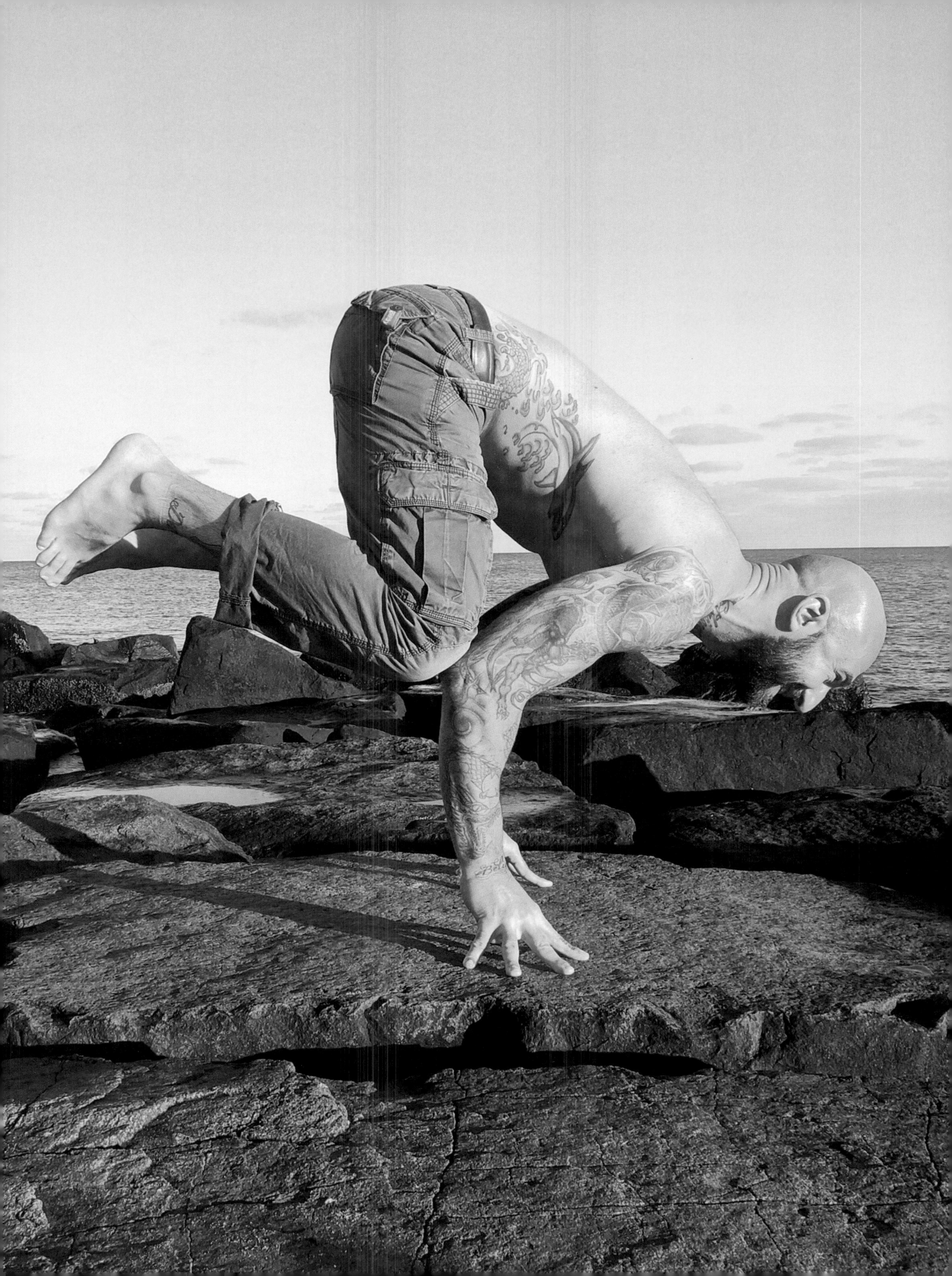

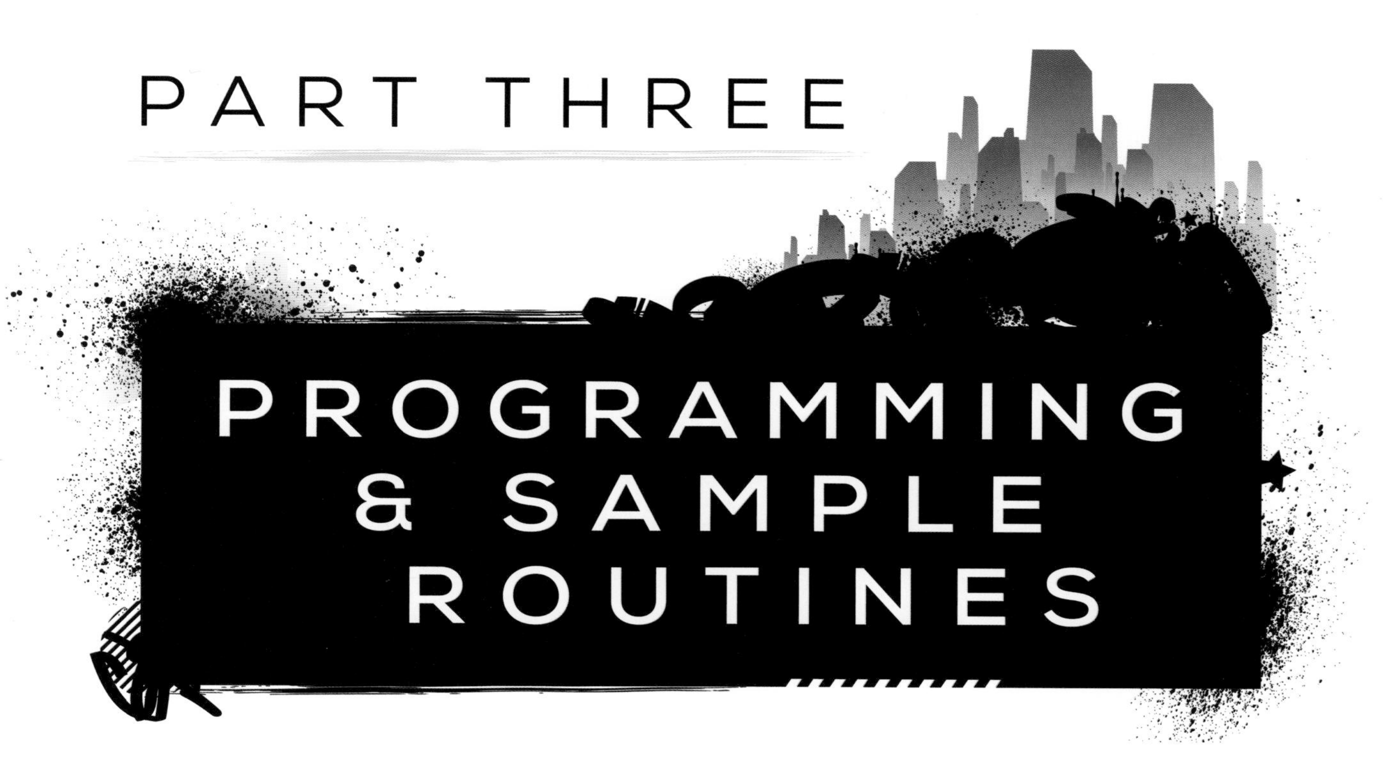

# PART THREE

# PROGRAMMING & SAMPLE ROUTINES

"The essence of education is not to transfer knowledge; it is to guide the learning process, to put responsibility into the students' own hands. It is the bestowal of keys that allow people to unlock the vault of knowledge on their own."

*-Tsunesaburo Makiguchi*

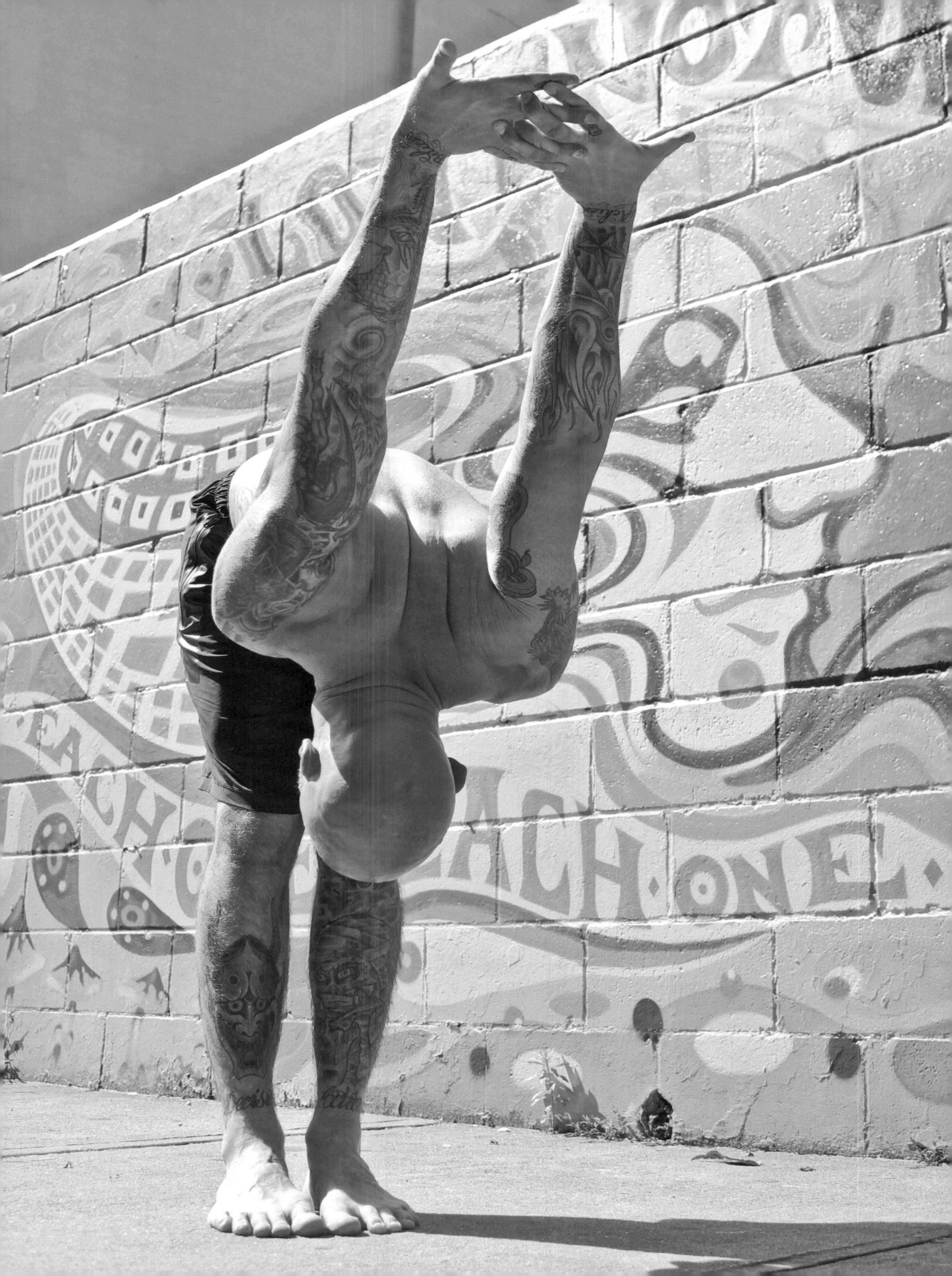
EACH·ONE

# STANDARDS OF PRACTICE

Genetics play a role in every aspect of how our bodies look and move - but don't use that as an excuse for inaction! Some people will be able to achieve a full straddle without much skill-specific work, while others may require years of dedicated practice. Some may never achieve a split no matter how diligently they train. This is fine. You must respect your body and work with it rather than against it if you wish to have a long-lasting, fruitful practice.

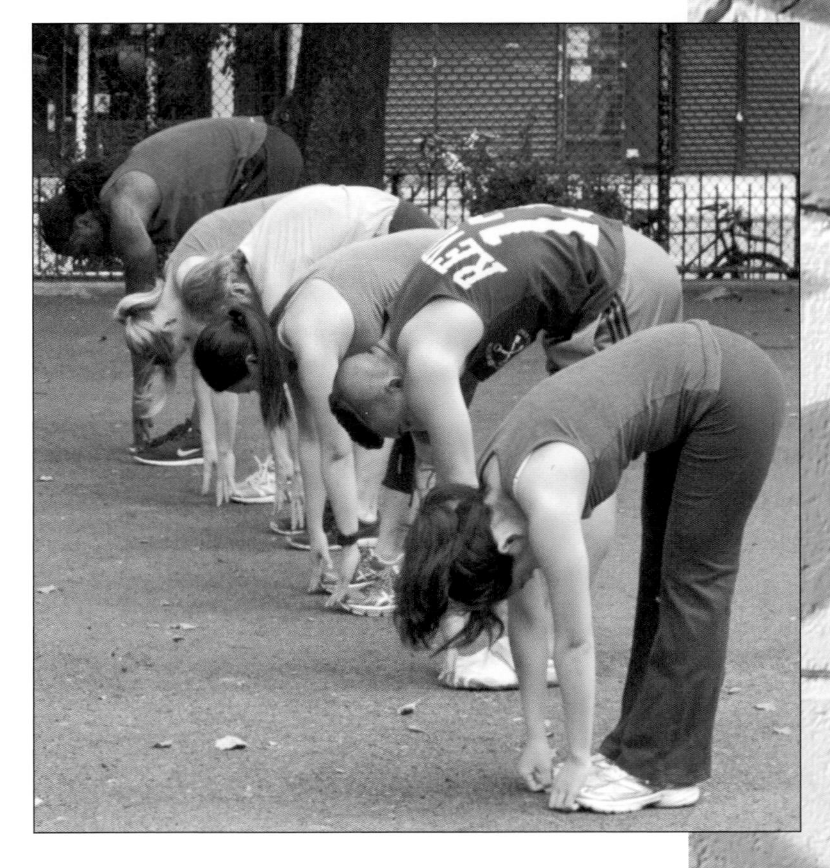

While some folks are naturally more "bendy" than others, there are certain minimum standards that one should aim to meet in order to possess the basic foundation of mobility that is required for healthy, functional movement patterns.

Any healthy, able-bodied person should work toward the following minimum standards of flexibility:

1. **Bend over and touch your toes with your knees locked.**

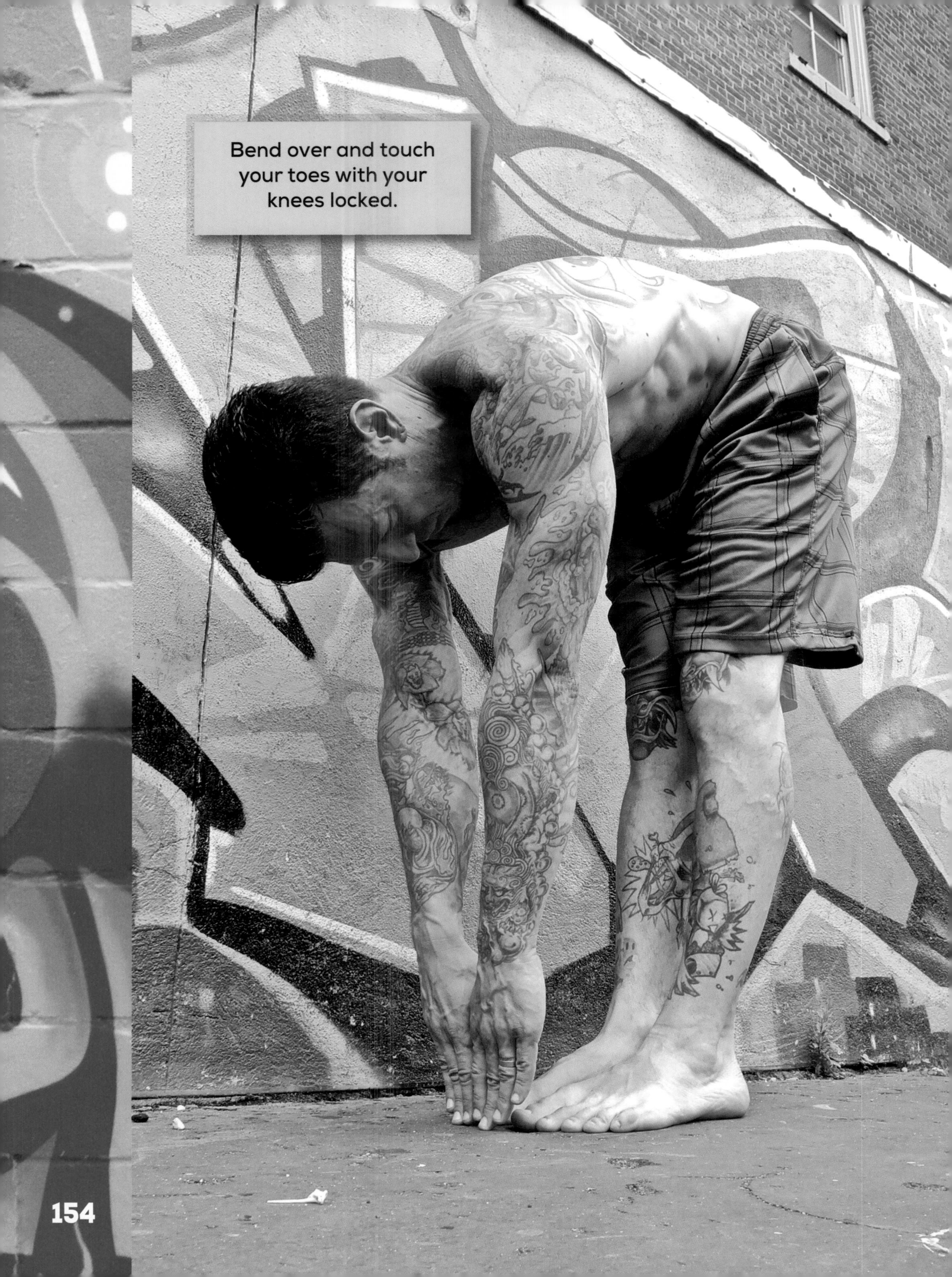
Bend over and touch
your toes with your
knees locked.

2. Get into a deep squat position with both heels flat on the floor and your calves and hamstrings in contact with one another.

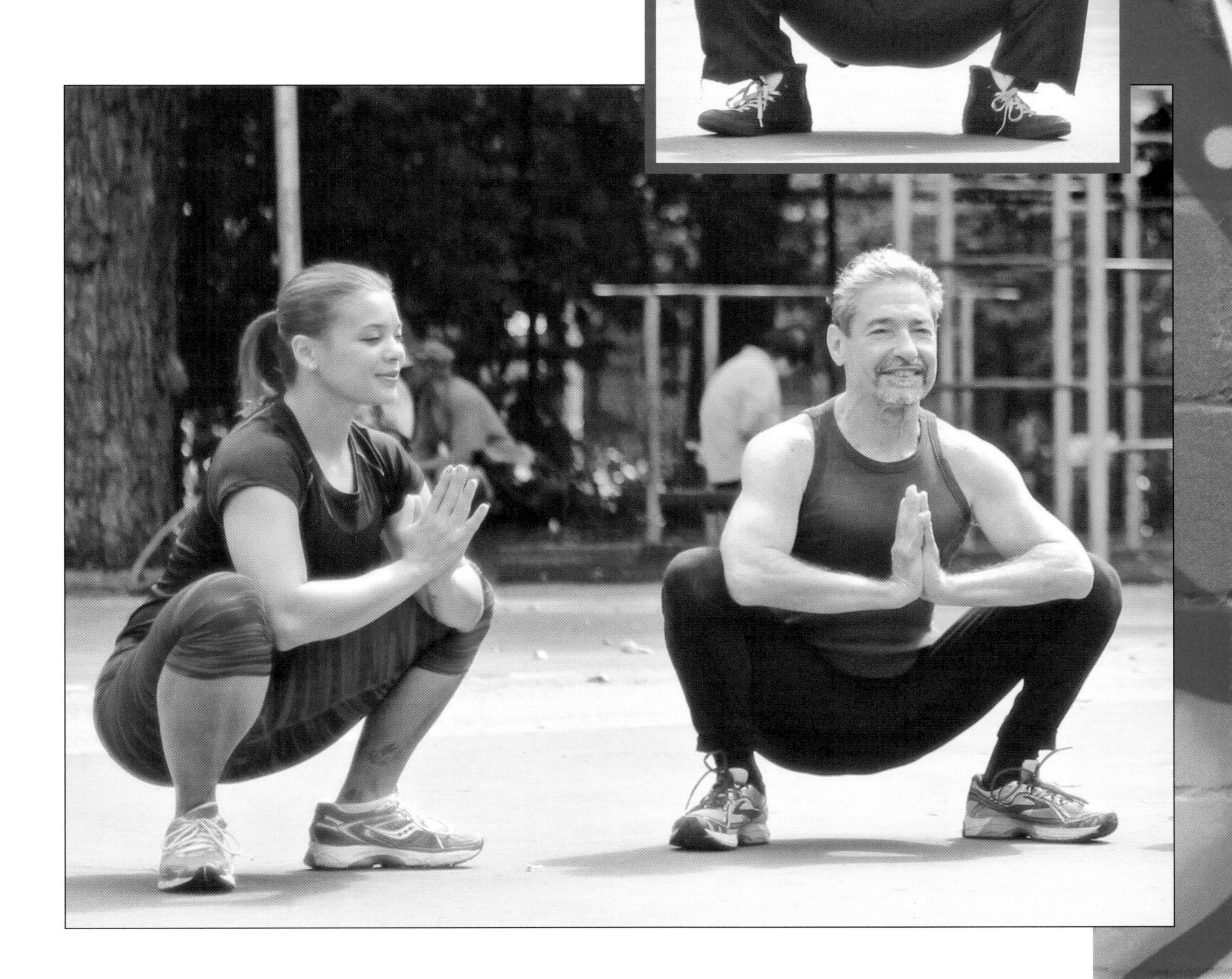

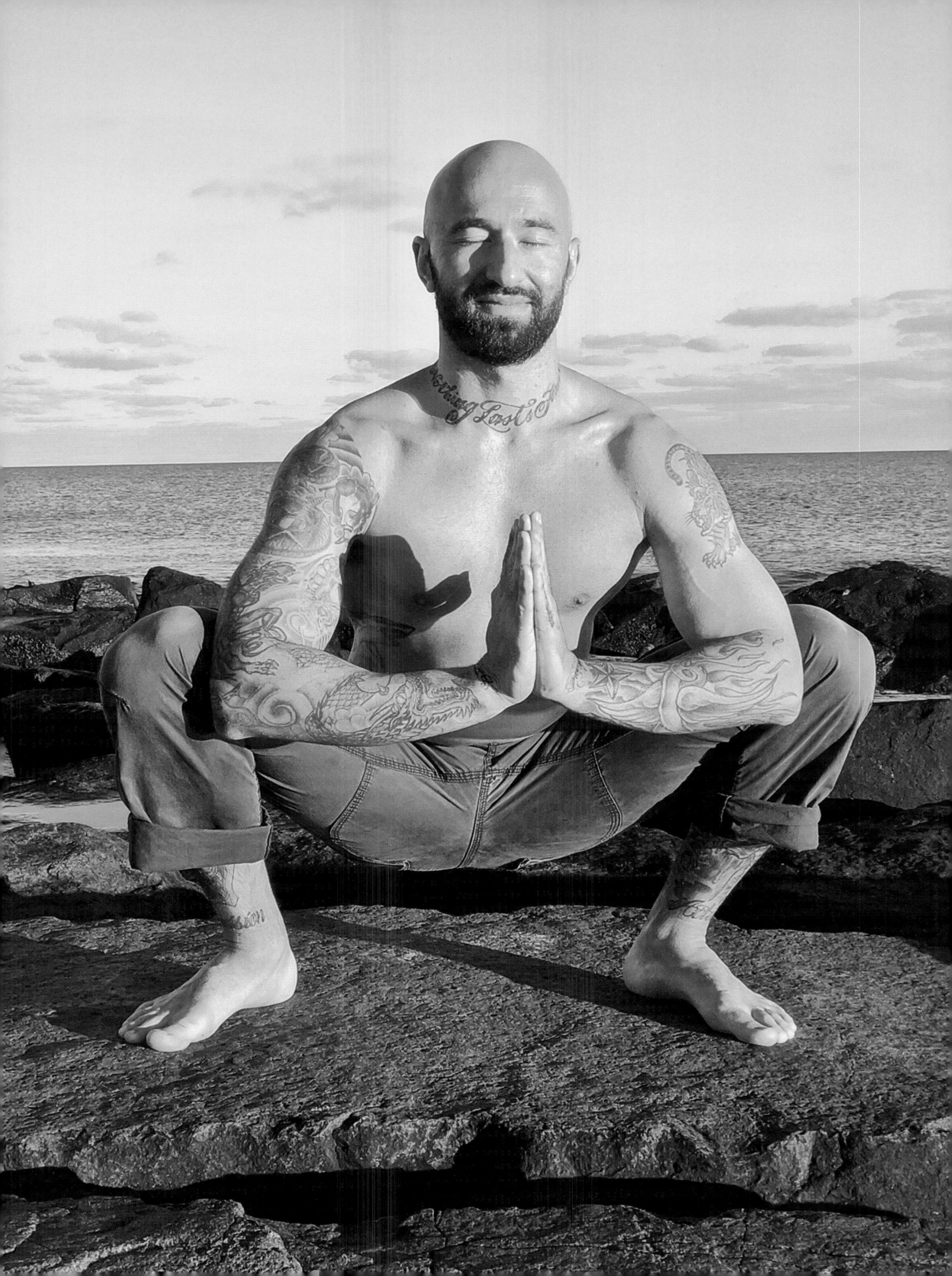

3. Lie flat on your back with your legs straight and lower back in contact with the ground. Reach your arms overhead with both wrists flat on the floor behind you with minimal flexion at the elbows.

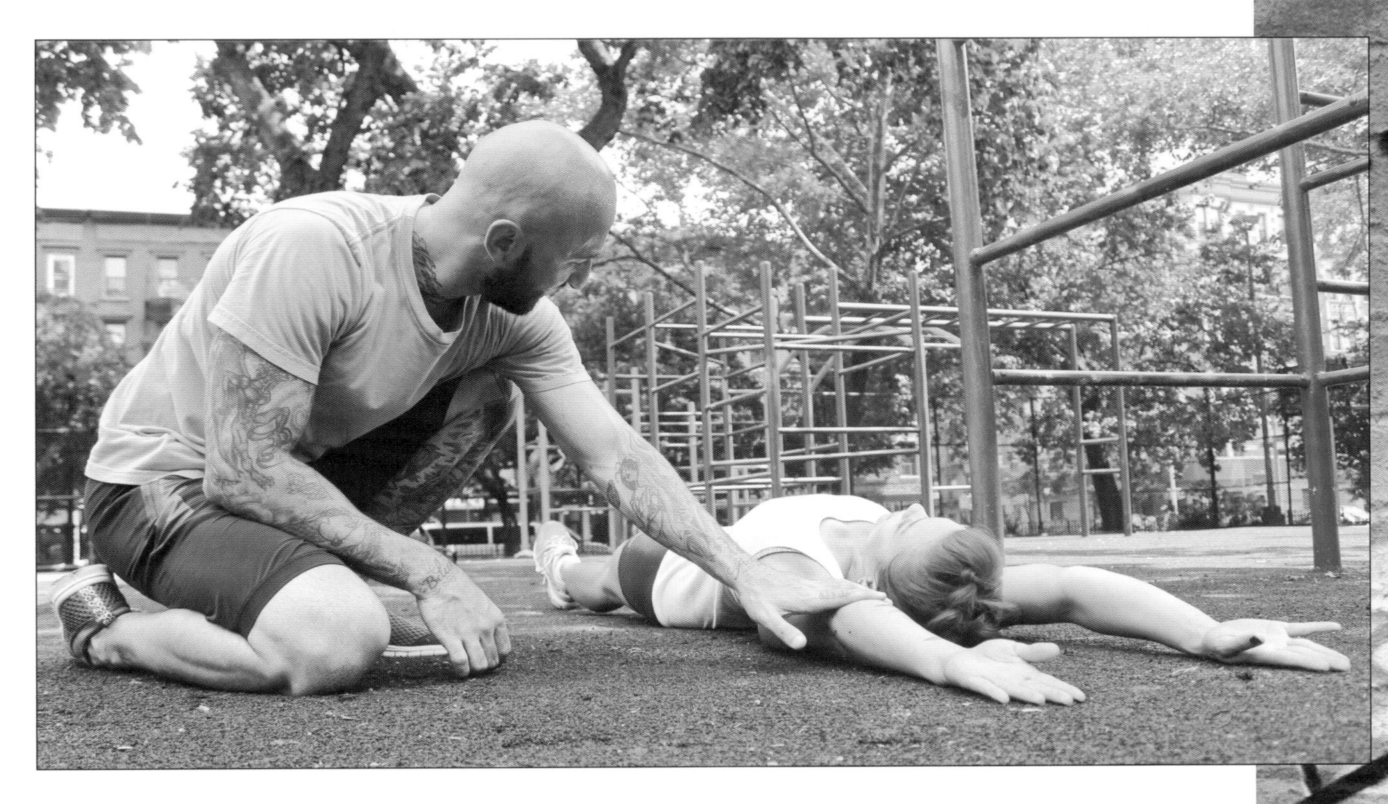

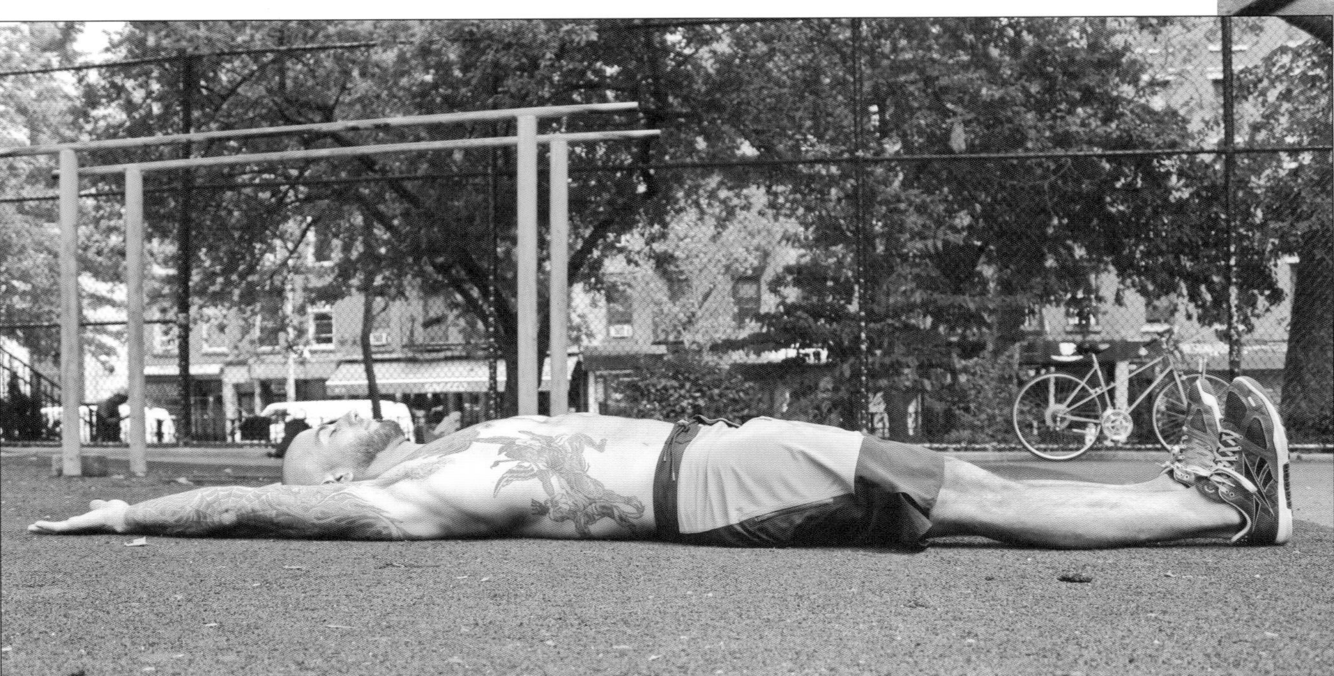

4. From a standing position, pick up one leg and place the outside of your ankle on a bench, bar or other object that is just below waist height. Now rotate your hip to try to touch your knee to the object as well (your shin should be perpendicular to your body.)

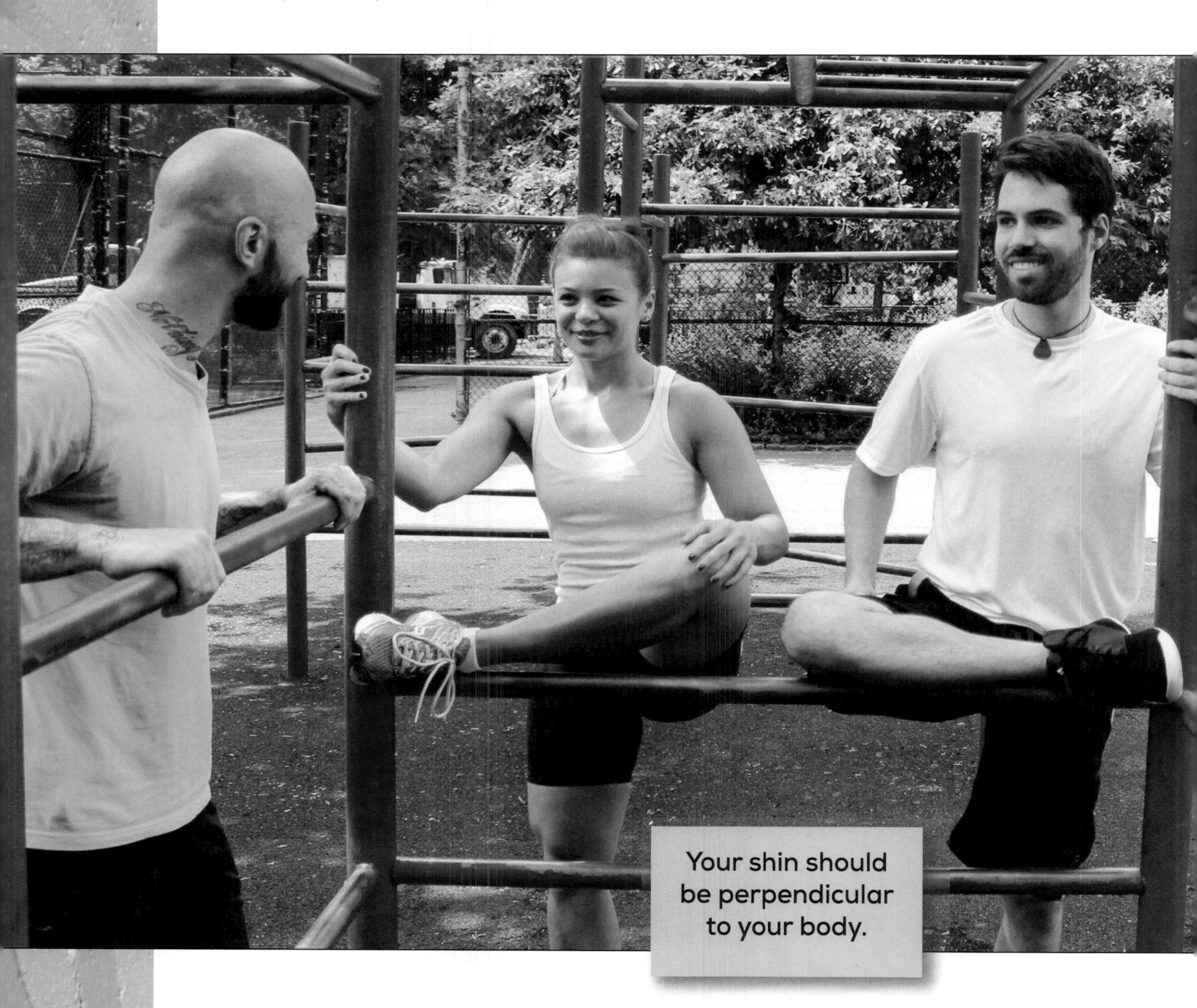

Your shin should be perpendicular to your body.

5. Reach both arms behind your back - one from above, one from below - and touch the tips of your middle fingers together..

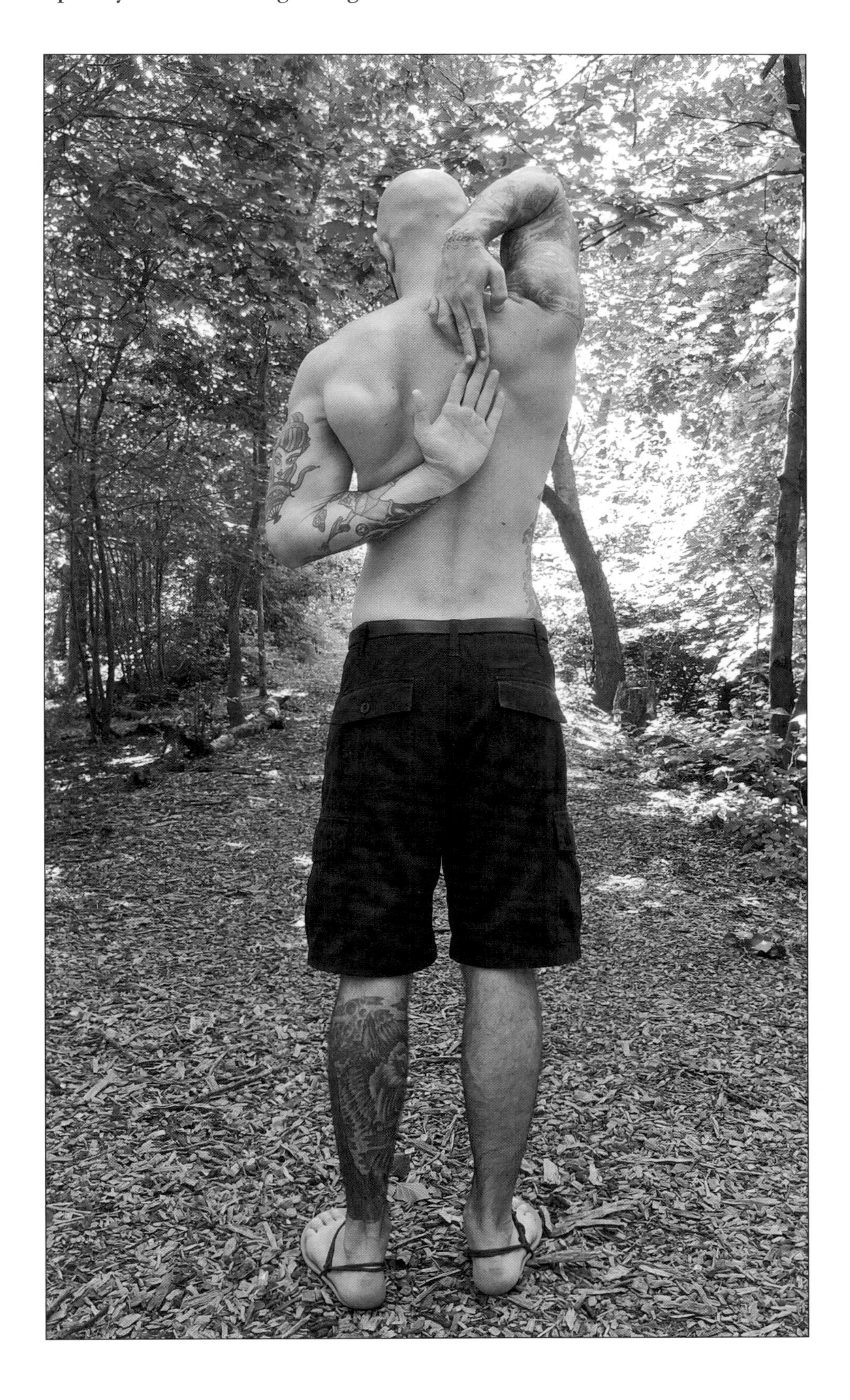

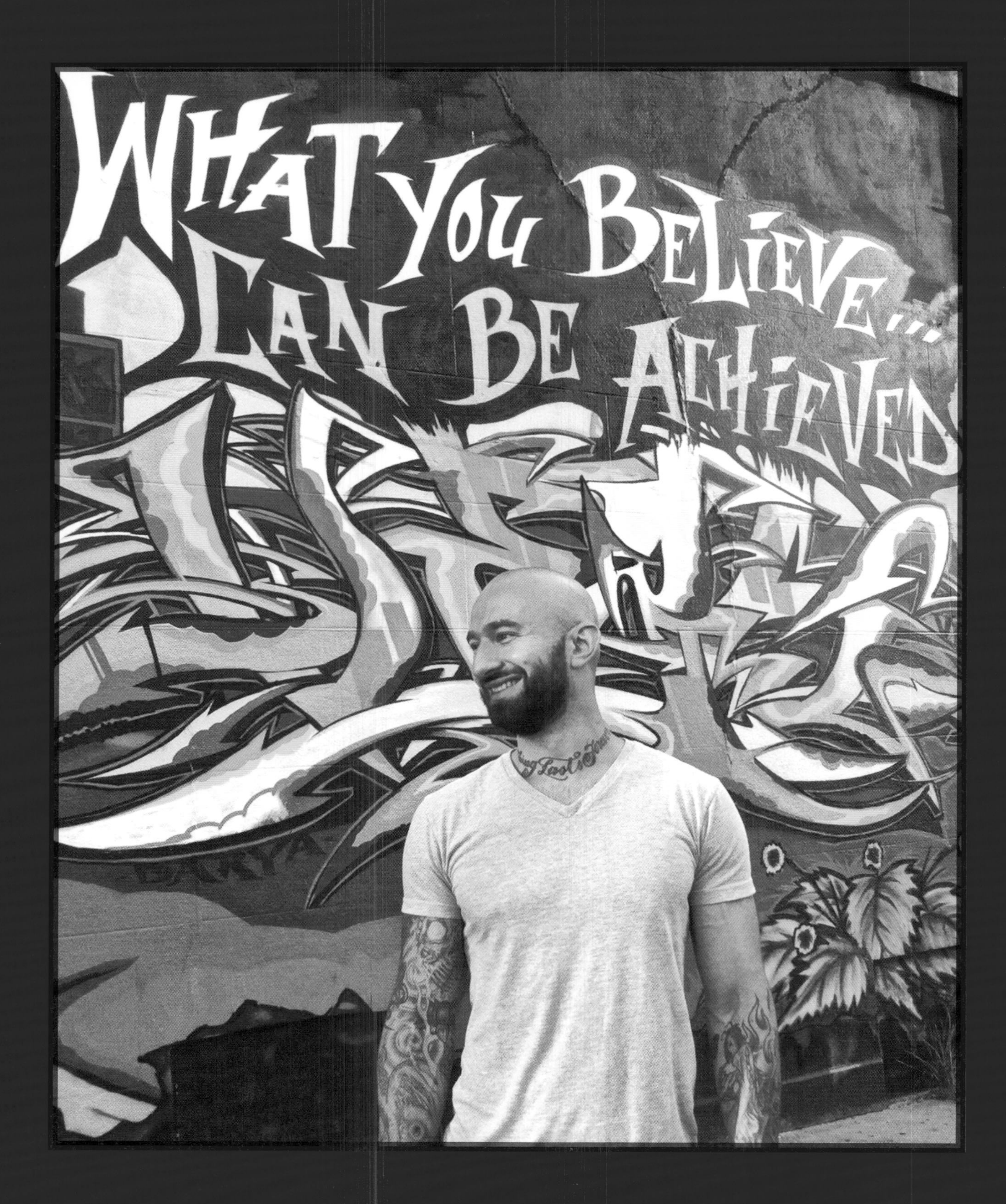
WHAT YOU BELIEVE...
CAN BE ACHIEVED

# ON MATS

As I aim to keep my training as minimalistic as possible, I try to avoid relying on equipment. With a few minor exceptions all the exercises in this book can be done with no equipment at all. You may, however, find it beneficial to use a yoga mat or other exercise mat in your practice, particularly if you are new to this style of movement.

A mat has many benefits, such as providing a soft surface for poses where you're kneeling or seated, as well as traction for when you are standing. Slippery surfaces can pose a challenge for many poses and while there are many surfaces that can provide stability, using a mat can give you the confidence that you'll be able to keep steady footing.

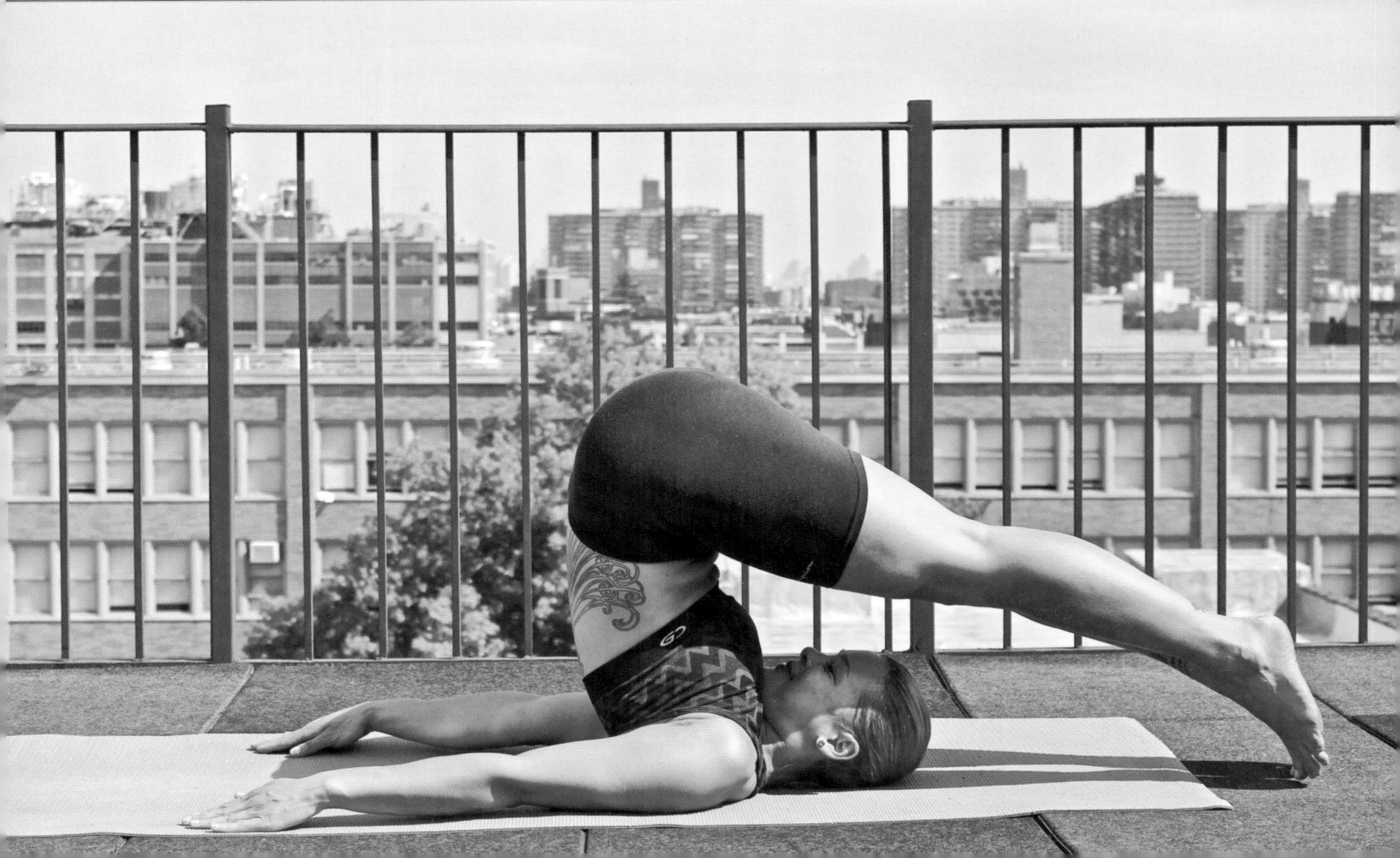

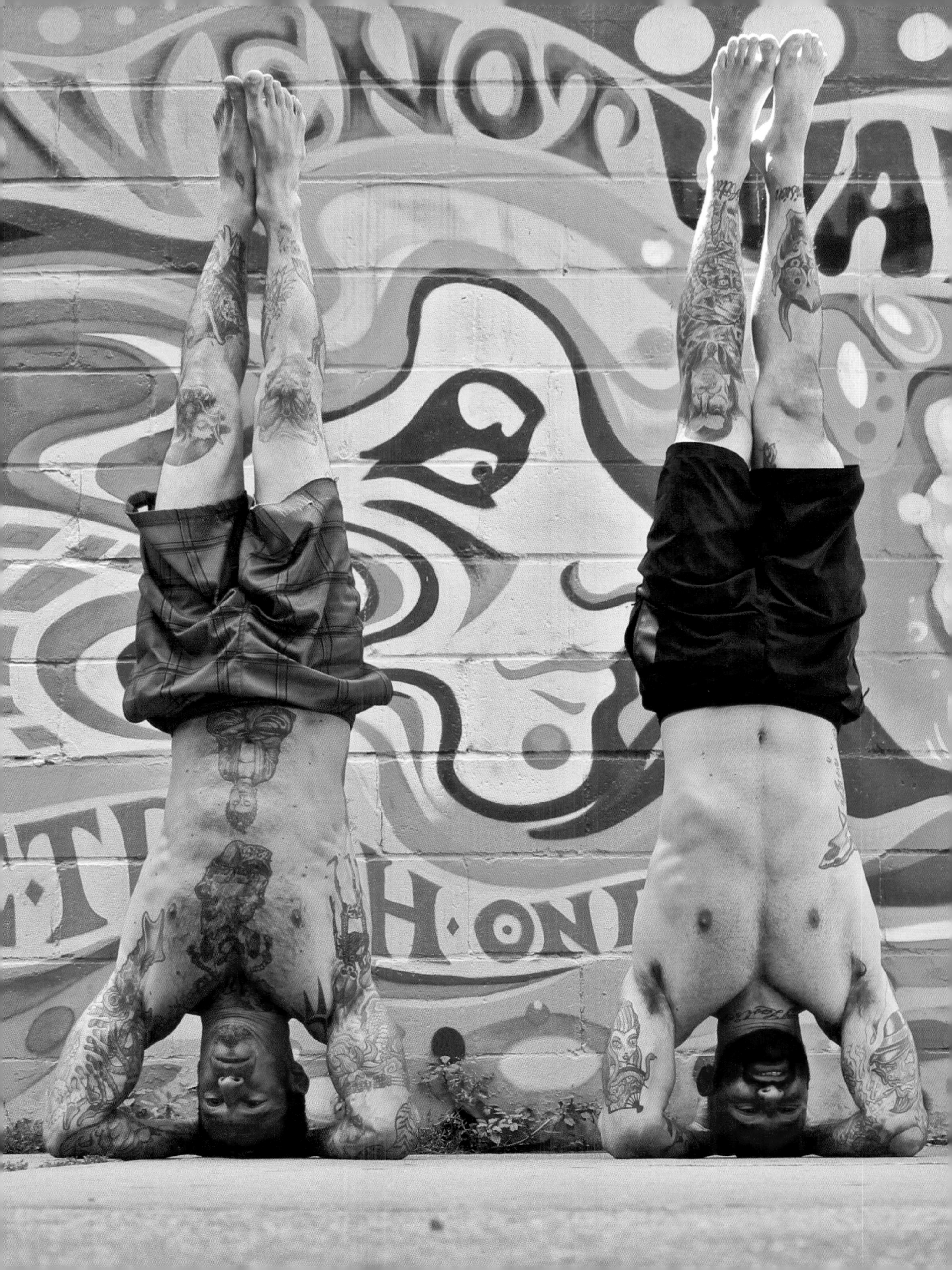

# SYMMETRY

Though muscle imbalances are common, striving for symmetry between both sides of your body will help keep you fit and injury-free.

Research has shown that people who are perceived as being the best-looking by their peers are those with nearly symmetrical sides to their faces. To achieve symmetry in your body is also a sign of beauty - calisthenic beauty!

The human body is never going to be perfectly symmetrical, however, it is still beneficial to work toward correcting imbalances by prioritizing your tighter/weaker side. If you have one side that is stronger or more flexible than the other, I suggest working that side first when performing iso-lateral movements.

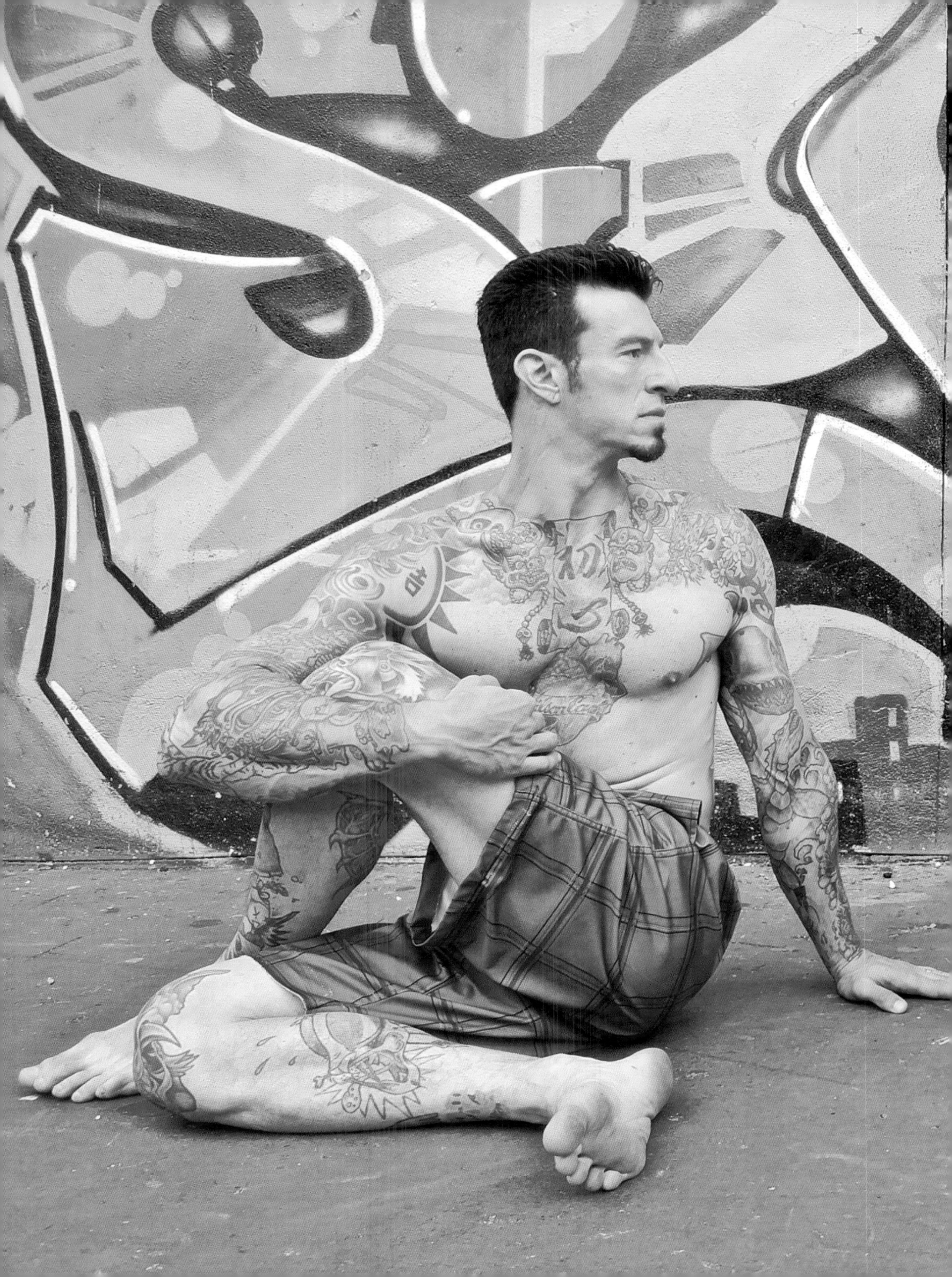

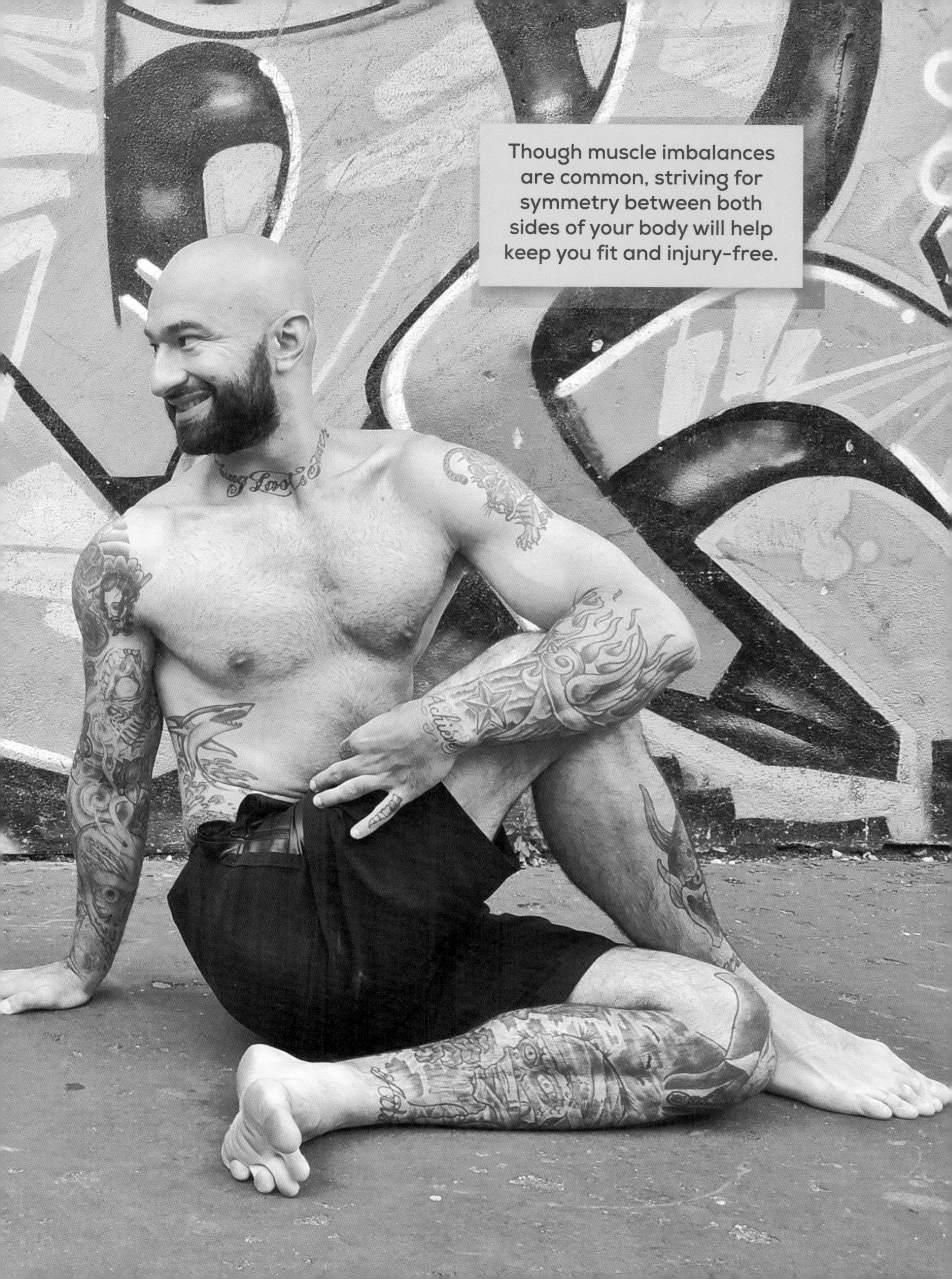

Though muscle imbalances are common, striving for symmetry between both sides of your body will help keep you fit and injury-free.

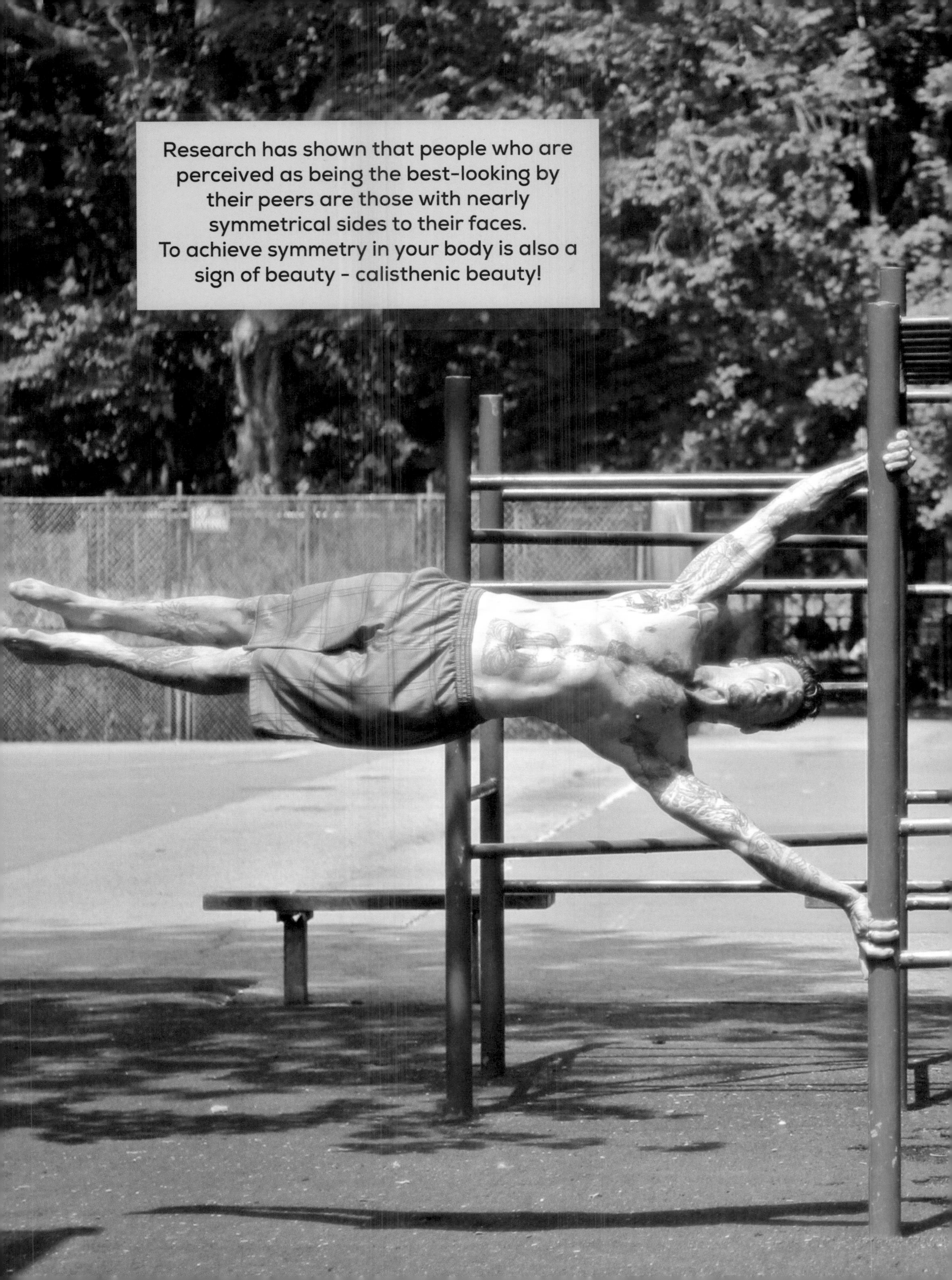
Research has shown that people who are perceived as being the best-looking by their peers are those with nearly symmetrical sides to their faces.
To achieve symmetry in your body is also a sign of beauty - calisthenic beauty!

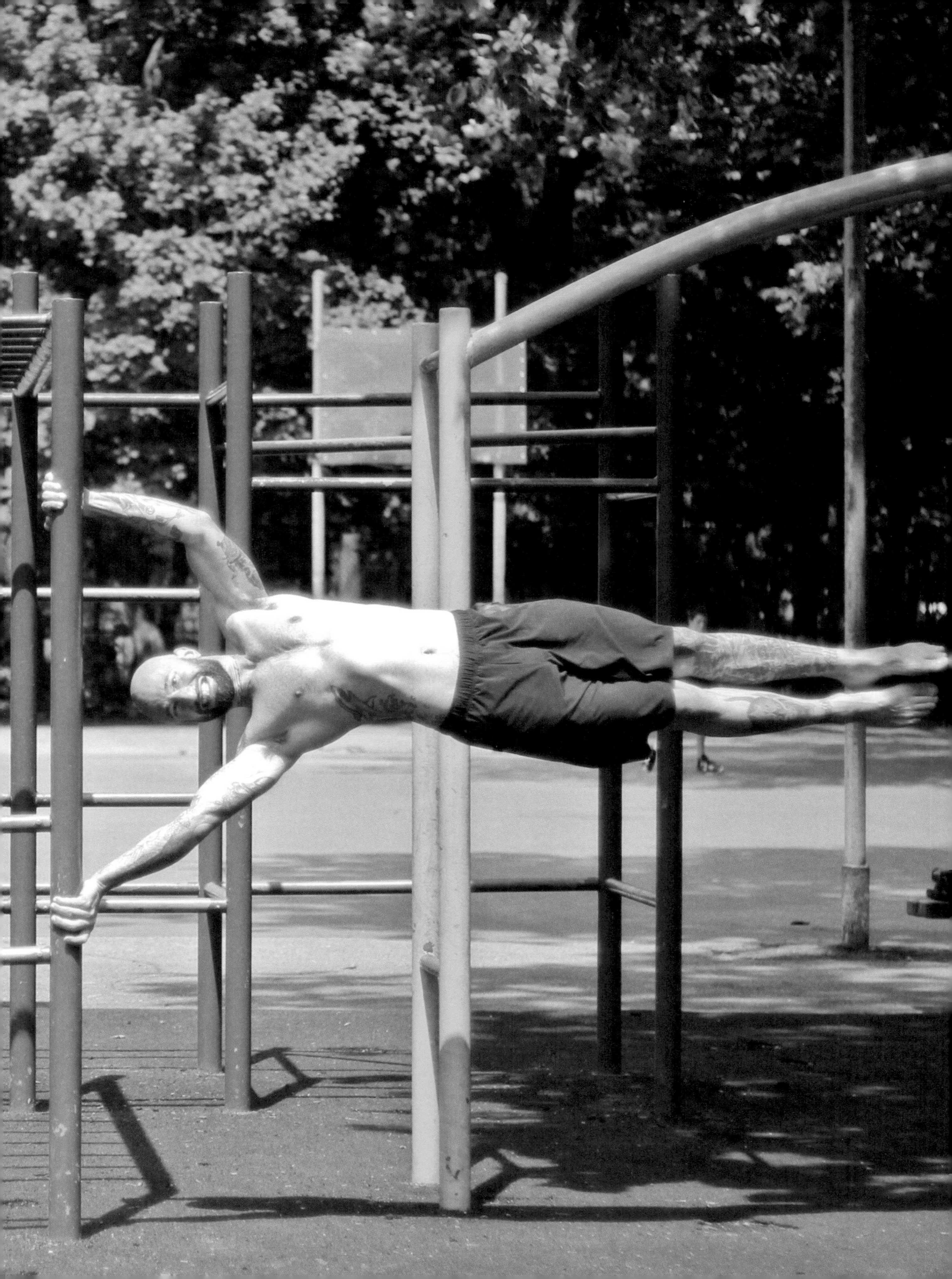

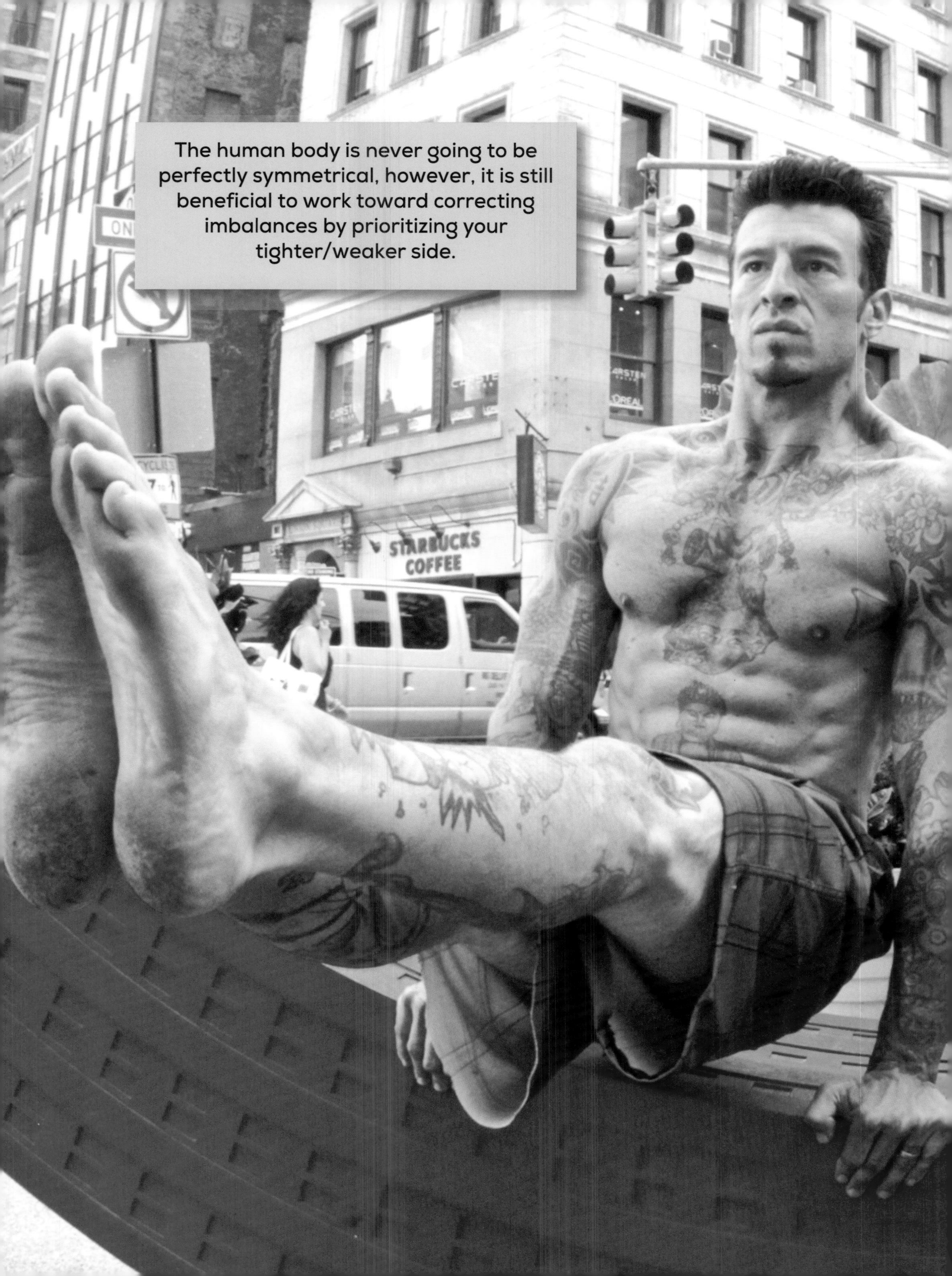


The human body is never going to be perfectly symmetrical, however, it is still beneficial to work toward correcting imbalances by prioritizing your tighter/weaker side.

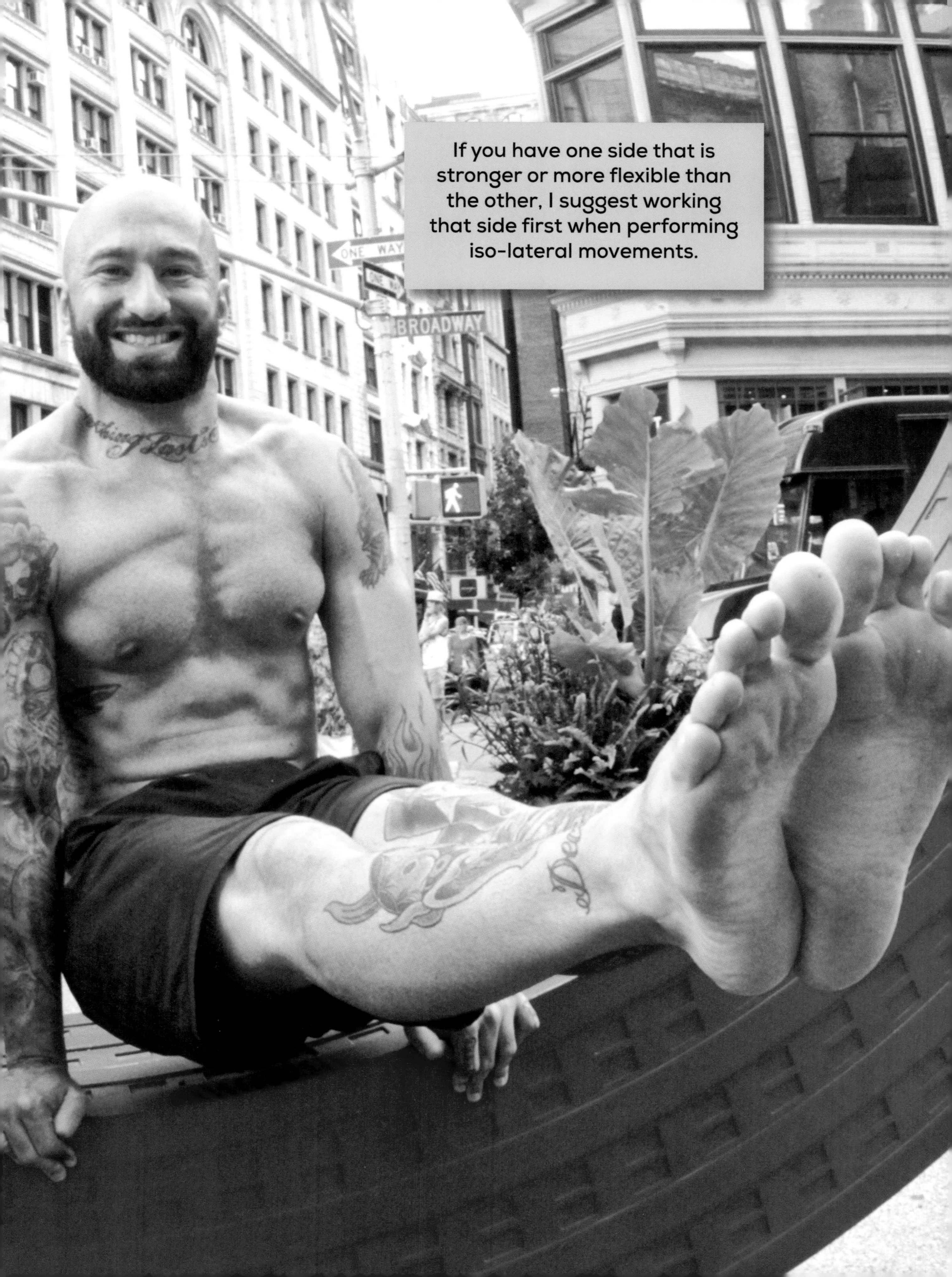


If you have one side that is stronger or more flexible than the other, I suggest working that side first when performing iso-lateral movements.

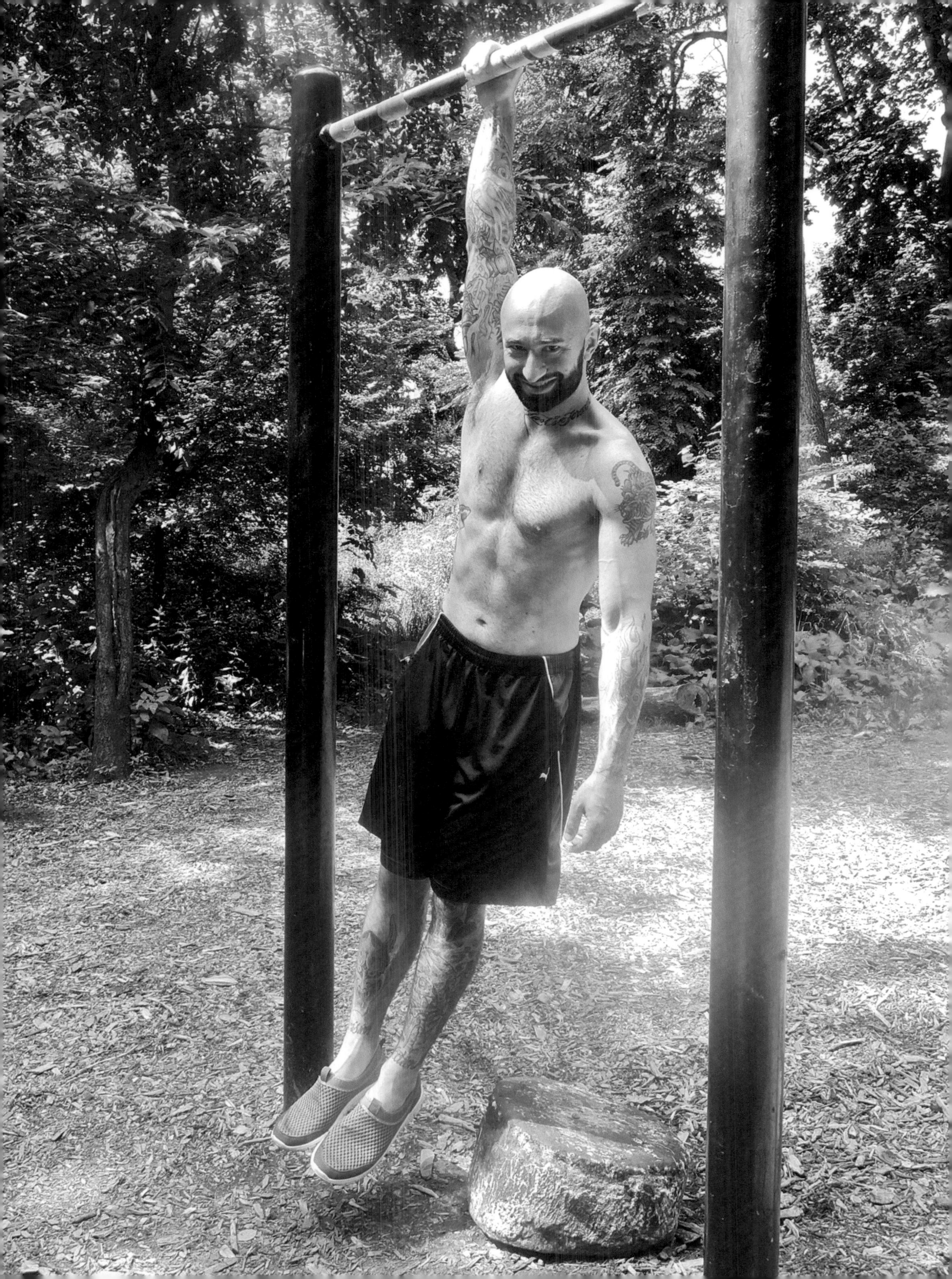

# HYPOTHETICAL TRAINING SPLITS

Split routines are exercise programs that involve working different exercises or body parts on different days. The idea is that by breaking your workouts up, you allow adequate rest time for your muscles without having to take a day off. For example, if your arms are sore on Tuesday from working them on Monday, you might work your legs to give your arms some rest. Since you're working fewer muscles per training session, the amount of volume done on each body part increases, and since the volume has increased, those muscles may require additional rest.

Though it can be helpful to follow a template of some sort, do not get sucked into the trap of adhering too strictly to what's on the schedule. There are a myriad of unpredictable factors that can affect your workout on any given day: what you've eaten recently, the amount of sleep you've had, stress levels – even the weather. When I train clients in person, I come into the session with an idea of what I am going to do with them, but I always wind up making changes and improvising based on what is actually happening in front of me.

A workout regimen on paper is a good idea, but it's still just an idea. You have to put your plan into action to get any benefits. And once you start doing that, it might not go exactly as predicted; you are inevitably going to need to make modifications. In theory, theory and practice are the same. In practice, they couldn't be more different.

## Hypothetical Training Split A:

Day 1 - Pull-ups, Push-ups, Dips, Hanging Leg Raises etc.
Day 2 - Squats, Lunges, Bridges, Handstands, etc.
Day 3 - Stretch
Day 4 - Rest, repeat or active recovery

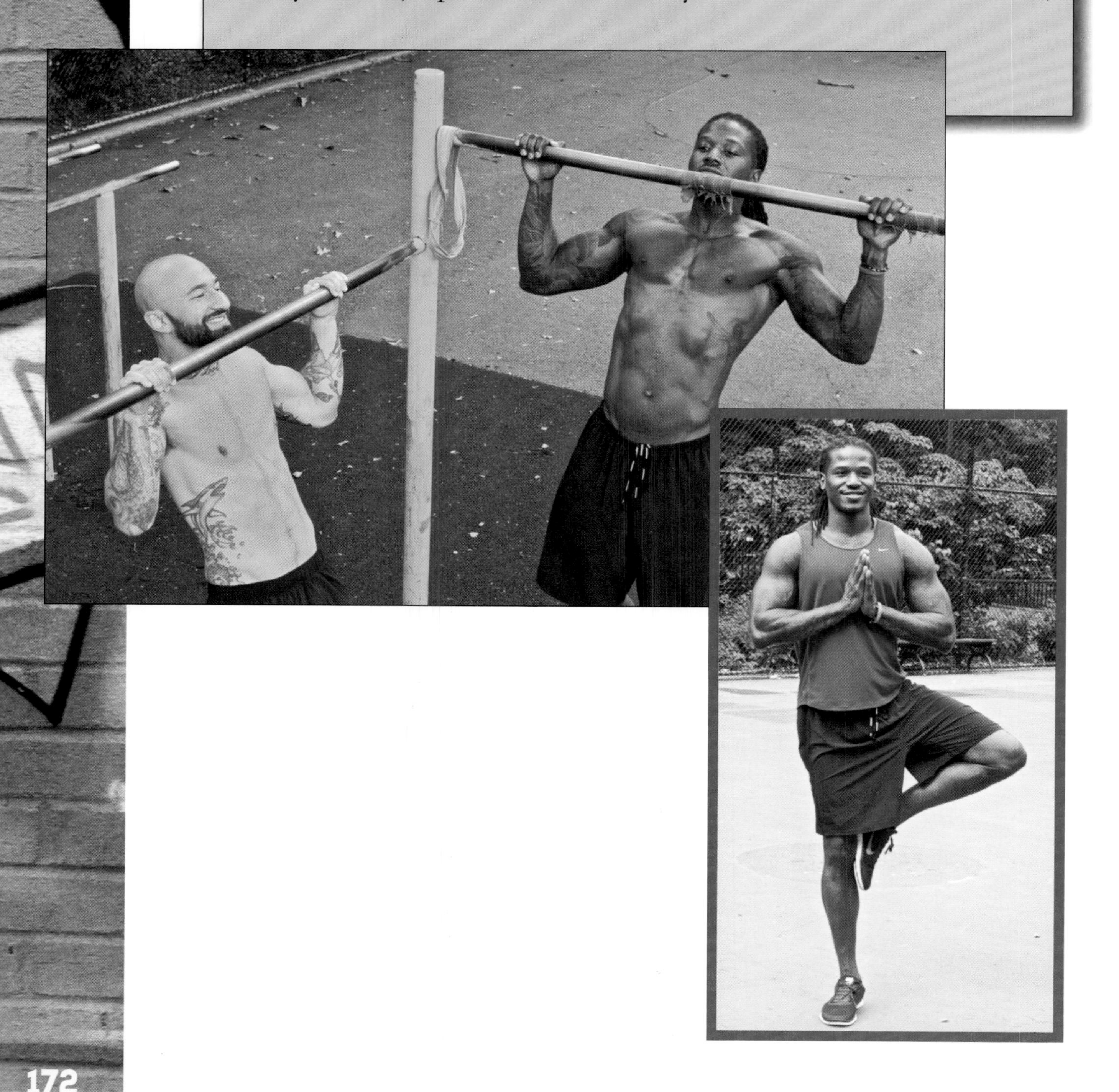

## Hypothetical Training Split B:

Day 1 - Full Body Calisthenics
Day 2 - Stretch
Day 3 - Rest, repeat or active recovery

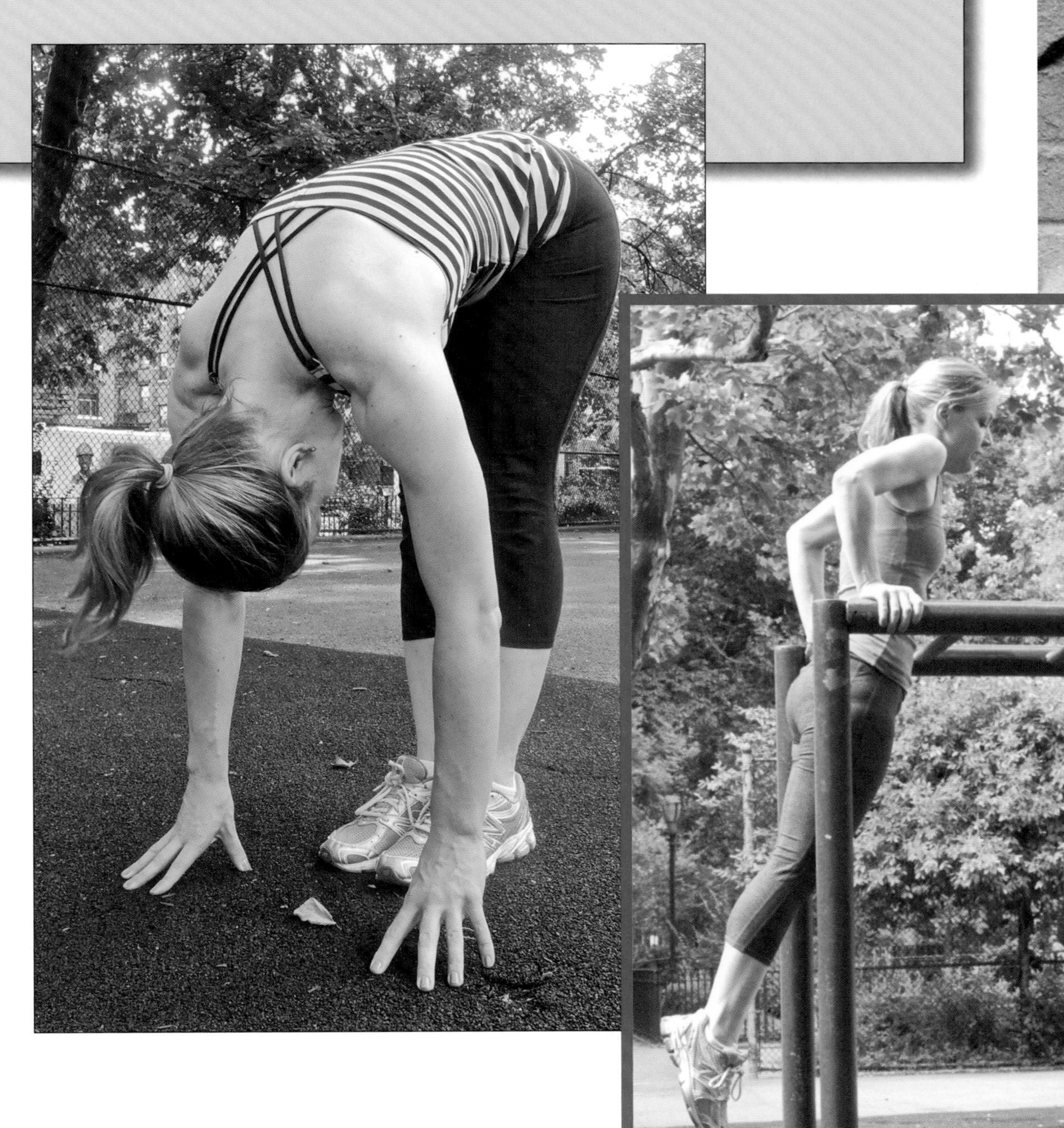

## Hypothetical Training Split C:

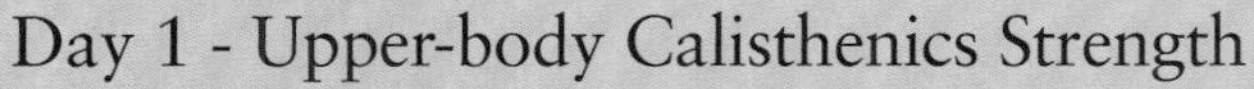

Day 1 - Upper-body Calisthenics Strength
Day 2 - Lower-body Calisthenics Strength
Day 3 - Upper-body Calisthenics Stretch
Day 4 - Lower-body Calisthenics Stretch
Day 5 - Rest, repeat or active recovery

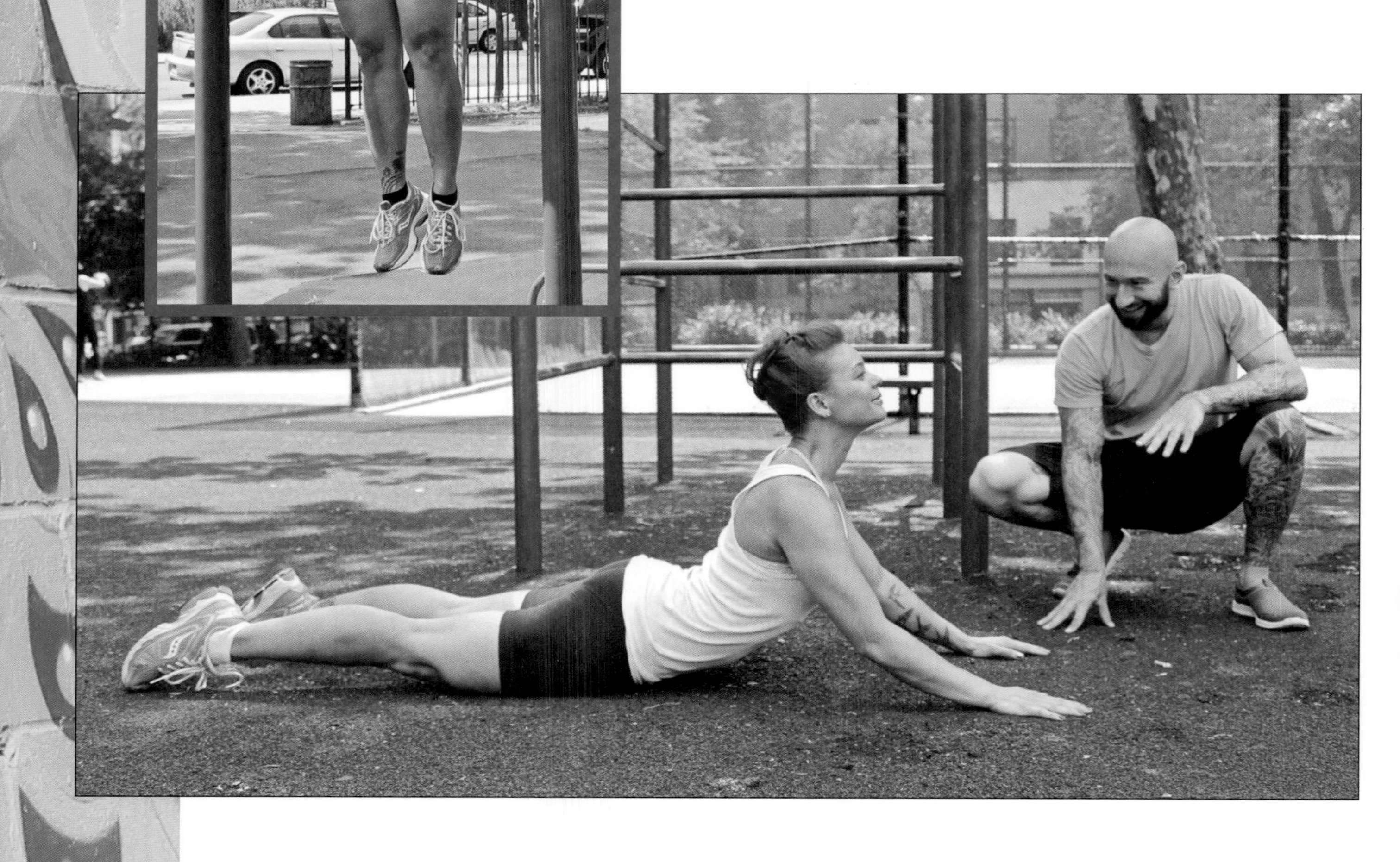

## Hypothetical Training Split D:

Day 1 - Upper-body Calisthenics Strength
Day 2 - Upper-body Calisthenics Stretch
Day 3 - Lower-body Calisthenics Strength
Day 4 - Lower-body Calisthenics Stretch
Day 5 - Rest, repeat or active recovery

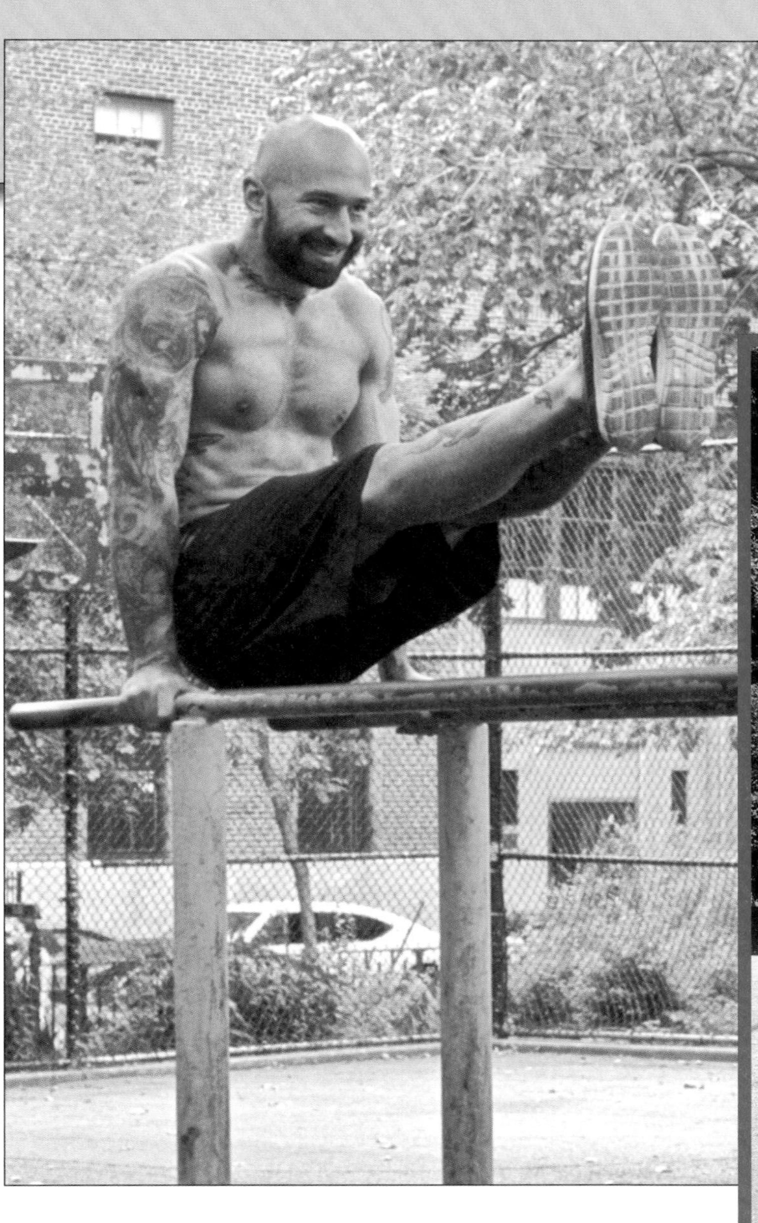

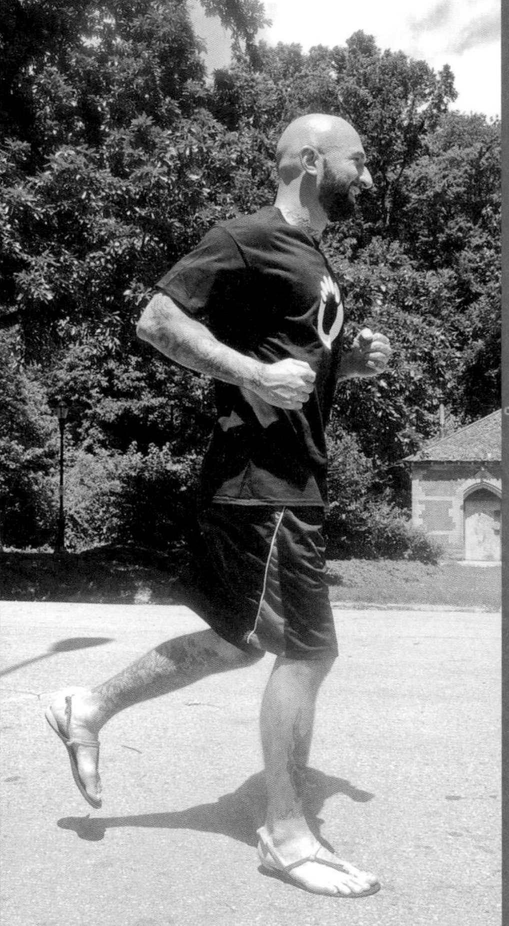

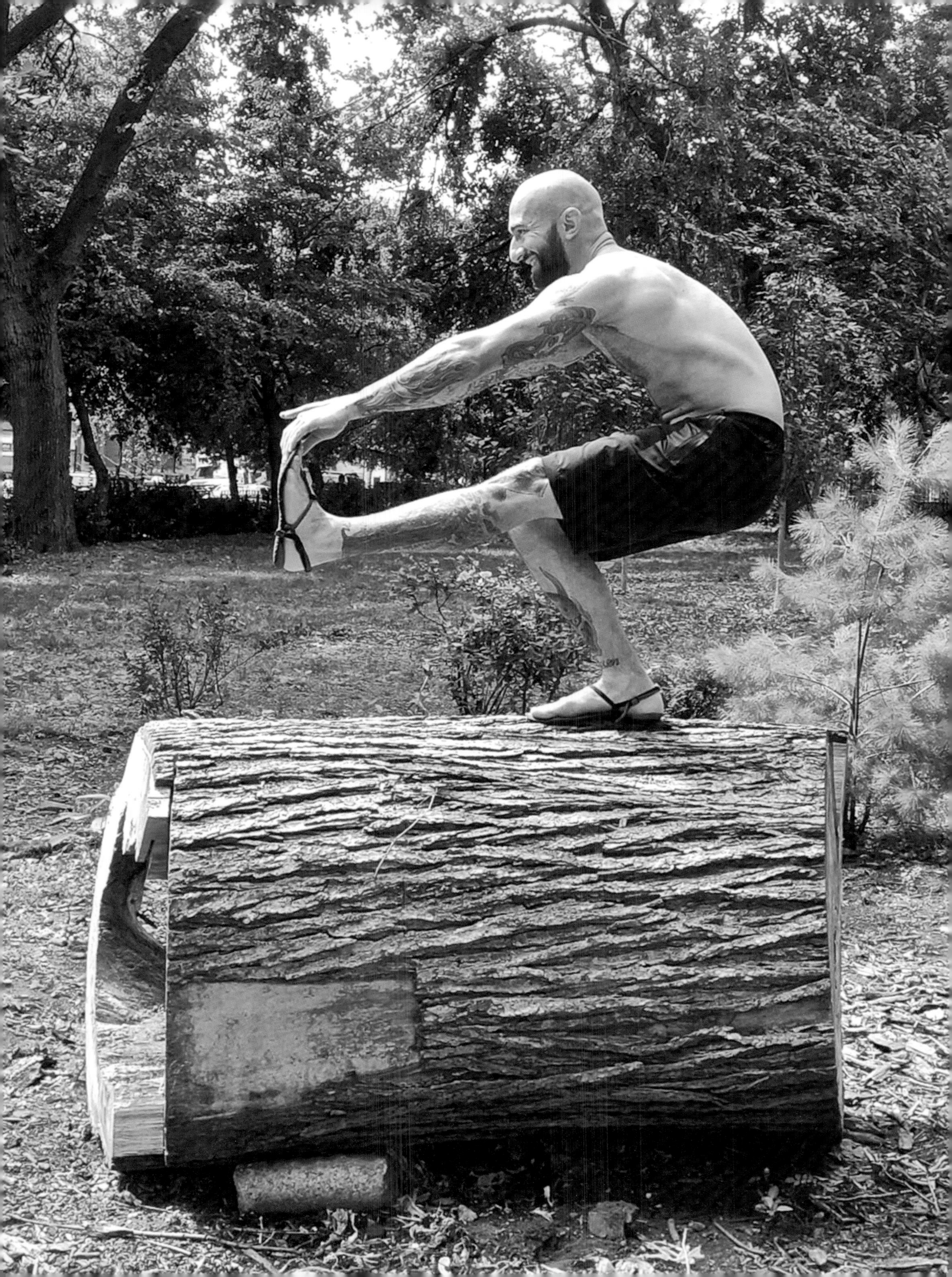

# SAMPLE ROUTINES

The following routines are based on things I've done in my own workouts or with my clients. I've tried to streamline them for general consumption, but feel free to make adjustments. These routines are basic guidelines meant to be tinkered with and explored. Don't feel tied down to following them as written.

For the dynamic stretches, I recommend 10-20 reps for each set with 2-3 sets per exercise. For the static holds, I suggest counting 5-10 slow breaths in each pose and repeating each pose twice (either back to back or as a circuit with the other poses in the series). You can perform these routines as warm-ups or cooldowns, or do them on separate days from your strength training altogether. You can make any substitutions that you need to or mix and match the routines in any way that you see fit. I don't expect anyone to follow these routines to the letter.

Though solitary practice has its benefits, I encourage you to attend a class or work one-on-one with a qualified teacher. There is no substitute for in-person experience.

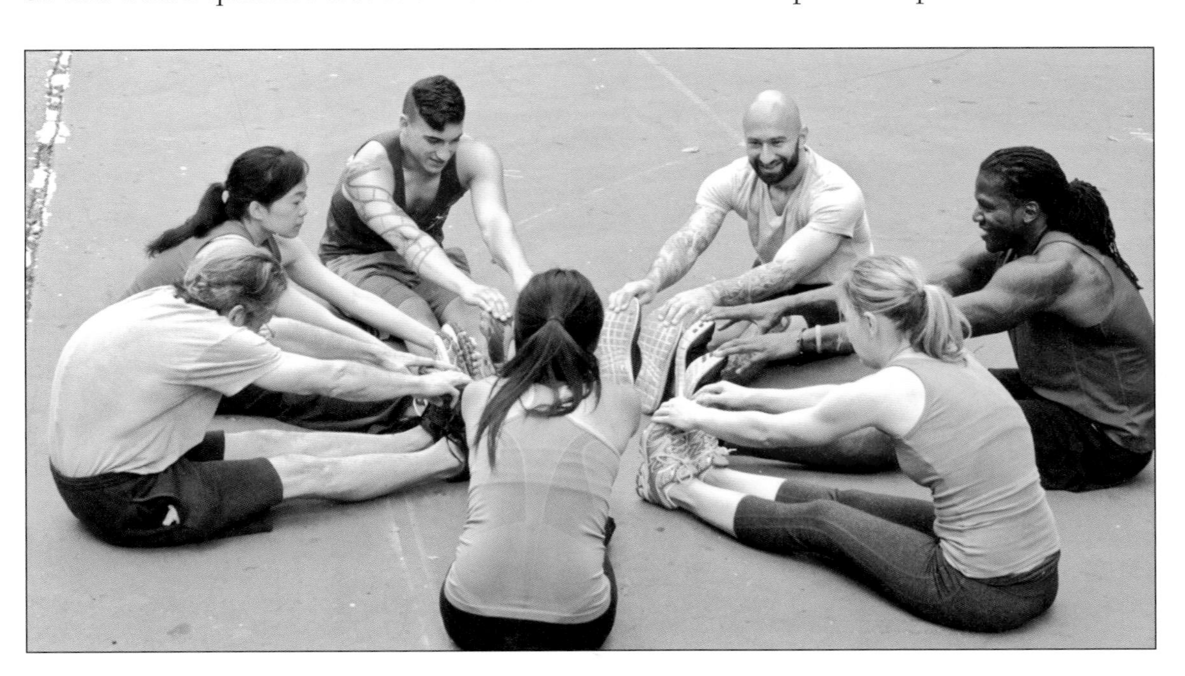

## Rise and Shine

Statue
Mountain
Crescent Moon (both sides)
Full Forward Bend
Half Forward Bend
Full Forward Bend
Yoga Lunge
Downward Dog
Yoga Lunge (other side)
Downward Dog
Cobra or Sphinx
Child's Pose or Inchworm

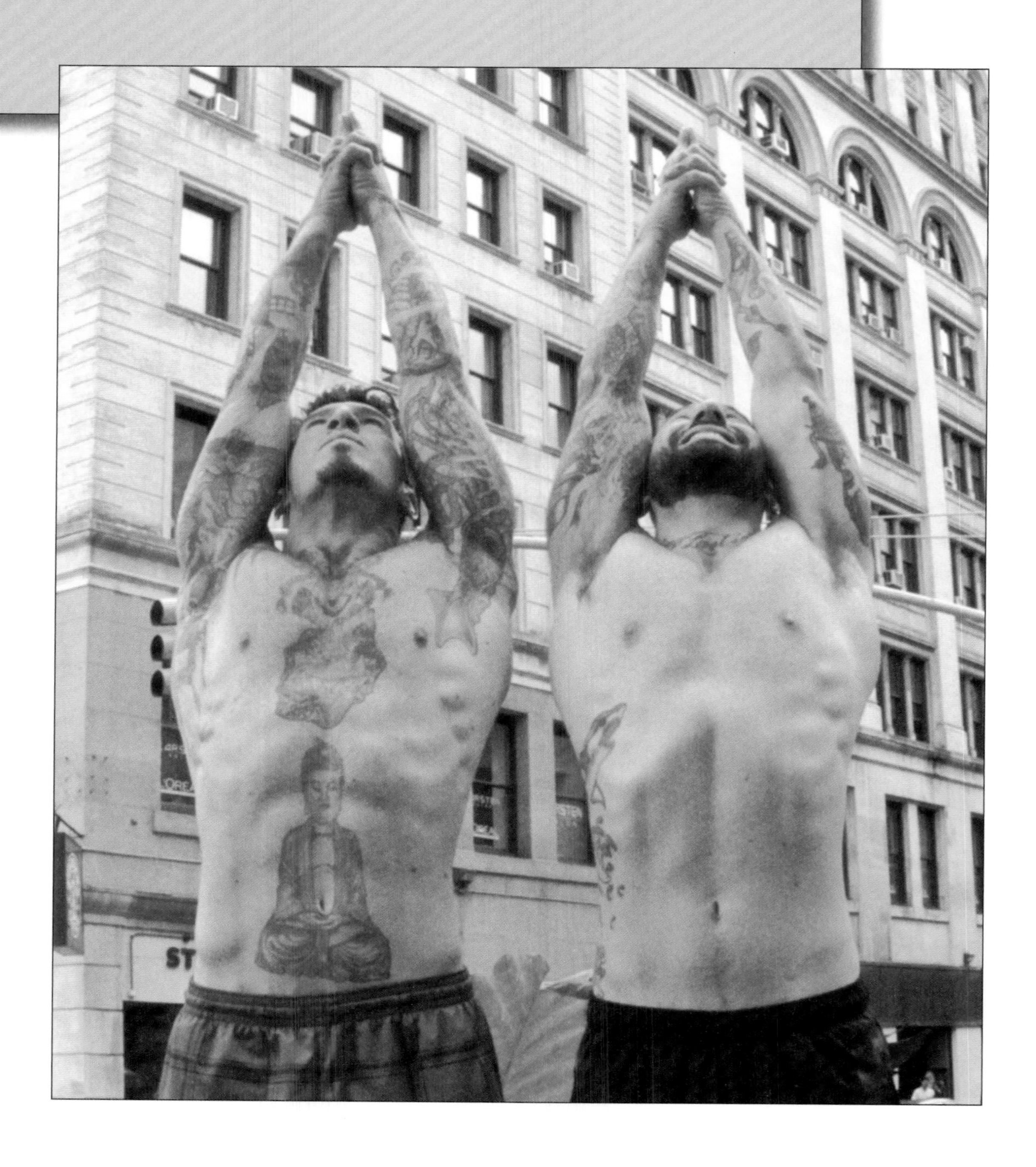

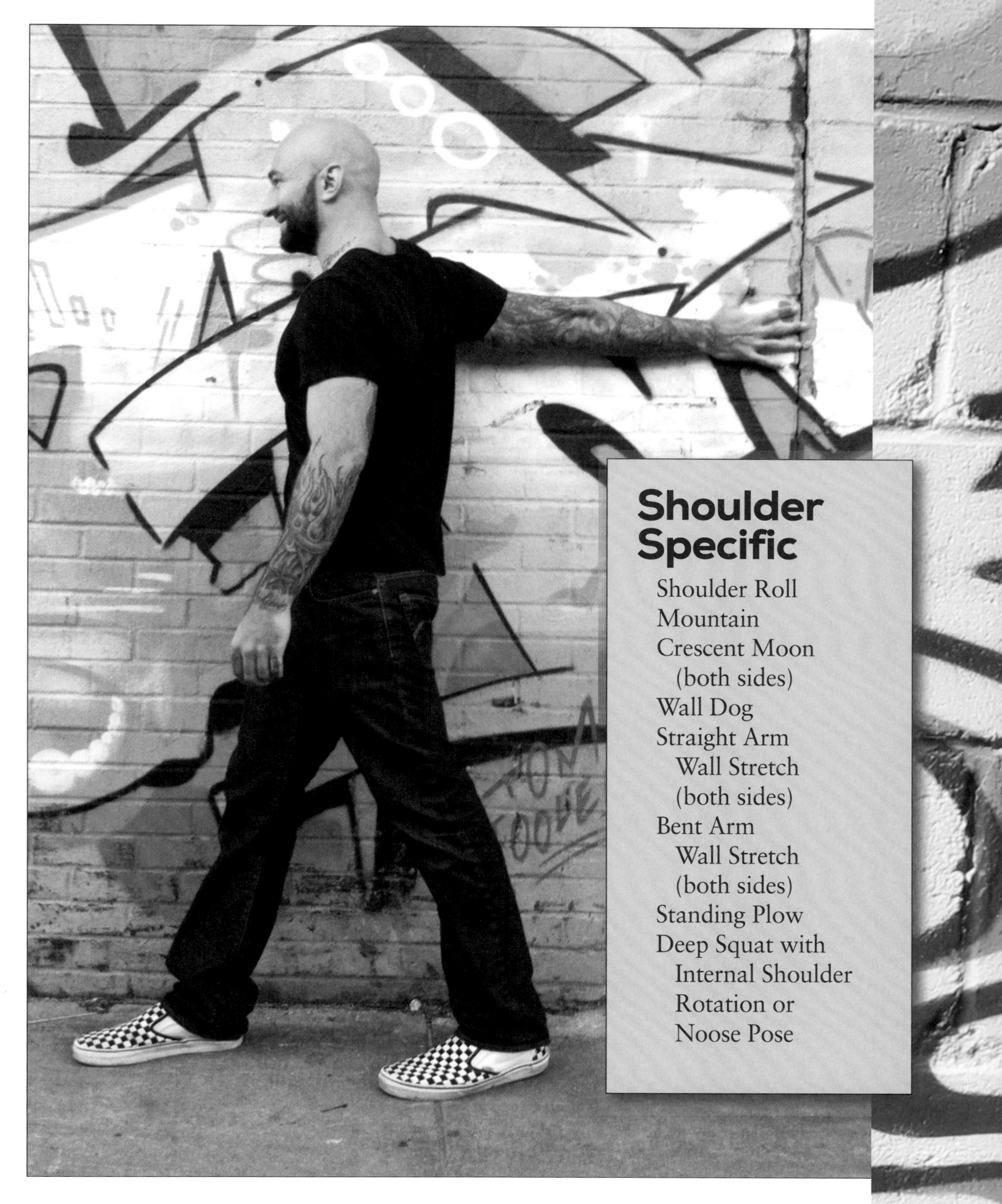

## Shoulder Specific

Shoulder Roll
Mountain
Crescent Moon
(both sides)
Wall Dog
Straight Arm
Wall Stretch
(both sides)
Bent Arm
Wall Stretch
(both sides)
Standing Plow
Deep Squat with
Internal Shoulder
Rotation or
Noose Pose

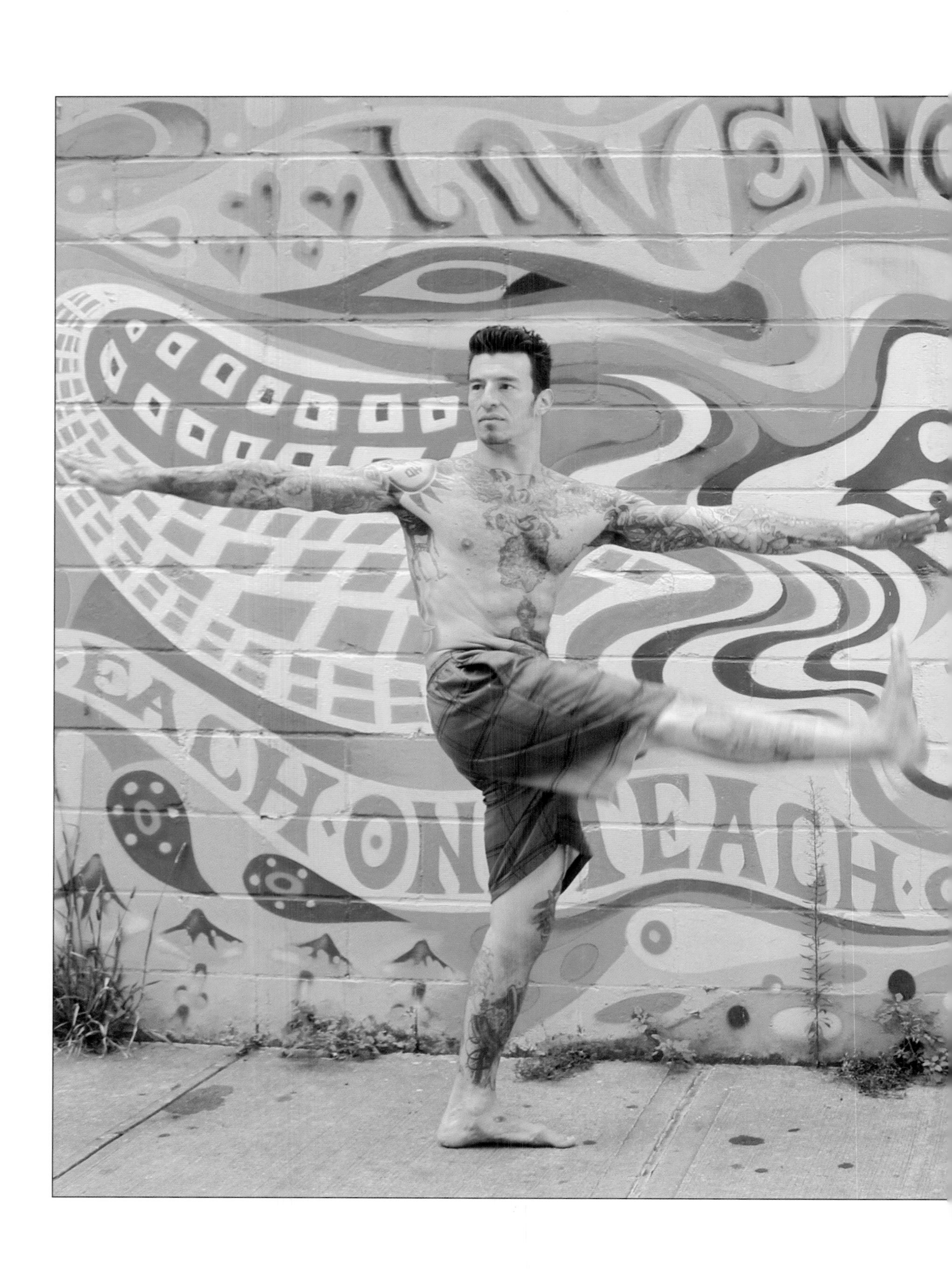

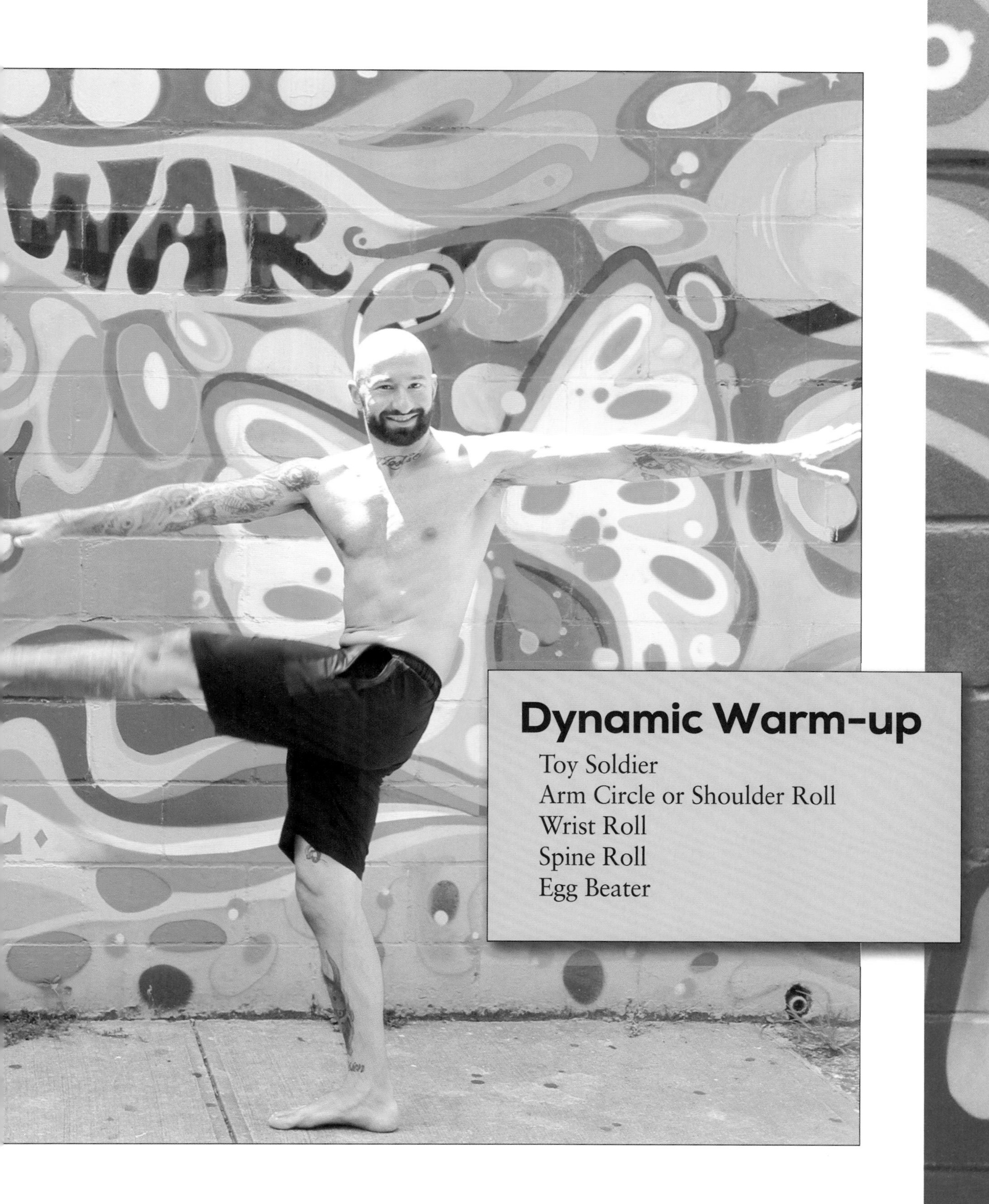


## Dynamic Warm-up

Toy Soldier
Arm Circle or Shoulder Roll
Wrist Roll
Spine Roll
Egg Beater

## Hips and Hammies

Mountain
Half Forward Bend
Full Forward Bend
Grounded Lunge
Downward Dog
Grounded Lunge (opposite side)
Lying Twist (both sides)
Seated Twist (both sides)
Half Straddle (both sides)
Full Straddle
Seated Forward Bend
Butterfly
Frog
Ankle to Knee Pose, Half Lotus or Lotus

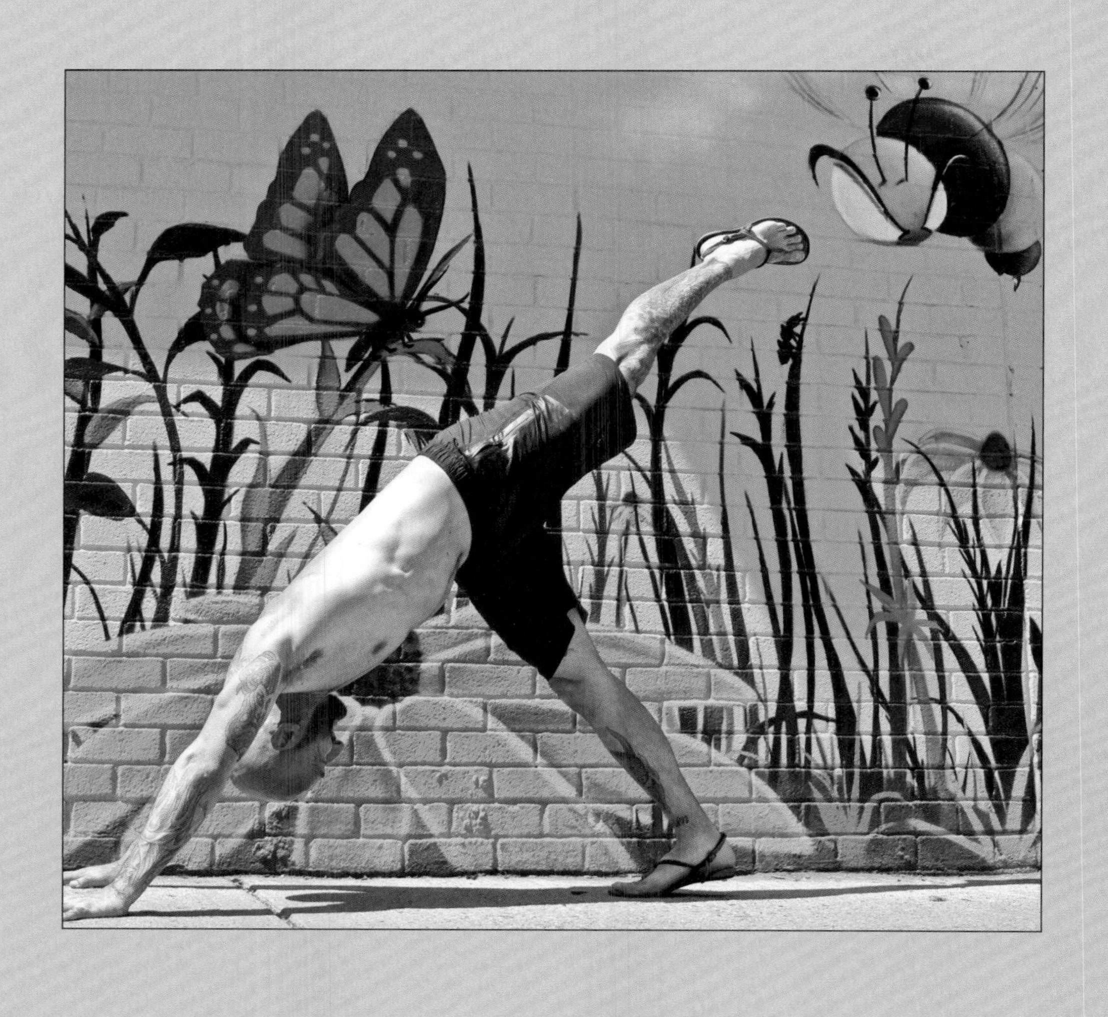

## The Complete Body

Statue
Mountain
Crescent Moon (both sides)
(Warrior I
Warrior II
Triangle) - repeat in order on both sides
Tree Pose
Bound Eagle
Standing Single Leg Foot Hold or Standing Head to Knee
Drinking Bird
Standing Quad Stretch or Standing Bow Pose
Downward Dog
Cobra, Sphinx or Updog
Child's Pose
Lying Knee to Chest
Lying Twist
Half Straddle (both sides)
Full Straddle
Seated Forward Bend
Butterfly
Shoulderstand
Plow
Camel
Wheel
Dead Man's Pose

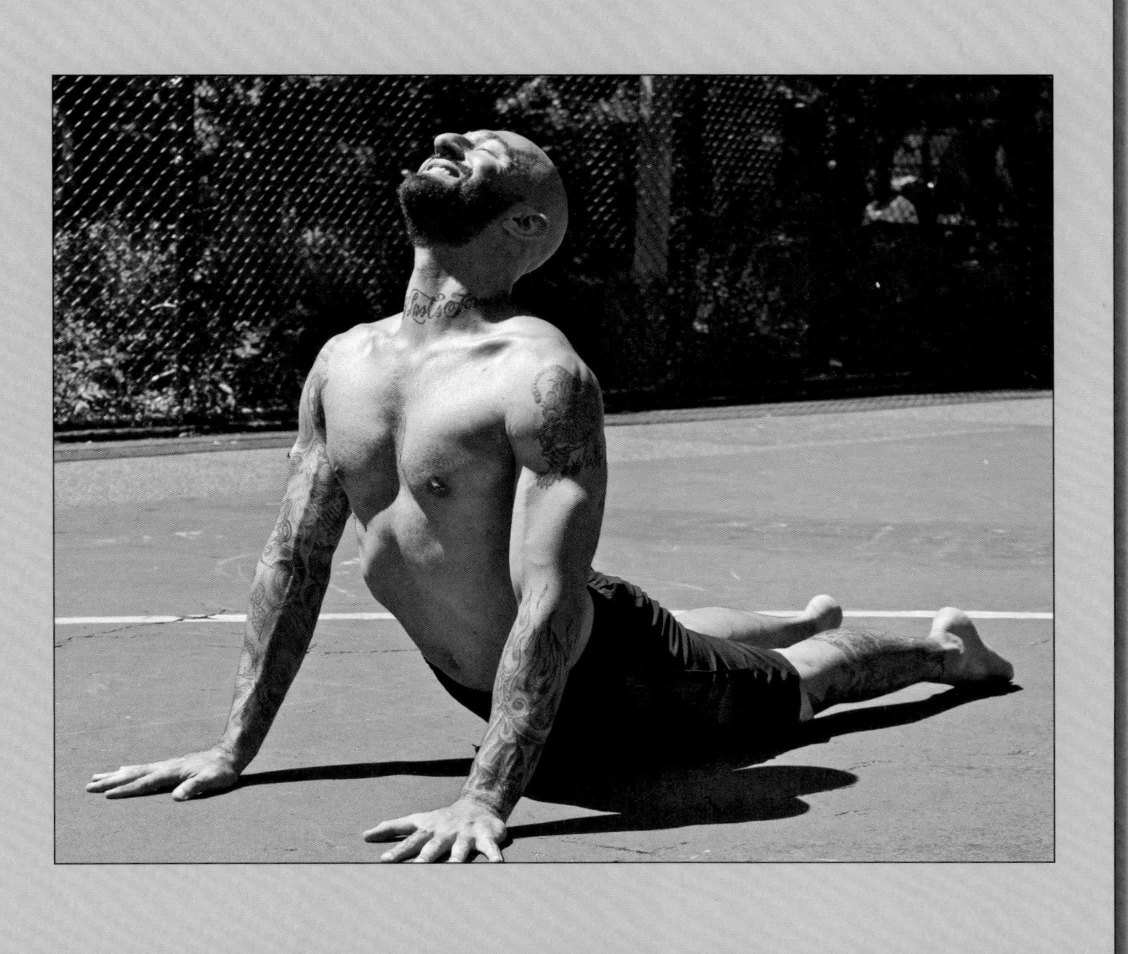

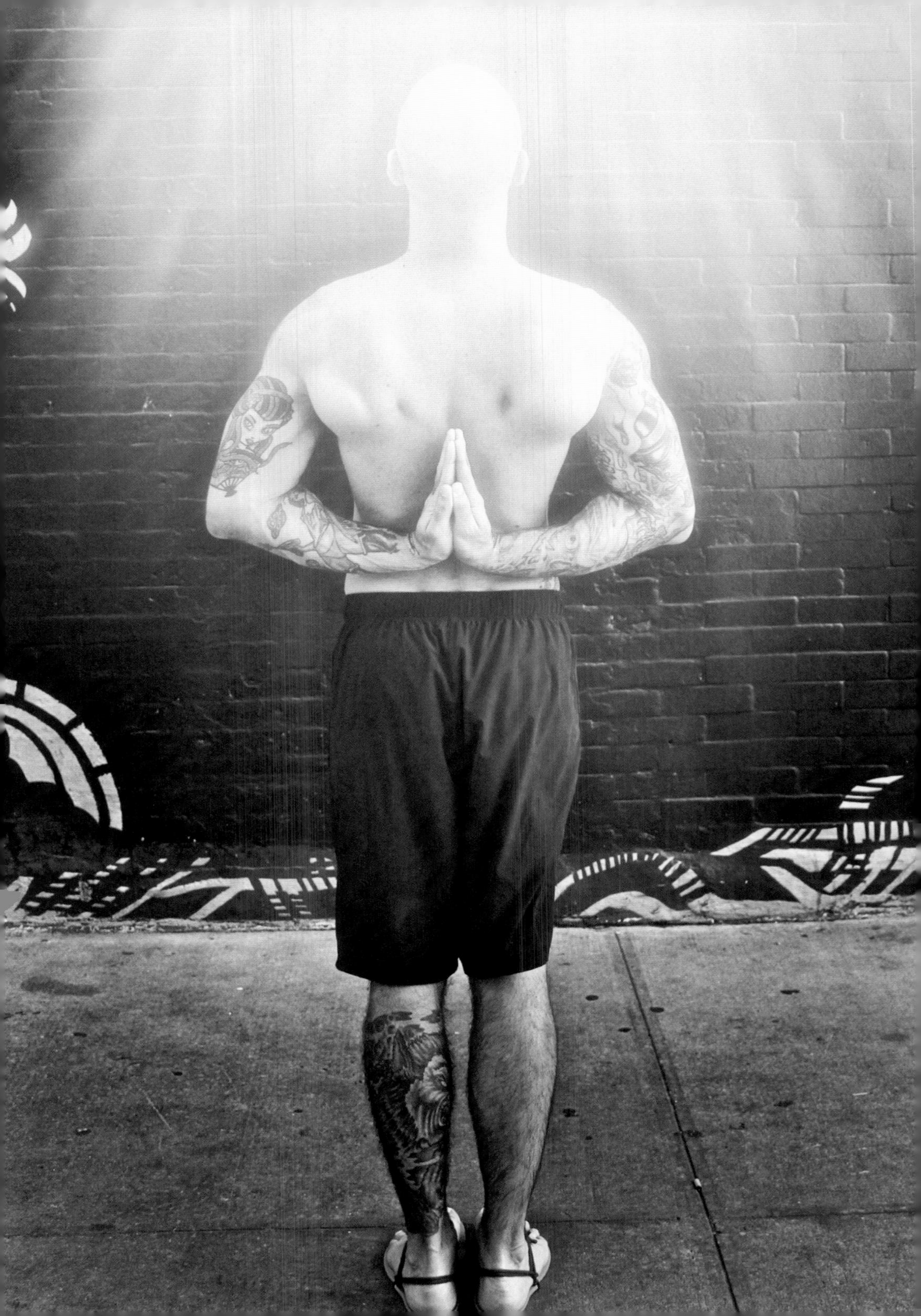

# ACKNOWLEDGEMENTS

Thank you to my amazing girlfriend, Rachel Kuhns, whose companionship, love and support helped make 2013 the best year of my life. Rachel is also a terrific editor, fitness model and photographer, and helped a ton with putting this book together. I love you, babe!

Thank you to my brother, training partner and best friend, Danny Kavadlo. Also a terrific editor, fitness model and photographer. This book would not have been possible without you, Danny!

Thanks to Derek Brigham, the best graphics guy in the business. Derek really outdid himself this time. You da man, Big D!

Thank you to Jordan Perlson, Lauren Sison, Meng He, Kiki Flynn and Wes Sanchez, all of whom have been a part of "Team Al" for a long time, providing invaluable behind-the-scenes help. You guys rock!

Thank you to John Du Cane, Dennis Armstrong, Rose Widell, Tammy Drury, Allison Olson, Mumtaz Walli-Ware and the rest of the Dragon Door team. I'm grateful for everything you have done (and continue to do) for me!

Thank you to Paul Wade, Adrienne Harvey, Steven Low, Angelo Gala, Beth Andrews, Andrew Read, Logan Christopher, Fredrik Högström, Anders Randin and everyone else who represents the Progressive Calisthenics Certification all over the world. You make me proud to be part of such a distinguished group of athletes!

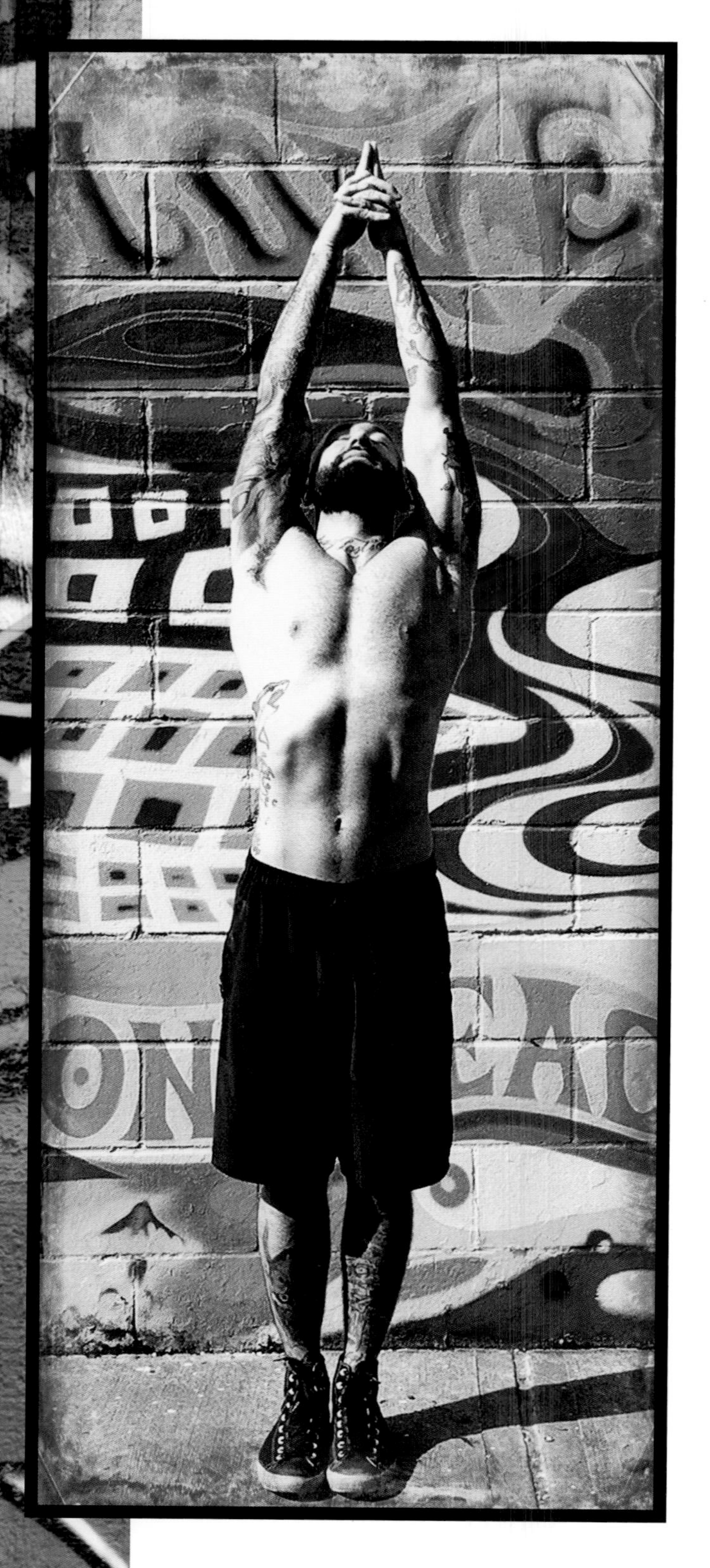

Thank you to Elliott Hulse for writing the wonderful foreword to this book. I've been a fan for a long time and it's an honor to have your endorsement, Elliott!

Thank you to Daniel Lucas, Keith Paine, Antonio Sini, Grace Shon and the rest of the team at Nimble Fitness in NYC. You guys have had my back since day one!

Thank you to Steven Sashen at Xero Shoes for all the cool minimalist footwear. If you like my sandals, go get yourself a pair at Xeroshoes.com!

And of course, a big thank you to every one of you who have bought my books, attended my workshops, watched my YouTube videos, liked me on Facebook or interacted with me in any other capacity. Without all of you, none of this would be possible!

We're Working Out!

Al Kavadlo

# About the Author

Al Kavadlo is one of the world's top experts in bodyweight strength training and the lead instructor for Dragon Door's Progressive Calisthenics Certification (PCC). A veteran of the fitness industry, Kavadlo has been featured in *The New York Times* and is well known for his appearance in the popular ***Convict Conditioning*** book series. As a trainer, Al has worked with all types of people from everyday working folks to Olympic medalists.

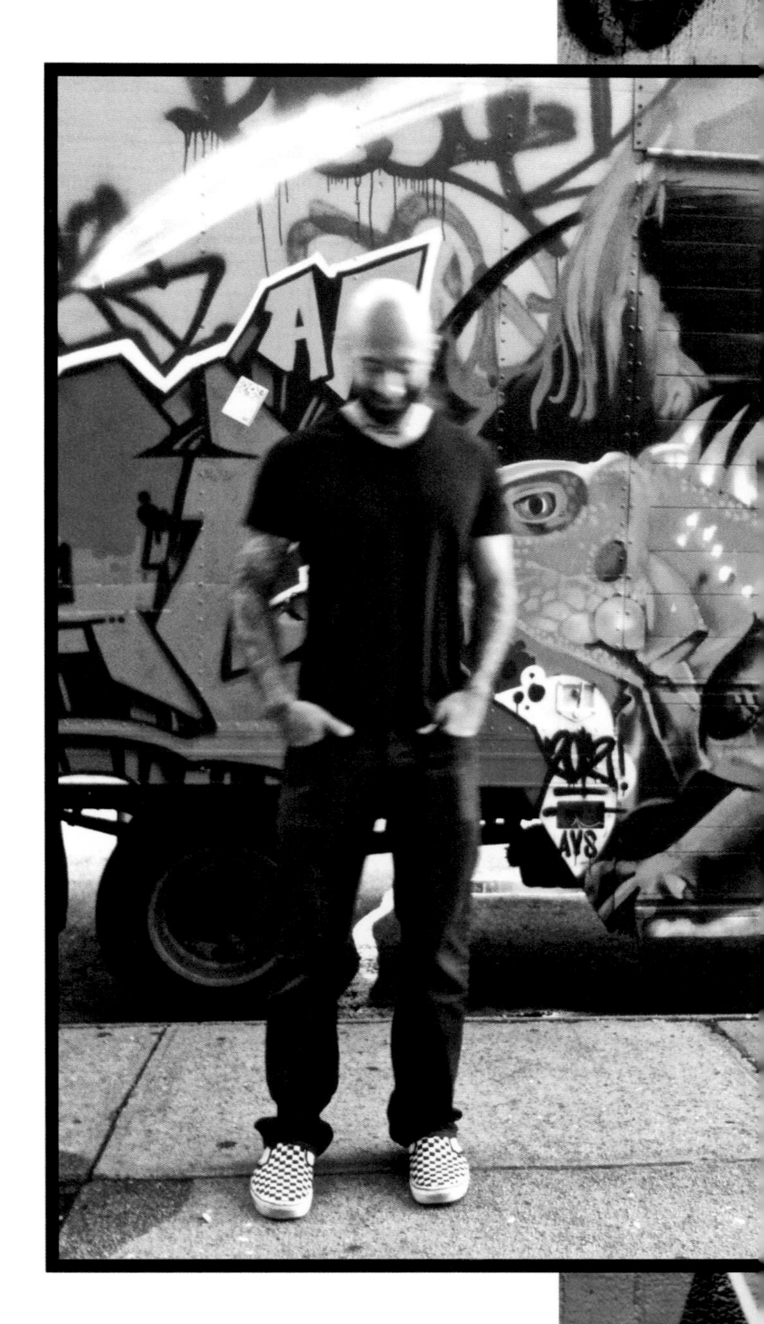

## Also available by Al Kavadlo:

*Pushing The Limits! -*
*Total Body Strength With No Equipment*
Dragon Door Publications, 2013

*Raising The Bar -*
*The Definitive Guide to Pull-up Bar Calisthenics*
Dragon Door Publications, 2012

*We're Working Out! -*
*A Zen Approach to Everyday Fitness,*
Muscle-up Publications, 2010

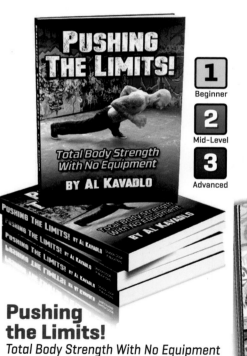

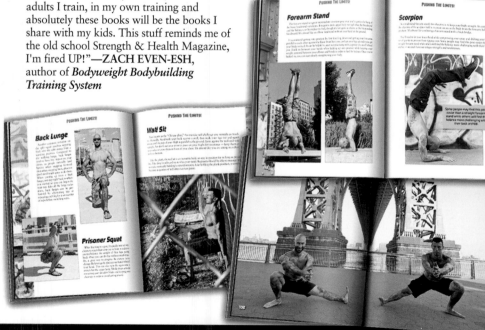

# Go Beyond Mere "Toughness"— When You Master The Art of Bar Athletics and Sculpt the Ultimate in Upper Body Physiques

"***Raising the Bar*** is very likely the most important book on strength and conditioning to be published in the last fifty years. If you only ever get your hands on one training manual in your life, make it this one. Buy it, read it, use it. This book has the power to transform you into the ultimate bar athlete."
**—Paul "Coach" Wade**, author of ***Convict Conditioning***

**Raising the Bar**

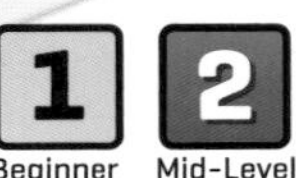

Beginner

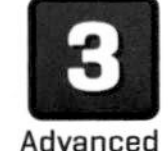

Mid-Level

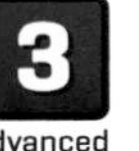

Advanced

***The Definitive Guide to Bar Calisthenics***
**By Al Kavadlo** **#B63 $39.95**
224 pages, 330 Photos

*Raising the Bar* breaks down every type of exercise you can do with a pull-up bar. From the basic two arm hang, to the mighty muscle-up, all the way to the elusive one arm pull-up, "bar master" Al Kavadlo takes you step by expert step through everything you need to do to build the chiseled frame you've always wanted.

Whether you're a die-hard calisthenics enthusiast or just looking to get in the best shape of your life, *Raising the Bar* will meet all your expectations—and then some!

**The message is clear:** you can earn yourself a stunning upper body with just 3 basic moves and 1 super-simple, yet amazingly versatile tool.

And what's even better, this 3 + 1 formula for upper body magnificence hides enough variety to keep you challenged and surging to new heights for a lifetime of cool moves and ever-tougher progressions!

Cast in the "concrete jungle" of urban scaffolding and graffiti-laden, blasted walls—and sourced from iconic bar-athlete destinations like Tompkins Square Park, NYC—*Raising the Bar* rears up to grab you by the throat and hurl you into an inspiring new vision of what the human body can achieve. Embrace Al Kavadlo's vision, pick up the challenge, share the Quest, follow directions—and the Holy Grail of supreme upper body fitness is yours for the taking.

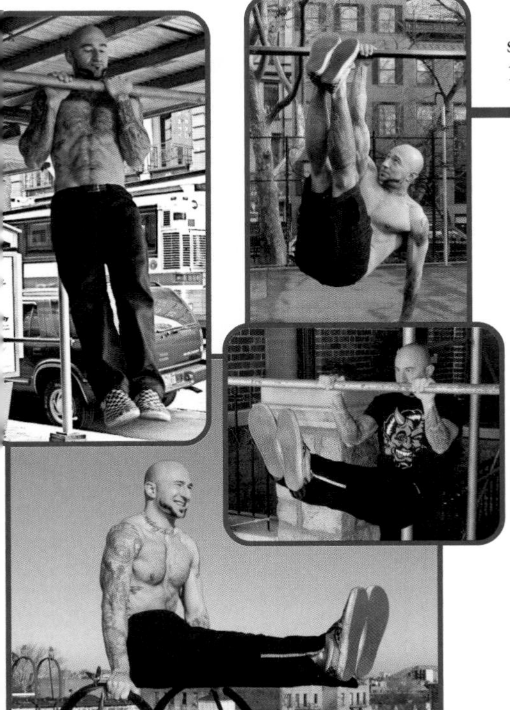

"With *Raising the Bar*, Al Kavadlo has put forth the perfect primal pull-up program. Al's progressions and demonstrations make even the most challenging exercises attainable. Anyone who is serious about pull-ups should read this book."—**Mark Sisson**, author of *The Primal Blueprint.*

**A Kick Ass Encyclopedia of Bodyweight Exercises**

"Al Kavadlo has put together a kick ass encyclopedia of the most powerful and most commonly used bodyweight exercises amongst the various groups of bodyweight masters.

From the most simple form of each exercise progressing to the most challenging form of each exercise, Al covers it. As a Coach and bodyweight training addict I loved all the variations shown.This book is far beyond just pull ups and there are countless exercises for upper body and abs. Al covers what is probably EVERY exercise he knows of, uses and teaches others, breaking down proper techniques, regressions and progressions. This is HUGE for the trainers out there who do NOT know how to adapt bodyweight exercises to each individual's fitness level.

If you're a fan of bodyweight training, between this book and *Convict Conditioning* you can turn your body into a deadly weapon!!!" **—Zach Even-Esh**, Manasquan, NJ

"Al has put together the companion manual for all the crazy bar calisthenics videos that you find yourself watching over and over again—a much needed resource. Within this book is a huge volume of bar exercises that will keep your pullup workouts fresh for years, and give you some insane goals to shoot for."
**—Max Shank, Senior RKC**

"The only tool required to fully train bodyweight is a bar or something to hang on. I believe that this amazing book by Al Kavadlo, contains everything that is ever possible to do with a bar, from entry level to 'mutant' level. Thanks to the information contained in this book you will have material to practice and improve your skills for years"**—Fabio Zonin, Senior RKC, Italian bodybuilding champion, Master Instructor FIF**

**www.dragondoor.com**
**1-800-899-5111**

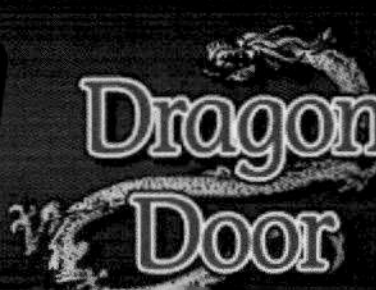


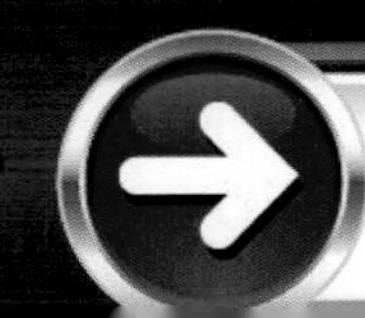

**Order *Raising The Bar* online:**
www.dragondoor.com/B63

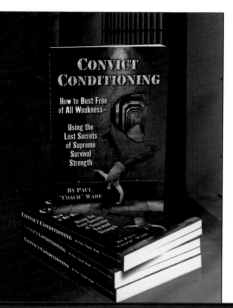

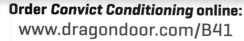

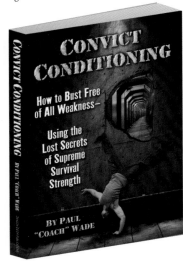

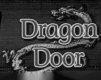

# The Experts Give High Praise to *Convict Conditioning 2*

"Coach Paul Wade has outdone himself. His first book *Convict Conditioning* is to my mind THE BEST book ever written on bodyweight conditioning. Hands down. Now, with the sequel *Convict Conditioning 2*, Coach Wade takes us even deeper into the subtle nuances of training with the ultimate resistance tool: our bodies.

In plain English, but with an amazing understanding of anatomy, physiology, kinesiology and, go figure, psychology, Coach Wade explains very simply how to work the smaller but just as important areas of the body such as the hands and forearms, neck and calves and obliques in serious functional ways.

His minimalist approach to exercise belies the complexity of his system and the deep insight into exactly how the body works and the best way to get from A to Z in the shortest time possible.

I got the best advice on how to strengthen the hard-to-reach extensors of the hand right away from this exercise Master I have ever seen. It's so simple but so completely functional I can't believe no one else has thought of it yet. Just glad he figured it out for me.

Paul teaches us how to strengthen our bodies with the simplest of movements while at the same time balancing our structures in the same way: simple exercises that work the whole body.

And just as simply as he did with his first book. His novel approach to stretching and mobility training is brilliant and fresh as well as his take on recovery and healing from injury. Sprinkled throughout the entire book are too-many-to-count insights and advice from a man who has come to his knowledge the hard way and knows exactly of what he speaks.

This book is, as was his first, an amazing journey into the history of physical culture disguised as a book on calisthenics. But the thing that Coach Wade does better than any before him is his unbelievable progressions on EVERY EXERCISE and stretch! He breaks things down and tells us EXACTLY how to proceed to get to whatever level of strength and development we want. AND gives us the exact metrics we need to know when to go to the next level.

Adding in completely practical and immediately useful insights into nutrition and the mindset necessary to deal not only with training but with life, makes this book a classic that will stand the test of time.

Bravo Coach Wade, Bravo." **—Mark Reifkind, Master RKC**, author of *Mastering the HardStyle Kettlebell Swing*

"I've been lifting weights for over 50 years and have trained in the martial arts since 1965. I've read voraciously on both subjects, and written dozens of magazine articles and many books on the subjects. This book and Wade's first, *Convict Conditioning*, are by far the most commonsense, information-packed, and result producing I've read. These books will truly change your life.

Paul Wade is a new and powerful voice in the strength and fitness arena, one that is commonsense, inspiring, and in your face. His approach to maximizing your body's potential is not the same old hackneyed material you find in every book and magazine piece that pictures steroid-bloated models screaming as they curl weights. Wade's stuff has been proven effective by hard men who don't tolerate fluff. It will work for you, too—guaranteed.

As an ex-cop, I've gone mano-y-mano with ex-cons that had clearly trained as Paul Wade suggests in his two *Convict Conditioning* books. While these guys didn't look like steroid-fueled bodybuilders (actually, there were a couple who did), all were incredibly lean, hard and powerful. Wade blows many commonly held beliefs about conditioning, strengthening, and eating out of the water and replaces them with result-producing information that won't cost you a dime." **—Loren W. Christensen**, author of *Fighting the Pain Resistant Attacker*, and many other titles

"The overriding principle of *Convict Conditioning* 2 is 'little equipment-big rewards'. For the athlete in the throwing and fighting arts, the section on Lateral Chain Training, Capturing the Flag, is a unique and perhaps singular approach to training the obliques and the whole family of side muscles. This section stood out to me as ground breaking and well worth the time and energy by anyone to review and attempt to complete. Literally, this is a new approach to lateral chain training that is well beyond sidebends and suitcase deadlifts.

The author's review of passive stretching reflects the experience of many of us in the field. But, his solution might be the reason I am going to recommend this work for everyone: The Trifecta. This section covers what the author calls The Functional Triad and gives a series of simple progressions to three holds that promise to oil your joints. It's yoga for the strength athlete and supports the material one would find, for example, in Pavel's *Loaded Stretching*.

I didn't expect to like this book, but I come away from it practically insisting that everyone read it. It is a strongman book mixed with yoga mixed with street smarts. I wanted to hate it, but I love it."
—Dan John, author of *Don't Let Go* and co-author of *Easy Strength*

"*Convict Conditioning* is one of the most influential books I ever got my hands on. *Convict Conditioning 2* took my training and outlook on the power of bodyweight training to the 10th degree—from strengthening the smallest muscles in a maximal manner, all the way to using bodyweight training as a means of healing injuries that pile up from over 22 years of aggressive lifting.

I've used both *Convict Conditioning* and *Convict Conditioning 2* on myself and with my athletes. Without either of these books I can easily say that these boys would not be the BEASTS they are today. Without a doubt *Convict Conditioning 2* will blow you away and inspire and educate you to take bodyweight training to a whole NEW level."
—Zach Even-Esh, Underground Strength Coach

**Convict Conditioning 2**
*Advanced Prison Training Tactics for Muscle Gain, Fat Loss and Bulletproof Joints*
**By Paul "Coach" Wade**
**#B59 $39.95**
Paperback 8.5 x 11 354 pages
261 photos, charts and illustrations

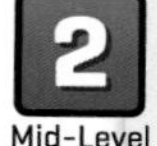


3
Advanced

www.dragondoor.com
1-800-899-5111

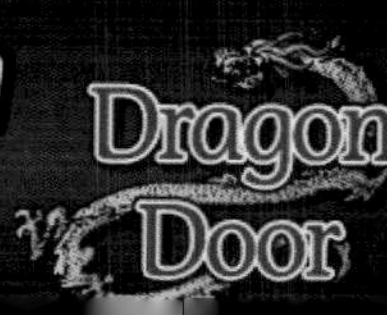


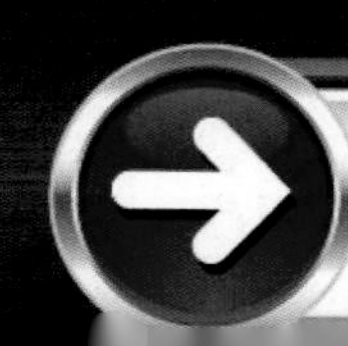

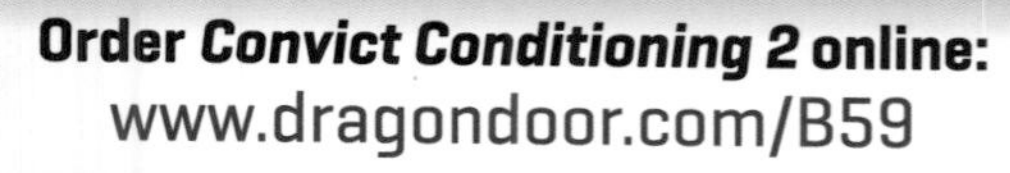

# —Table of Contents—

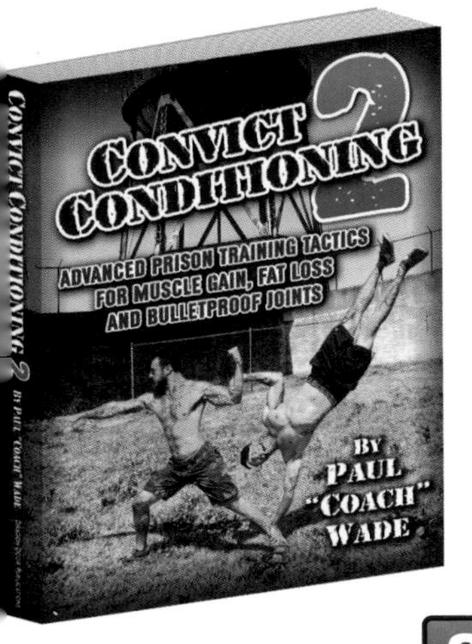


## Convict Conditioning 2

*Advanced Prison Training Tactics for Muscle Gain, Fat Loss and Bulletproof Joints*

**By Paul "Coach" Wade**

**#B59 $39.95**

Paperback 8.5 x 11 354 pages

261 photos, charts and illustrations

**2** Mid-Level

**3** Advanced

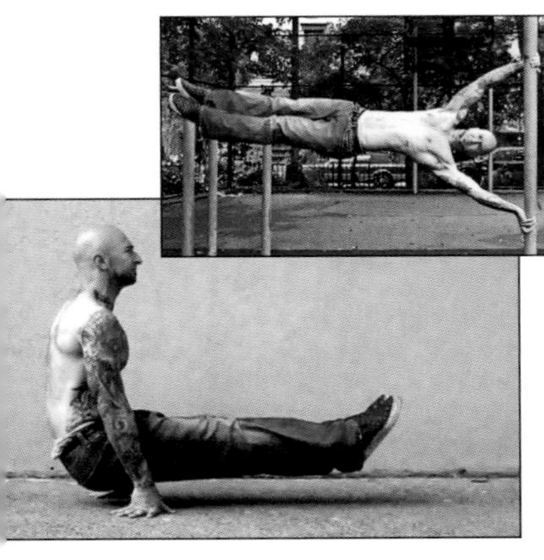

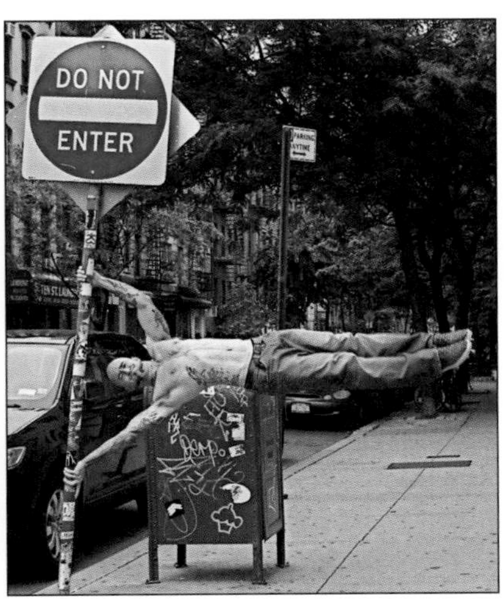


**Foreword**
*The Many Roads to Strength by Brooks Kubik*

Opening Salvo: *Chewing Bubblegum and Kicking Ass*

1. Introduction: *Put Yourself Behind Bars*

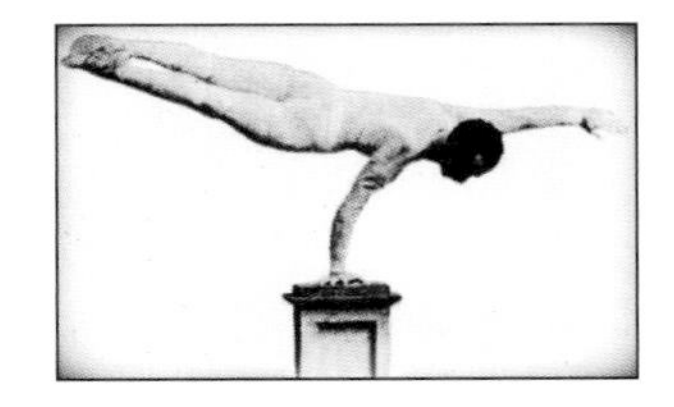

**PART I: SHOTGUN MUSCLE**

**Hands and Forearms**

2: Iron Hands and Forearms: *Ultimate Strength —with Just Two Techniques*

3: The Hang Progressions: *A Vice-Like Bodyweight Grip Course*

4: Advanced Grip Torture: *Explosive Power + Titanium Fingers*

5: Fingertip Pushups: *Keeping Hand Strength Balanced*

6: Forearms into Firearms: *Hand Strength: A Summary and a Challenge*

**Lateral Chain**

7: Lateral Chain Training: *Capturing the Flag*

8: The Clutch Flag: *In Eight Easy Steps*

9: The Press Flag: *In Eight Not-So-Easy Steps*

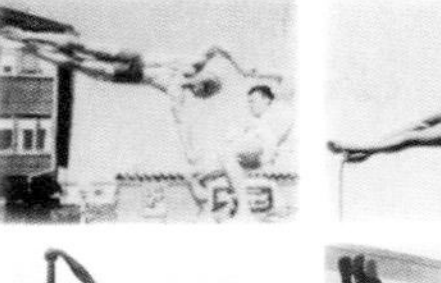

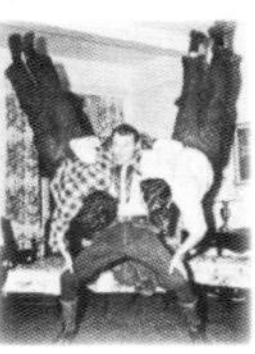

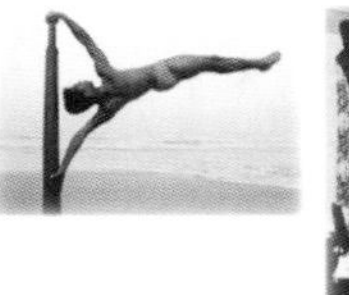

**Neck and Calves**

10. Bulldog Neck: *Bulletproof Your Weakest Link*

11. Calf Training: *Ultimate Lower Legs—No Machines Necessary*

**PART II: BULLETPROOF JOINTS**

12. Tension-Flexibility: *The Lost Art of Joint Training*

13. Stretching—the Prison Take: *Flexibility, Mobility, Control*

14. The Trifecta: *Your "Secret Weapon" for Mobilizing Stiff, Battle-Scarred Physiques—for Life*

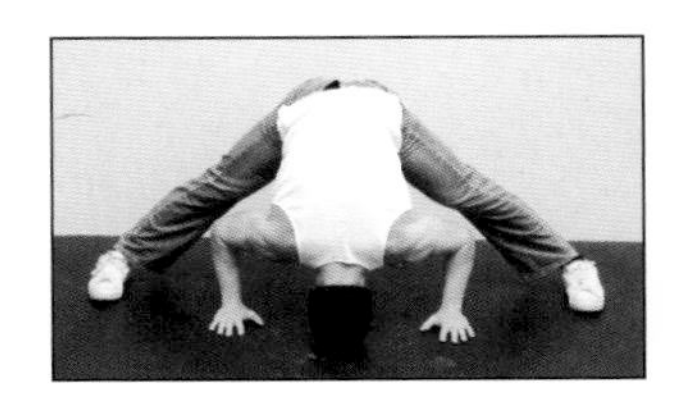

15: The Bridge Hold Progressions: *The Ultimate Prehab/Rehab Technique*

16: The L-Hold Progressions: *Cure Bad Hips and Low Back—Inside-Out*

17: Twist Progressions: *Unleash Your Functional Triad*

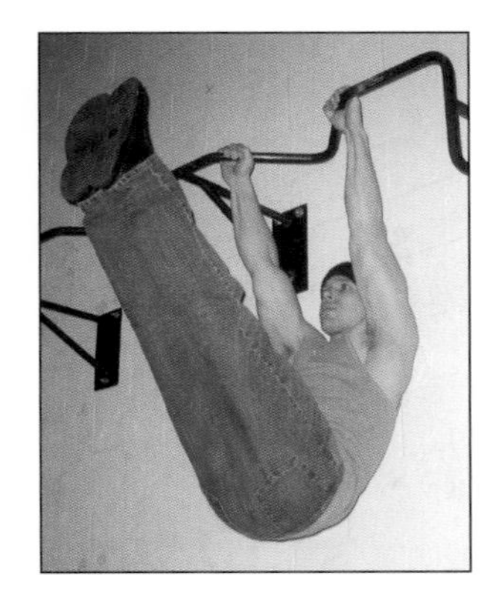

**PART III: WISDOM FROM CELLBLOCK G**

18. Doing Time Right: *Living the Straight Edge*

19. The Prison Diet: *Nutrition and Fat Loss Behind Bars*

20. Mendin' Up: *The 8 Laws of Healing*

21. The Mind: *Escaping the True Prison*

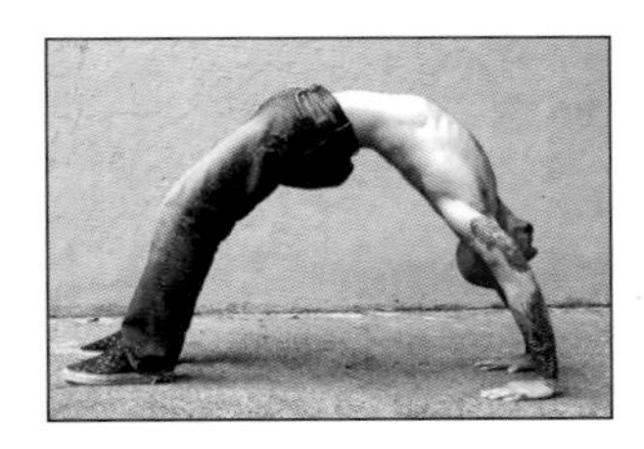

**!BONUS CHAPTER!**

Pumpin' Iron in Prison: *Myths, Muscle and Misconceptions*

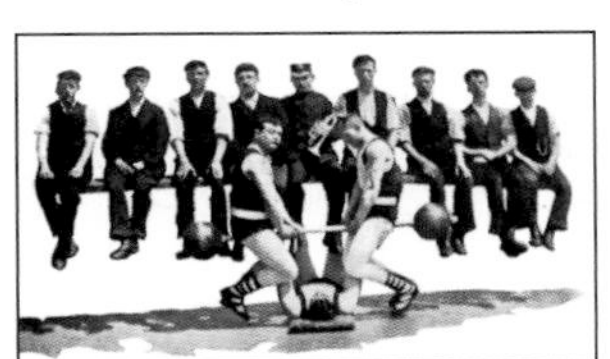

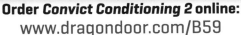

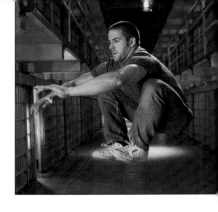

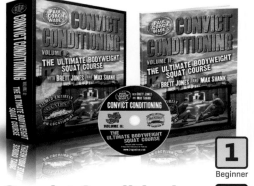

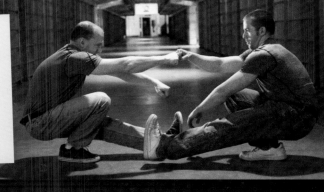

# Demonic Abs Are a Man's Best Friend—Discover How to Seize a Six-Pack from Hell and OWN the World...

# Leg Raises

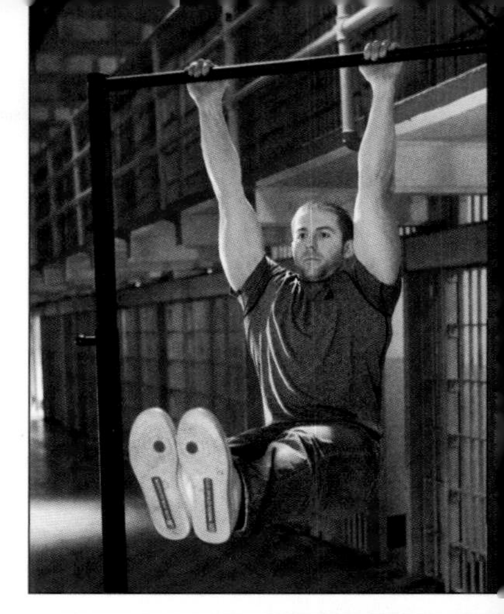

Paul Wade's *Convict Conditioning 3, Leg Raises: Six Pack from Hell* teaches you in absolute detail how to progress from the ease of a simple Knee Tuck—to the magnificent, "1-in-1,000" achievement of the Hanging Straight Leg Raise. Ten progressive steps guide you to inevitable mastery of this ultimate abs exercise. Do it, seize the knowledge—but beware—the Gods will be jealous!

This home-study course in ultimate survival strength comes replete with bonus material not available in **Paul Wade's** original *Convict Conditioning* book—and numerous key training tips that refine and expand on the original program.

Prowl through the heavily and gorgeously-illustrated 80-plus-page manual and devour the entire film script at your animal leisure. Digest the brilliant, precise photographs and reinforce the raw benefits you absorbed from the DVD.

Paul Wade adds a bonus **Ten Commandments for Perfect Bodyweight Squats**—which is worth the price of admission alone. And there's the additional bonus of **4 major Variant drills** to add explosivity, fun and super-strength to your core practice.

Whatever you are looking for when murdering your abs—be it a fist-breaking, rock-like shield of impenetrable muscle, an uglier-is-more-beautiful set of rippling abdominal ridges, or a monstrous injection of lifting power—it's yours for the progressive taking with *Convict Conditioning, Volume 3, Leg Raises: Six Pack from Hell*

## Prison-Style Midsection Training—For an All Show AND All Go Physique

When convicts train their waists, they want real, noticeable results—and by "results" we don't mean that they want cute, tight little defined abs. We mean that they want thick, strong, muscular midsections. They want *functionally* powerful abs and hips they can use for heavy lifting, kicking, and brawling. They want guts so strong from their training that it actually hurts an attacker to punch them in the belly. Prison abs aren't about all show, no go—a prison-built physique has to be all show and all go. Those guys don't just want six-packs—they want six-packs from Hell.

And, for the first time, we're going to show you how these guys get what they want. We're not going to be using sissy machines or easy isolation exercises—we're going straight for the old school secret weapon for gut training; progressive leg raises.

If you want a six-pack from Hell, the first thing you need to do is focus your efforts. If a weightlifter wanted a very thick, powerful chest in a hurry, he wouldn't spread his efforts out over a dozen exercises and perform them gently all day long. No—he'd pick just one exercise, probably the bench press, and just focus on getting stronger and stronger on that lift until he was monstrously strong. When he reached this level, and his pecs were thick slabs of meat, only then would he maybe begin sculpting them with minor exercises and higher reps.

It's no different if you want a mind-blowing midsection. Just pick one exercise that hits all the muscles in the midsection—the hip flexors, the abs, the intercostals, the obliques—then blast it.

And the one exercise we're going to discover is the best midsection exercise known to man, and the most popular amongst soldiers, warriors, martial artists and prison athletes since men started working out—the leg raise.

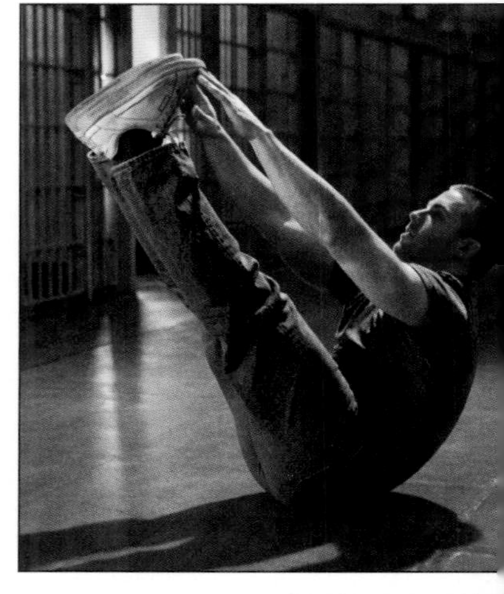

You'll discover ten different leg raise movements, each one a little harder than the last. You'll learn how to get the most out of each of these techniques, each of these ten steps, before moving up to the next step. By the time you get through all ten steps and you're working with the final Master Step of the leg raise series, you'll have a solid, athletic, stomach made of steel, as well as powerful hips and a ribcage armored with dense muscle. You'll have abs that would've made Bruce Lee take notice!

## The Ten Commandments You Must Obey to Earn a Real Monster of an Athletic Core

Paul Wade gives you ten key points, the "Ten Commandments" of leg raises, that will take your prison-style core training from just "okay" to absolutely phenomenal. We want the results to be so effective that they'll literally shock you. This kind of accelerated progress can be achieved, but if you want to achieve it you better listen carefully to these ten key pointers you'll discover with the DVD.

Bodyweight mastery is a lot like high-level martial arts. It's more about *principles* than individual techniques. Really study and absorb these principles, and you'll be on your way to a six-pack from Hell in no time.

The hanging straight leg raise, performed strictly and for reps, is the Gold Standard of abdominal strength techniques. Once you're at the level where you can throw out sets of twenty to thirty rock solid reps of this exercise, your abs will be thick and strong, but more importantly, they'll be functional—not just a pretty six-pack, but a real monster of an athletic core, which is capable of developing high levels of force.

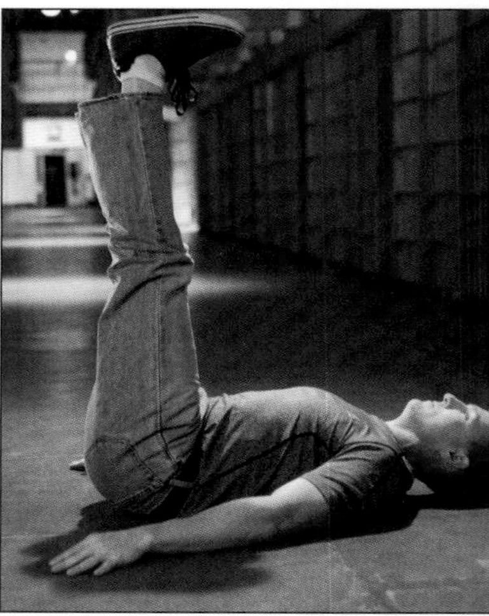

Hanging will work your serratus and intercostals making these muscles stand out like fingers, and obliques and flank muscles will be tight and stro from holding your hips in place. Your lumbar sp will achieve a gymnastic level of flexibility, like fl steel, and your chances of back pain will be grea reduced.

The bottom line: If you want to be stronger and athletic than the next guy, you need the edge that straight leg raises can give you.

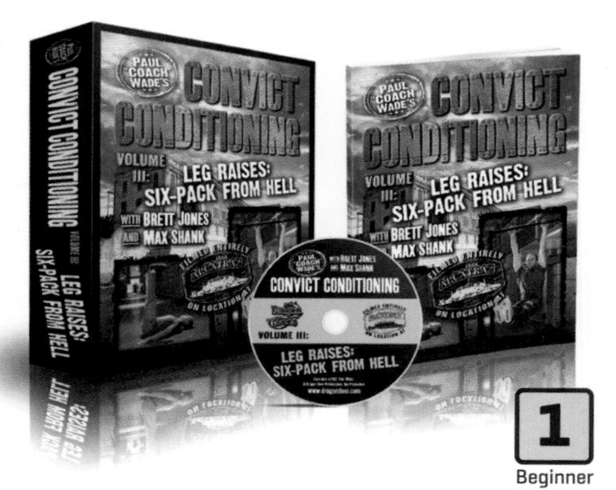


1 Beginner

2 Mid-Level

3 Advanced

**Convict Conditioning**

*Volume 3: Leg Raises*
*Six Pack from Hell*

**By Paul "Coach" Wade featuring Brett Jones and Max Shank**

**#DV085 $59.95**

DVD 57 minutes with full color Companion Manual, 82 pages

# Erect Twin Pythons of Coiled Beef Up Your Spine and Develop Extreme, Explosive Resilience—With the Dynamic Power and Flexible Strength of Advanced Bridging

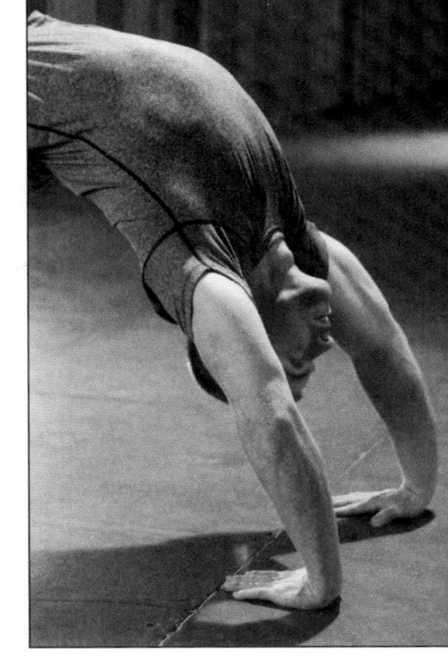

Paul Wade's *Convict Conditioning* system represents the ultimate distillation of hardcore prison bodyweight training's most powerful methods. What works was kept. What didn't, was slashed away. When your life is on the line, you're not going to mess with less than the absolute best. Many of these older, very potent solitary training systems have been on the verge of dying, as convicts begin to gain access to weights, and modern "bodybuilding thinking" floods into the prisons. Thanks to Paul Wade, these ultimate strength survival secrets have been saved for posterity. And for you...

Filmed entirely—and so appropriately— on "The Rock", Wade's *Convict Conditioning Volume 4, Advanced Bridging: Forging an Iron Spine* explodes out of the cellblock to teach you in absolute detail how to progress from the relative ease of a Short Bridge—to the stunning, "1-in-1,000" achievement of the Stand-to-Stand Bridge. Ten progressive steps guide you to inevitable mastery of this ultimate exercise for an unbreakable back.

This home-study course in ultimate survival strength comes replete with bonus material not available in **Paul Wade's** original *Convict Conditioning* book—and numerous key training tips that refine and expand on the original program.

Prowl through the heavily and gorgeously-illustrated 80-plus-page manual and devour the entire film script at your animal leisure. Digest the brilliant, precise photographs and reinforce the raw benefits you absorbed from the DVD.

Paul Wade adds a bonus **Ten Commandments for Perfect Bridges**—which is worth the price of admission alone. And there's the additional bonus of **4 major Variant drills** to add explosivity, fun and super-strength to your core practice.

Whatever you are looking for from your pushups—be it supreme functional strength, monstrous muscle growth or explosive upper-body power—it's yours for the progressive taking with *Convict Conditioning Volume 4: Advanced Bridging: Forging an Iron Spine.*

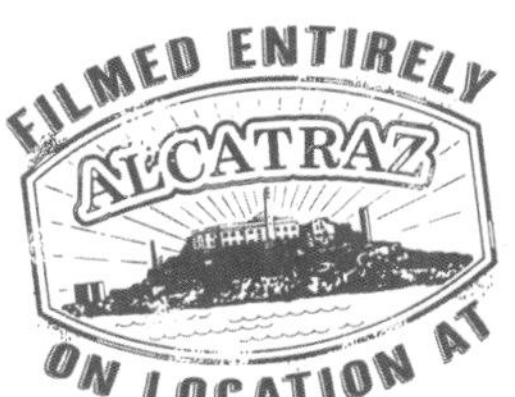


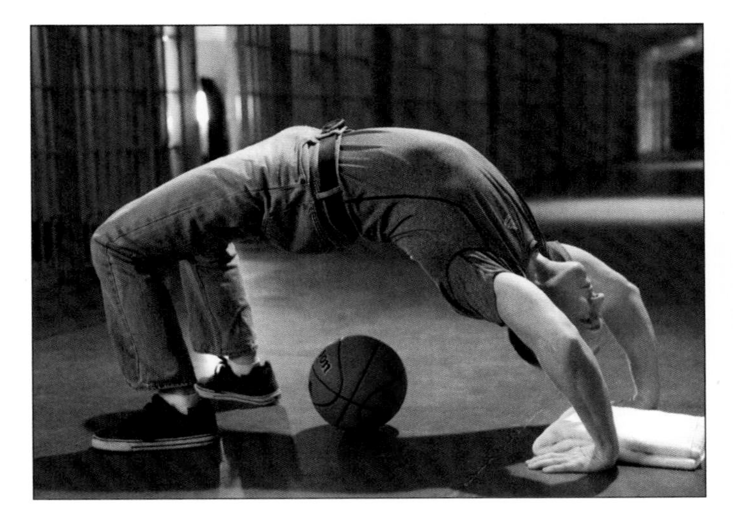

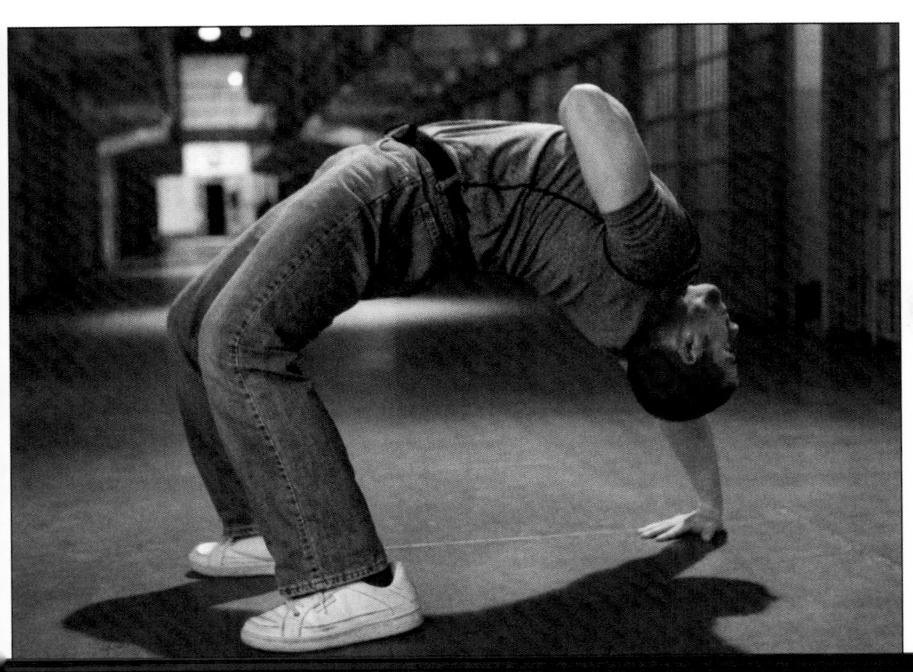

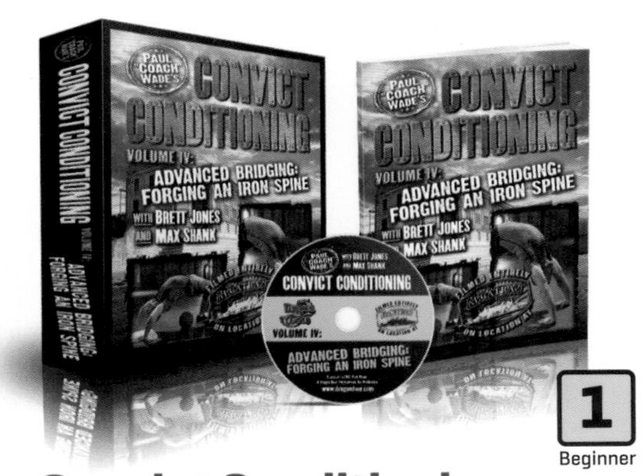


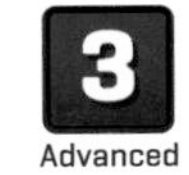


**Convict Conditioning**
*Volume 4: Advanced Bridging: Forging an Iron Spine*
**By Paul "Coach" Wade featuring Brett Jones and Max Shank**
**#DV087 $59.95**
DVD 59 minutes with full color Companion Manual, 88 pages

# WHEN IT COMES TO SERIOUS TRAINING, YOU KEEP A LOG OR YOU FAIL

## Save Yourself From Failure—With The Ultimate Bodyweight Training Log

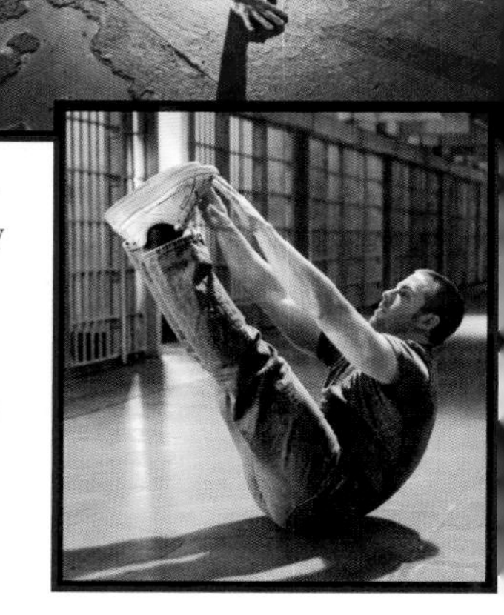

T*he Convict Conditioning Ultimate Bodyweight Training Log* is the first-ever training log designed specifically for bodyweight athletes. Other logs are structured to contain sections where you detail the amount of weight you used, the type of equipment or machine you worked out on, even what your heart-rate was and what vitamins you took today. You won't find any of this distracting information in this log. It's a log for pure, unadulterated, hardcore bodyweight training. We provide the inspiration and the structure—you provide the perspiration and bloody-mindedness to seize the plan and make it happen.

We've all heard the phrase "the spirit is willing but the flesh is weak". And never was this more true than in the quest for strength!

So, what are the two golden keys, or secrets to bending the flesh to the spirit's desire?

### The first secret is the system—and the system is dedicated, organized application over time.

The first secret is the system—and the system is dedicated, organized application over time. And in the hard world of strength that means keeping track of your goals and measuring your progress. When it comes to serious training, you keep a log or you fail. The sins of sloppiness, haphazardness, laziness and disorganization lay waste to our dreams of physical achievement—and sabotage the best intentions to beat our flesh into righteous steel. We invite you to exorcize the demons of weakness from your flesh—with a "religious" dedication to tracking and measuring—Convict Conditioning style.

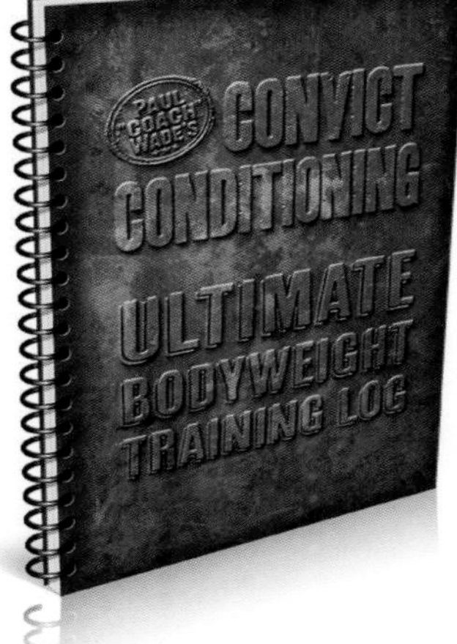


**Convict Conditioning**
*Bodyweight Training Log*
**By Paul "Coach" Wade**
**#B67 $59.95**
290 pages. Paperback (spiral bound)

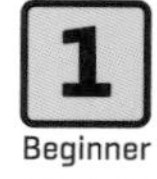

Beginner

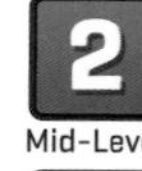

Mid-Level

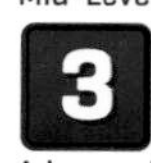

Advanced

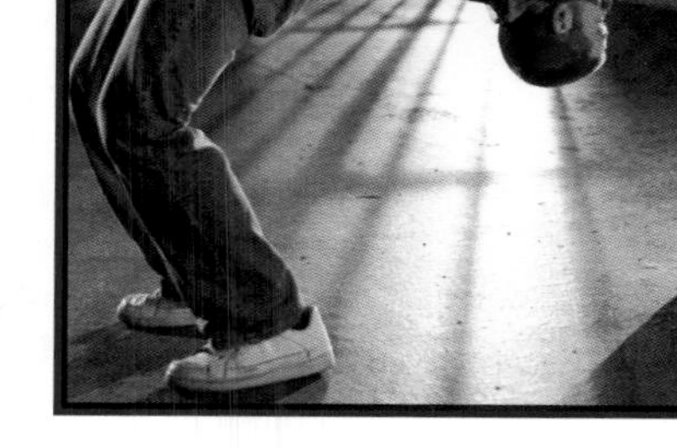

### The second secret for strength success is inspiration.

In this stunning companion to his bestselling bodyweight exercise masterpiece, Convict Conditioning author Paul Wade, goes far, far beyond the traditional log book—by delivering a bucket-load of inspiring stories and jewel-like training tips to push you forward in your quest for ever-greater strength.

This book is the first-ever training log designed specifically for bodyweight athletes. Other logs are structured to contain sections where you detail the amount of weight you used, the type of equipment or machine you worked out on, even what your heart-rate was and what vitamins you took today. You won't find any of this distracting information in this log. It's a log for pure, unadulterated, hard core bodyweight training. We provide the inspiration and the structure—you provide the perspiration and bloody-mindedness to seize the plan and make it happen.

There is a window of opportunity awaiting you. The strength gains that have continued to elude you can finally be yours. That window of opportunity lies within these pages and within your heart. Bring it!

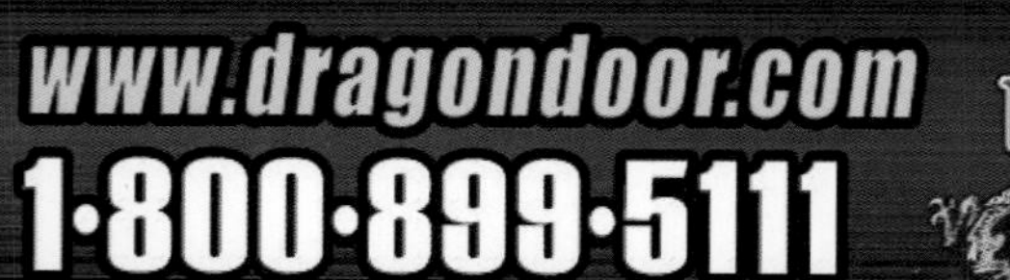


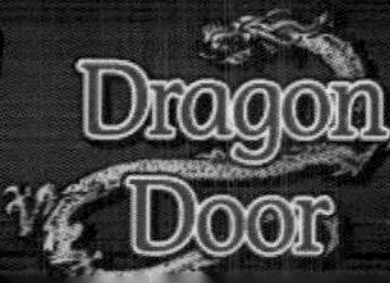


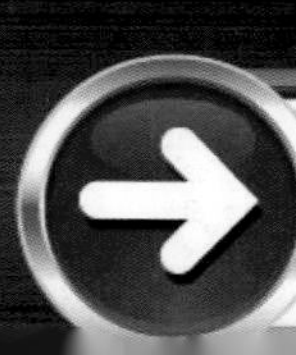

**Order *CC Ultimate Bodyweight Training Log* online:**
www.dragondoor.com/B67

# Does Anyone Else Want to Be a Highly Successful Personal Trainer—And Truly Live Your Dream?

Most folk who embark on a career as a trainer, do so initially out of a personal passion for fitness and a strong desire to help other achieve results. Be it weight loss, conditioning, strength gains, flexibility or enhanced performance.

But a passion for working out and an earnest desire to help others—alone—does not a successful personal trainer make. The sad fact is that the turn over rate for personal trainers after one year is over 80%. Why? It's almost always because the trainer didn't have a proper understanding of the BUSINESS of being a fitness professional.

The bottom line is that without the appropriate success blueprint, the most skilled and knowledgeable personal trainer is usually doomed to failure. Unfortunately, until now, there has been no such battle-tested blueprint available either to the novice trainer or the professional struggling to stay alive. Now, however that's all changed, thanks to Danny Kavadlo's *Everybody Needs Training*. Follow the hard-earned wisdom within these pages and failure will no longer be an option.

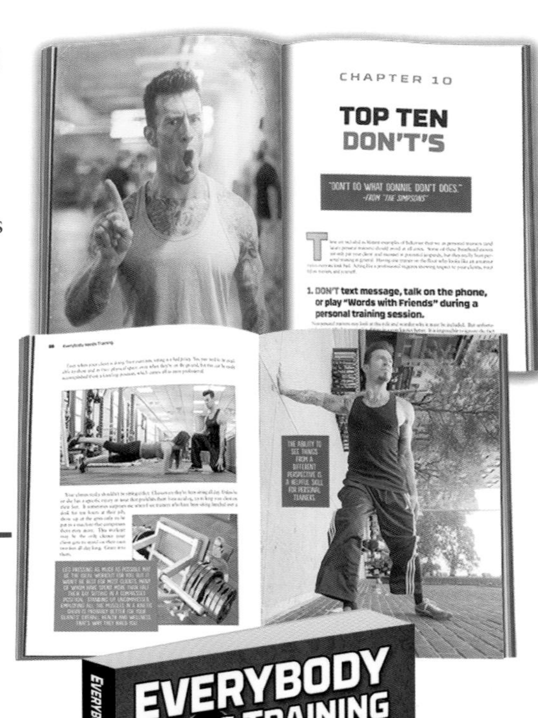


---

"Danny Kavadlo's training helped me to discover strengths I never knew I had, and I can take those lessons with me wherever I go, for the rest of my life. The wisdom and insight contained in *Everybody Needs Training* not only relates to being a successful fitness trainer, but can be applied for peace and success in many of life's ventures. Danny is the best!"—ELIZABETH GILBERT, #1 New York Times Best Selling Author, ***Eat, Pray, Love.*** One of TIME Magazine's 100 Most Influential People in the World

---

"Everybody Needs Training is quite 'something.' I don't think I have ever seen this kind of depth in the field. It's both obvious and 'wow' as you read it. Amazing stuff. It fills a gap in the community that, frankly, surprises me no one has really filled."—DAN JOHN, author, *Never Let Go*

---

"Christmas wishes DO come true….Danny Kavadlo has written a training book! Imagine if you could squeeze all the hard-earned wisdom, secrets and tactics of one of the world's hottest personal trainers between the covers of a beautifully illustrated tell-all manual, and you have imagined *Everybody Needs Training*.

Like Danny himself, this groundbreaking book is incredibly smart, brutally honest, laugh-out-loud funny, and totally out of left field…if you train others (casually or professionally), want a career training others, or if you just love the now-famous "Kavadlo approach" to getting in shape, you owe it to yourself to grab a copy of this masterpiece. I cannot recommend it highly enough."—PAUL WADE, author of *Convict Conditioning*

---

"Danny Kavadlo strikes the right tone: if you are built for it, personal training is one hell-of-a-satisfying career: do it right and you are literally transforming people's bodies and lives. So if you think you're built for it and considering jumping into the shark tank of personal training, *Everybody Needs Training* will be invaluable. And the tattooed Gonzo vibe is priceless."—MARTY GALLAGHER, author of ***The Purposeful Primitive***, 3-time World Masters Powerlifting Champion

---

## Everybody Needs Training

*Proven Success Secrets for the Professional Fitness Trainer—How to Get More Clients, Make More Money, Change More Lives*

**By Danny Kavadlo**

**#B72 $34.95**

Paperback 216 pages, 235 photos

Beginner

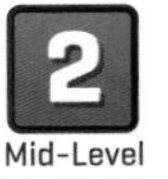
Mid-Level

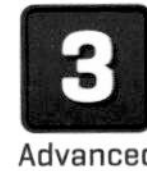
Advanced

www.dragondoor.com
1-800-899-5111

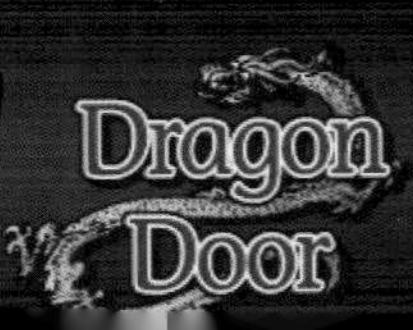
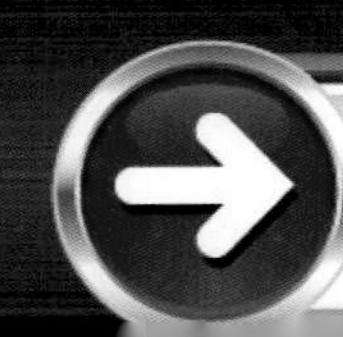

**Order *Everybody Needs Training* online:**
www.dragondoor.com/B72

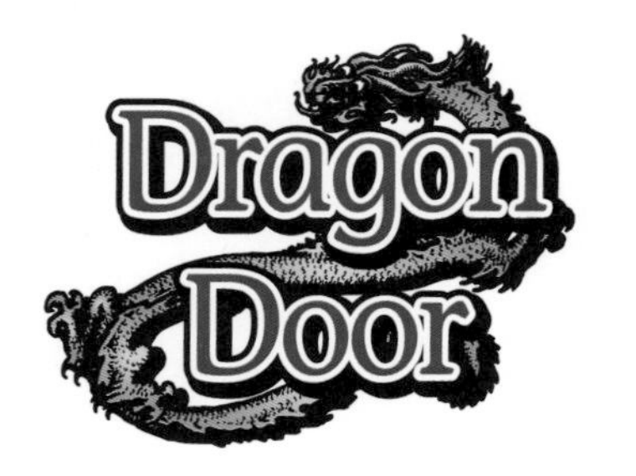

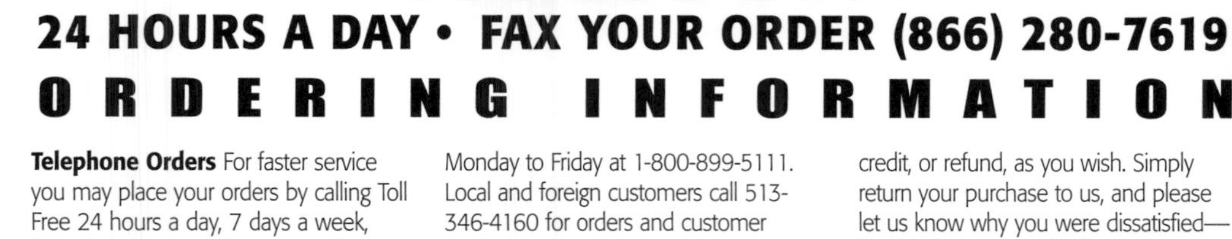

# 1·800·899·5111

## 24 HOURS A DAY • FAX YOUR ORDER (866) 280-7619

## ORDERING INFORMATION

**Telephone Orders** For faster service you may place your orders by calling Toll Free 24 hours a day, 7 days a week, 365 days per year. When you call, please have your credit card ready.

**Customer Service Questions?** Please call us between 9:00am– 11:00pm EST Monday to Friday at 1-800-899-5111. Local and foreign customers call 513-346-4160 for orders and customer service

**100% One-Year Risk-Free Guarantee.** If you are not completely satisfied with any product—we'll be happy to give you a prompt exchange, credit, or refund, as you wish. Simply return your purchase to us, and please let us know why you were dissatisfied—it will help us to provide better products and services in the future. *Shipping and handling fees are non-refundable.*

**Complete and mail with full payment to: Dragon Door Publications, 5 County Road B East, Suite 3, Little Canada, MN 55117**

**Please print clearly**

**Sold To:** **A**

*Name* ______________________

*Street* ______________________

*City* ______________________

*State* ______________ *Zip* ________

*Day phone** ______________________

* *Important for clarifying questions on orders*

**Please print clearly**

**SHIP TO:** ***(Street address for delivery)*** **B**

*Name* ______________________

*Street* ______________________

*City* ______________________

*State* ______________ *Zip* ________

*Email* ______________________

***Warning to foreign customers***

**The Customs in your country may or may not tax or otherwise charge you an additional fee for goods you receive. Dragon Door Publications is charging you only for U.S. handling and international shipping. Dragon Door Publications is in no way responsible for any additional fees levied by Customs, the carrier or any other entity.**

| ITEM # | QTY. | ITEM DESCRIPTION | ITEM PRICE | A OR B | TOTAL |
|---|---|---|---|---|---|
| | | | | | |
| | | | | | |
| | | | | | |
| | | | | | |
| | | | | | |
| | | | | | |
| | | | | | |
| | | | | | |
| | | | | | |
| | | | | | |
| | | | | | |
| | | | | | |

| | |
|---|---|
| *Total of Goods* | |
| *Shipping Charges* | |
| *Rush Charges* | |
| *Kettlebell Shipping Charges* | |
| *OH residents add 6.5% sales tax* | |
| *MN residents add 6.5% sales tax* | |
| *TOTAL ENCLOSED* | |

**HANDLING AND SHIPPING CHARGES • NO COD'S**

**Total Amount of Order Add (Excludes kettlebells and kettlebell kits):**

| | | | |
|---|---|---|---|
| $00.00 to 29.99 | Add $6.00 | $100.00 to 129.99 | Add $14.00 |
| $30.00 to 49.99 | Add $7.00 | $130.00 to 169.99 | Add $16.00 |
| $50.00 to 69.99 | Add $8.00 | $170.00 to 199.99 | Add $18.00 |
| $70.00 to 99.99 | Add $11.00 | $200.00 to 299.99 | Add $20.00 |
| | | $300.00 and up | Add $24.00 |

*Canada and Mexico add $6.00 to US charges. All other countries, flat rate, double US Charges. See Kettlebell section for Kettlebell Shipping and handling charges.*

**METHOD OF PAYMENT** ❐ CHECK ❐ M.O. ❐ MASTERCARD ❐ VISA ❐ DISCOVER ❐ AMEX

Account No. *(Please indicate all the numbers on your credit card)* EXPIRATION DATE

□□□□ □□□□ □□□□ □□□□ □□/□□

**Day Phone:** (___) ____________

**Signature:** ______________________ **Date:** ____________

**NOTE:** *We ship best method available for your delivery address. Foreign orders are sent by air. Credit card or International M.O. only. For* **RUSH** *processing of your order, add an additional $10.00 per address. Available on money order & charge card orders only.*

*Errors and omissions excepted. Prices subject to change without notice.*

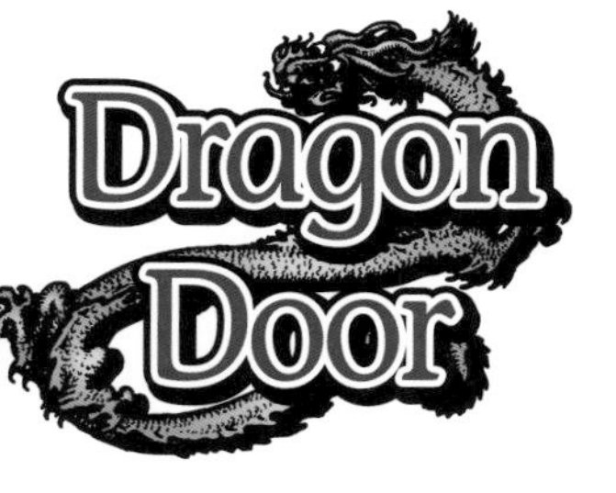


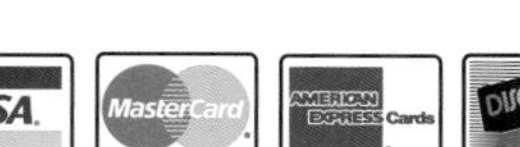


# 1·800·899·5111

## 24 HOURS A DAY • FAX YOUR ORDER (866) 280-7619

## ORDERING INFORMATION

**Telephone Orders** For faster service you may place your orders by calling Toll Free 24 hours a day, 7 days a week, 365 days per year. When you call, please have your credit card ready.

**Customer Service Questions?** Please call us between 9:00am– 11:00pm EST Monday to Friday at 1-800-899-5111. Local and foreign customers call 513-346-4160 for orders and customer service

**100% One-Year Risk-Free Guarantee.** If you are not completely satisfied with any product—we'll be happy to give you a prompt exchange, credit, or refund, as you wish. Simply return your purchase to us, and please let us know why you were dissatisfied—it will help us to provide better products and services in the future. *Shipping and handling fees are non-refundable.*

**Complete and mail with full payment to: Dragon Door Publications, 5 County Road B East, Suite 3, Little Canada, MN 55117**

**lease print clearly**

**old To:** **A**

ame____________________________

reet ____________________________

ty ____________________________

ate __________________ Zip ________

ay phone*__________________________

**mportant for clarifying questions on orders*

**Please print clearly**

**SHIP TO:** ***(Street address for delivery)*** **B**

Name____________________________

Street ____________________________

City ____________________________

State __________________ Zip ________

Email ____________________________

***Warning to foreign customers:***

**The Customs in your country may or may not tax or otherwise charge you an additional fee for goods you receive. Dragon Door Publications is charging you only for U.S. handling and international shipping. Dragon Door Publications is in no way responsible for any additional fees levied by Customs, the carrier or any other entity.**

| ITEM # | QTY. | ITEM DESCRIPTION | ITEM PRICE | A OR B | TOTAL |
|---|---|---|---|---|---|
| | | | | | |
| | | | | | |
| | | | | | |
| | | | | | |
| | | | | | |
| | | | | | |
| | | | | | |
| | | | | | |
| | | | | | |
| | | | | | |
| | | | | | |
| | | | | | |

**ANDLING AND SHIPPING CHARGES • NO COD'S**

**tal Amount of Order Add (Excludes kettlebells and kettlebell kits):**

| | | | |
|---|---|---|---|
| **0.00 to 29.99** | **Add $6.00** | **$100.00 to 129.99** | **Add $14.00** |
| **0.00 to 49.99** | **Add $7.00** | **$130.00 to 169.99** | **Add $16.00** |
| **0.00 to 69.99** | **Add $8.00** | **$170.00 to 199.99** | **Add $18.00** |
| **0.00 to 99.99** | **Add $11.00** | **$200.00 to 299.99** | **Add $20.00** |
| | | **$300.00 and up** | **Add $24.00** |

*nada and Mexico add $6.00 to US charges. All other countries, flat rate, double Charges. See Kettlebell section for Kettlebell Shipping and handling charges.*

| | |
|---|---|
| *Total of Goods* | |
| *Shipping Charges* | |
| *Rush Charges* | |
| *Kettlebell Shipping Charges* | |
| *OH residents add 6.5% sales tax* | |
| *MN residents add 6.5% sales tax* | |
| *TOTAL ENCLOSED* | |

**ETHOD OF PAYMENT** ❐ CHECK ❐ M.O. ❐ MASTERCARD ❐ VISA ❐ DISCOVER ❐ AMEX

count No. *(Please indicate all the numbers on your credit card)* EXPIRATION DATE

☐☐☐☐ ☐☐☐☐ ☐☐☐☐ ☐☐☐☐ ☐☐/☐☐

**ay Phone:** (____)______________

**gnature:** ____________________________ **Date:** ____________

**TE:** *We ship best method available for your delivery address. Foreign orders are sent by air. Credit card or rnational M.O. only. For* **RUSH** *processing of your order, add an additional $10.00 per address. Available on ney order & charge card orders only.*

*rs and omissions excepted. Prices subject to change without notice.*

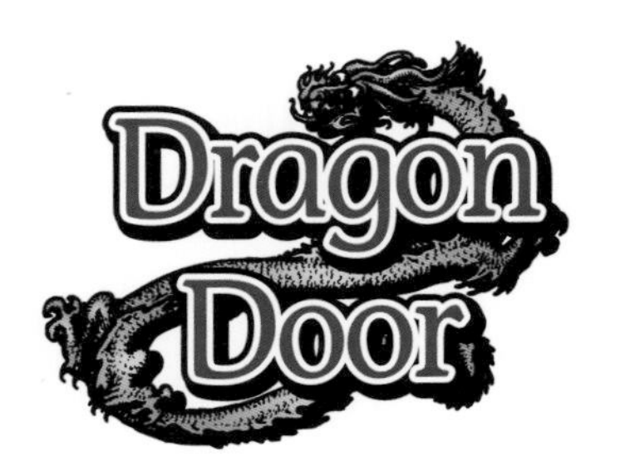

# 1·800·899·5111

## 24 HOURS A DAY • FAX YOUR ORDER (866) 280-7619

## ORDERING INFORMATION

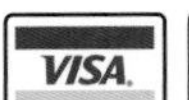
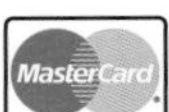
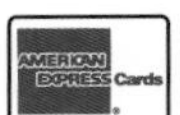
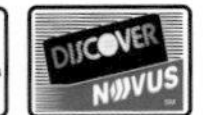

**Telephone Orders** For faster service you may place your orders by calling Toll Free 24 hours a day, 7 days a week, 365 days per year. When you call, please have your credit card ready.

**Customer Service Questions?** Please call us between 9:00am– 11:00pm EST Monday to Friday at 1-800-899-5111. Local and foreign customers call 513-346-4160 for orders and customer service

**100% One-Year Risk-Free Guarantee.** If you are not completely satisfied with any product—we'll be happy to give you a prompt exchange, credit, or refund, as you wish. Simply return your purchase to us, and please let us know why you were dissatisfied—it will help us to provide better products and services in the future. *Shipping and handling fees are non-refundable.*

**Complete and mail with full payment to: Dragon Door Publications, 5 County Road B East, Suite 3, Little Canada, MN 55117**

**Please print clearly**

**Sold To:** **A**

*Name* ______________________

*Street* ______________________

*City* ______________________

*State* ______________ *Zip* ________

*Day phone** ______________________

** Important for clarifying questions on orders*

**Please print clearly**

**SHIP TO:** ***(Street address for delivery)*** **B**

*Name* ______________________

*Street* ______________________

*City* ______________________

*State* ______________ *Zip* ________

*Email* ______________________

***Warning to foreign customers:***
**The Customs in your country may or may not tax or otherwise charge you an additional fee for goods you receive. Dragon Door Publications is charging you only for U.S. handling and international shipping. Dragon Door Publications is in no way responsible for any additional fees levied by Customs, the carrier or any other entity.**

| ITEM # | QTY. | ITEM DESCRIPTION | ITEM PRICE | A OR B | TOTAL |
|---|---|---|---|---|---|
| | | | | | |
| | | | | | |
| | | | | | |
| | | | | | |
| | | | | | |
| | | | | | |
| | | | | | |
| | | | | | |
| | | | | | |
| | | | | | |
| | | | | | |
| | | | | | |

| | |
|---|---|
| *Total of Goods* | |
| *Shipping Charges* | |
| *Rush Charges* | |
| *Kettlebell Shipping Charges* | |
| *OH residents add 6.5% sales tax* | |
| *MN residents add 6.5% sales tax* | |
| *TOTAL ENCLOSED* | |

**HANDLING AND SHIPPING CHARGES • NO COD'S**

**Total Amount of Order Add (Excludes kettlebells and kettlebell kits):**

| | | | |
|---|---|---|---|
| **$00.00 to 29.99** | **Add $6.00** | **$100.00 to 129.99** | **Add $14.00** |
| **$30.00 to 49.99** | **Add $7.00** | **$130.00 to 169.99** | **Add $16.00** |
| **$50.00 to 69.99** | **Add $8.00** | **$170.00 to 199.99** | **Add $18.00** |
| **$70.00 to 99.99** | **Add $11.00** | **$200.00 to 299.99** | **Add $20.00** |
| | | **$300.00 and up** | **Add $24.00** |

*Canada and Mexico add $6.00 to US charges. All other countries, flat rate, double US Charges. See Kettlebell section for Kettlebell Shipping and handling charges.*

**METHOD OF PAYMENT** ❒ CHECK ❒ M.O. ❒ MASTERCARD ❒ VISA ❒ DISCOVER ❒ AMEX

Account No. *(Please indicate all the numbers on your credit card)* EXPIRATION DATE

□□□□ □□□□ □□□□ □□□□ □□/□□

**Day Phone:** (____) ____________

**Signature:** ______________________ **Date:** ____________

**NOTE:** *We ship best method available for your delivery address. Foreign orders are sent by air. Credit card or International M.O. only. For* **RUSH** *processing of your order, add an additional $10.00 per address. Available on money order & charge card orders only.*

*Errors and omissions excepted. Prices subject to change without notice.*